Logic
of the
Living Brain

Logic

of the

Living Brain, 1974.

GERD SOMMERHOFF,
Department of Anatomy and Embryology,
University College, London

JOHN WILEY & SONS

LONDON · NEW YORK · SYDNEY · TORONTO

Library of Congress catalog card number
73–8198

ISBN 0 471 81305 2

Made and printed in Great Britain by
William Clowes & Sons, Limited, London, Beccles and Colchester

Preface

The general problem of the nature of the mind and the specific problems of the neural mechanisms concerned in particular mental functions have a fascination which tempts us time and again to try and fit the available pieces of the jigsaw puzzle together even though we know that they are woefully incomplete. Why then go on trying rather than wait? One reason, no doubt, is sheer curiosity. A second and more pertinent reason is that no part of the brain acts in isolation and no aspect of brain function is unrelated to another or to the organization of the brain as a whole. Hence no matter how narrow a range of phenomena the specialist may study, the questions he asks and the directions in which he looks for an answer are bound to be influenced by his private vision of how one aspect of brain function relates to another and by preconceptions of many different kinds. It is therefore important that the work of the specialists should concurrently be supplemented by studies which take a global view of the brain and a critical interest in fundamental concepts. It is also important that these studies should be related to the work done in the laboratories so that either side can benefit from the impact of the other.

The critical examination and clarification of fundamental concepts and presuppositions has become particularly urgent in our time. For the progress made in the computer sciences and in the studies of artificial intelligence continues to raise many questions of a very fundamental nature, and often at a very abstract level of thought.

The greater part of this volume is therefore devoted to the analysis of basic concepts, issues and assumptions. Even when in Part II we come to look at the 'hardware' of the brain and a number of hypothetical model networks are introduced in Chapter 7, my primary object is merely to elucidate some of the implications of basic neural properties. Only after this chapter does the analysis give way to an attempt to achieve a coherent synthesis. At this point the book becomes frankly speculative and I hope I have done nothing to disguise this fact. I trust that the reader to whom speculation on this scale is repugnant will find enough in the earlier chapters to stimulate his own thoughts and his own, perhaps rather more cautious excursions of the imagination. For me the question of how the higher functions of the brain are at all *conceivable* in

v

neural terms has an abiding fascination even though it will yet be a while before we can hope to arrive at firm conclusions. I also believe that the persistent exercise of the imagination has an important part to play in our advance towards that goal.

The degree of diversification and specialization in brain research and in the allied disciplines is such that no one mind can keep abreast of all that is relevant. In consequence anyone who steps out of the frame of established research, either to take a fresh look at fundamental concepts or to speculate about the special capabilities of the human brain, is likely to draw the fire of specialists in each of the many territories he is likely to cross. In view of what I have said above it is clear that this is a risk one must learn to take in one's stride. Hence I make no apologies for what some may regard as blatant omissions; nor, on the other hand, do I claim finality for my conclusions.

The interest that has now come to be taken in the brain, not only by philosophers and psychologists but also by cyberneticists, automation engineers and computer scientists, made it especially difficult to decide on the best level of exposition. After some deliberation I decided to follow the example of a number of other authors and write the book with the intelligent general reader in mind. I am fully aware of the drawbacks of this solution. Like the 'average man' the 'general reader' is no more than a convenient fiction. I can only hope that in the present case it will turn out also to have been a moderately expedient one.

I am indebted to Professor B. Boycott, Dr. B. Delisle Burns, Dr. J. O'Keefe and Mr. David Murray, who were good enough to read the whole manuscript, and to Professor Sir Alfred Ayer, Professor J. Z. Young and Professor P. Wall who read specific sections of it. While I bear sole responsibility for the views expressed I owe much to their helpful suggestions and critical comments. I should also like to thank Mrs. Astafiev who did the illustrations and Miss Vanda Salmon who gave her valuable time to do all the typing. Last but not least I must acknowledge my debt to Professor Sir Peter Medawar for his constant encouragement and to the Nuffield Foundation for a generous grant.

University College   G. Sommerhoff
London

Contents

PART I

1. Introduction

  1.1 Analysis before synthesis   3

  1.2 Brains and computers 11

2. Selected brain functions

  2.1 The nature of goal-directed activity 16

  2.2 Internal representations of the outside world . . 25

  2.3 Language 38

  2.4 Rational thought 46

3. Mind, brain and behaviour

  3.1 Semantic divisions 51

  3.2 Science and purposive behaviour 55

  3.3 The dichotomy between mental and physical events . . 58

  3.4 Internal representations and consciousness . . . 67

4. Teleological systems

  4.1 The concept of directive correlation 73

  4.2 Major types of directive correlation 88

  4.3 Information theory and cybernetics 91

  4.4 Postscript and preview 93

5. Clarification of some critical concepts and relations

  5.1 Introduction 97

  5.2 Hierarchies of goals and subgoals 98

  5.3 Instinct and drive 103

  5.4 The nature of expectation 108

  5.5 The question of explicit error-signals . . . 116

  5.6 The question of explicit goal-signals 124

  5.7 Summary of Part I 128

PART II

6. Outlines of the nervous system

6.1 Introduction 135
6.2 The neuron 135
6.3 The central organization of the nervous system . . . 143
6.4 Properties of the afferent pathways 153
6.5 Attention and arousal 159
6.6 Learning (1): Criteria of success and failure . . . 166
6.7 Learning (2): Conditional versus unconditional synaptic
      changes 170
6.8 Learning (3): Reinforcement and extinction . . . 173
6.9 Reward and punishment systems 177
6.10 Short-circuiting 180
6.11 Concluding remarks 182

7. Significant operations and network configurations

7.1 Introduction 183
7.2 The power of recurrent inhibition and complementary coding 187
7.3 The lambda configuration as a possible learning system . 197
7.4 Response modulation, adequate stimulus substitution and
      forced acquisition 201
7.5 The recognition and reproduction of temporal sequences . 206
7.6 Reproductive memory circuits and 'imagination'. . . 211
7.7 The principle of reafference 215
7.8 The recognition of properties 217
7.9 The recognition of relations 221
7.10 The neural representation of properties and relations:
      Summary 225
7.11 Some relevant physiological observations . . . 228
7.12 Concluding remarks 230

8. Selected structures

8.1 The cerebellum 233
8.2 Lambda configurations in the cerebellum . . . 238
8.3 The allocortex and limbic system 240
8.4 Lambda configurations in the hippocampus . . . 246
8.5 The neocortex 249
8.6 Lambda elements in the neocortex 253
8.7 Concluding remarks 260

9. Shape recognition and internal models

9.1 Perception and movement 261
9.2 Shape recognition and contour-following 265
9.3 Shape recognition in central and peripheral vision . . 273
9.4 The stability of the visual scene 281
9.5 Internal models of the outside world 283
9.6 Models and memories in the temporal lobes . . . 289
9.7 The parietal lobes and the body schema 294
9.8 Summary 297

10. Central organizational relationships

10.1 What–where separation and attention 300
10.2 The internal representation of goals 309
10.3 The evaluating functions of the frontotemporal system . 311
10.4 The hedonic drive system 320
10.5 Major functions of the limbic system 323
10.6 Short-term and long-term memory 326
10.7 Motor integration 333
10.8 The ground plan 337

11. Thought and language

11.1 Perception and consciousness 344
11.2 Memory and imagination 351
11.3 Language functions 355

Appendixes

A. The basic concepts of information theory 378
B. The lambda system as a maximum intensity filter . . . 382
C. The distribution of learning changes 385

Bibliography 394

Index 407

PART I

CHAPTER 1

Introduction

1.1 ANALYSIS BEFORE SYNTHESIS

The peculiar fascination of the brain lies in the fact that there is probably no other object of scientific enquiry about which we know at once so much and yet understand so little. It has been said that ever since Descartes ejected 'mind' from 'matter' philosophers have struggled to bring them together again. This in itself is a shadowy question which must ultimately bow to the rather more down-to-earth and precise questions I shall deal with in this volume, but it epitomizes our state of ignorance.

The distance we still have to go is not always appreciated by the layman. From the many publicized advances in the field of 'artificial intelligence' and 'brainlike mechanisms' it is easy to form the impression that the mysteries of the brain are all but solved. The true picture, as we know, is very different— certainly so far as concerns the neural mechanisms of the higher brain functions, the neural correlates of the various facets of our mental life, such as seeing and hearing, learning and remembering, thinking, imagining, reasoning and the pursuit of rational goals.

These are all competences which the brain acquires only when it functions as an integral system, as an organic whole. None resides in a single separable mechanism. Our questions, therefore, are global questions. They touch upon all that is known about the brain. They also make us acutely aware of how much is still unknown. Over the years the fast growth of our knowledge of anatomical and physiological details has not been paralleled by equal advances in our understanding of the functional organization of the brain as a whole and of the mechanisms of the higher brain functions. If neurophysiologists devote so little space to thinking, concept formation and the like, it is because, as some will frankly acknowledge, there is still relatively little to say about them. The mystery that surrounds the neural correlates of our mental functions is one of the great remaining challenges in the life sciences.

The literature on different aspects of brain function is so vast that one of my first concerns must be to indicate the particular slot into which this volume fits and the particular contribution it attempts to make. Briefly, the slot is defined by the observation that the more sophisticated the brain functions the scientist has tried to model, the less he has generally been able to say about the neural networks involved. These links, therefore, are still waiting to be forged. Conversely, the more he has tried to think in terms of neural networks, the less sophisticated have been the functions he has managed to model.

In a sense, of course, this is what one would expect in view of the complexity of the subject. However, complexity is generally mastered by moving to higher levels of abstraction, and this is a question of concept formation. The question therefore arises whether we are doing enough to find the best concepts for tackling the problem. I contend that we are not. We may ask, for example, whether the abstract concepts we use are genuine abstractions from the phenomena we study or whether we have perhaps somewhat imprudently rushed in with abstractions taken from other fields of research. I believe we have.

Attempts to model the nervous system range over a very wide spectrum. A great deal of fruitful work has been done on the functional organization of small networks of neurons which are either taken to represent the entire nervous system of simple invertebrate organisms or relatively isolated components of a complex nervous system. Some of this work is reviewed by Harmon and Lewis[100] and by Kennedy, Selverston and Remler[132]. Advanced examples are Young's work on the brain of the octopus[277] and Marr's theoretical analysis of the possible action of the Purkinje cells in the cerebellum[160].

Other workers have considered particular network configurations regardless of their anatomical context and examined some particular aspect, for example their theoretical learning capacity. Thus Brindley[28] has proposed a classification of modifiable synapses and has attempted to examine mathematically what types would yield realistic memory functions. Uttley[259] has explored certain probabilistic theses concerning the associations formed during conditioning in networks of a given structure. By contrast, Beurle[19] has examined the theoretical properties of randomly connected networks. Other examples are Rosenblatt's networks of simulated neurons capable of generating sequences of inputs[209]. This is a development of his earlier work on 'perceptrons', theoretical models which were primarily concerned with pattern recognition[208].

One step removed from structurally detailed networks we have studies which assume that the brain (or parts of it) contain certain primary organized units and then investigate the holistic functions that may result from aggregates of such units. Probably the best-known example of this line of approach is the model proposed by Kilmer, McCulloch and Blum[134] for the reticular formation of the brain. This model took the form of a computer program written on the tentative assumption that the primary function of the reticular formation is to switch the animal from one mode of behaviour to another, e.g. from eating to fleeing, and that this function is mediated by a number of semi-independent modules. One of the objects of the program was to examine how such modules could 'argue' with each other until a majority decision resulted.

Further along the spectrum, when we reach studies of higher, 'mental' functions (comprehension of the spoken word, thought, insight and problem solving, mental associations, etc.), the link with the 'hardware' of the brain tends to become completely severed. The nature of this separation is best understood in terms of the notion of a Turing machine.

Turing showed how the organization of any computer or automaton may be thought of in terms of an ordered collection of *logical states* which can be completely specified in a *machine table* by their relations to each other and to the inputs and outputs of the machine, but whose physical realizations in terms of 'hardware' are left open [136, 257]. A 'Turing machine' then is any system for which a machine table can be specified—a system, therefore, which is specified by the functional interrelation of its logical states regardless of its physical constitution. A *particular* Turing machine might therefore be built in a variety of ways. It might employ electronics and transistor logic or hydraulics and fluid logic—or it might be simulated on a computer.

These notions are relevant here because they show that the higher competences of the brain can be simulated and investigated in studies which are independent of the 'hardware' and in consequence shed little or no light on the 'hardware' employed by the brain, i.e. on the networks of the nervous system and the underlying physiological mechanism. To say this, of course, is not to diminish the intrinsic value of these studies and of the computer simulations which many of them have developed. The reader will find many interesting examples of such studies in the successive volumes of *Machine Intelligence** edited by Michie and others.

Eventually, however, the link with neural networks must be found. It is my contention that our progress towards this goal has been held up by the fact that the growing scope and precision of our technology has not been matched by equal advances in the scope, precision and selection of the concepts we use in formulating our questions and interpreting our observations, especially when these concern the higher brain functions. Many of the traditional concepts of the behavioural and mental sciences are still too far removed from the standards of precision and clarity which the exact sciences have long since learnt to respect. Thus a large part of our efforts must be bent on finding more precise formulations for the phenomena we seek to explain and for the questions we wish to ask. These are problems of analysis which must precede any attempt at synthesis. Mechanics in the days before Newton, and cosmology in the days before Einstein, were held up by the same failure to examine and analyse with sufficient rigour the concepts necessary for a scientific description of the phenomena it is sought to explain, the same failure to make sufficiently precise the concepts we apply to our observations.

* Oliver and Boyd, Edinburgh, 1967 onwards.

Mechanics was held up by the failure to distinguish between velocity and acceleration; cosmology by a failure to realize the ambiguities inherent in the orthodox notions of time and distance. The history of science shows that progress may be held up by deadlocks which are only resolved when we reach out for higher standards of accuracy in our thinking.

The simplicity of even the most elementary concepts that form the stock-in-trade of the behavioural sciences turns out to be somewhat deceptive when we take a closer look at the organism as an integral physical or physiological system and when we try to describe in precise terms the observable properties of this system. The elementary notion of 'response' may be taken as a simple example. Consider the case in which a monkey has been taught to press a lever whenever it hears the sound of a buzzer. Within the framework of experimental psychology the notion of an acquired 'response' here seems definite enough, and it plainly relates to observable events. But when we think of the organism as a physical or physiological system whose current states and transactions are to be specified in terms of physical or physiological variables, the 'response' acquired by the monkey no longer denotes an easily definable set of events—even at the purely observational level. The action of pressing the lever does not define a single sequence of physical movements. There is more than one way in which an arm can reach out and move a lever. In fact, 'pressing the lever' may define merely a family of movements whose only common feature is that they are directed towards the same particular goal. Now to say that an action is directed towards a particular goal implies a multitude of things. It implies for example that the action is variable and that the manner of its execution is matched to the prevailing circumstances in a particular way. It implies that the action is adaptive in the sense that it is subject to systematic changes as a function of changing circumstances. In the present case we know not only that the monkey moves the arm in the manner we have actually observed in previous trials but also, for example, that the animal is now so conditioned that if we shift the position of the lever from one trial to the next the animal will produce the appropriate modifications of its movements even though it may never before have experienced the lever in that position. It has acquired a 'conditional readiness' to meet certain contingencies in a certain way. In formal terms the 'response' which here came into being thus really consists of a set of potential movement sequences of which, at any one trial, the animal selects the appropriate one as a function of the circumstances prevailing at the time. The set is definable only in terms of the domain and form of these functions and in terms of the goal of the action. In Chapter 4 these formal relationships will be made explicit in terms of the mathematical concept of 'directive correlation'. We shall then see more clearly that the goal-directedness of an action represents an objective system-property which can be expressed in terms of mathematical equations and which does not necessarily presuppose ideation and conscious 'purposes'.

These then are the kind of formal system-properties any learning theory must seek to explain. It is clear from the start that these learning changes cannot be explained simply in terms of some new set of neural pathways having been formed or facilitated between specific sensory input stations on the one hand and specific motor output stations on the other, as the 'stimulus–response theorists' often seem to suggest.

The 'responses' studied in physiology are concrete and specific physical events; a twitch of a muscle, a set of recordable neural discharges. But, with the exception of simple reflexes and stereotyped emotional responses, this is not usually the case in experimental psychology. The 'responses' investigated here tend to be complex units of behaviour which are categorized according to their goals. The animal is 'approaching the foodbox', 'searching for water', 'building a nest' etc. When the animal performs any of these responses its movements rarely follow precisely the same stereotyped pattern and, even when they do, they tend to be produced by constantly varying combinations of the muscles involved. On a large scale these differences may become radical. When a rat which has mastered a maze is injured it will change to dragging itself or crawling to the foodbox. If the maze is inundated it will swim to the foodbox. To list the 'responses' of animals in different experimental situations, therefore, is to list the goals rather than the movements. Adequate definitions of these responses cannot be translated into the language of the exact sciences until we have succeeded in making explicit the exact spatiotemporal and causal relations which are implied in the general notion of an action being directed towards a specific goal.

The notion of 'stimulus' too, is a more determinate concept in physiology than in psychology. Physiological stimuli are precisely definable physical events: a voltage applied at one point of the nervous system, a given quantity of a drug introduced at another. The 'stimuli' used by the psychologist are less definite in physical terms: an object is shown to the animal, a command spoken, a figure is flashed onto a screen. Stimuli of this kind are not usually identifiable with unique physical events and do not have definite sets of neural inputs. In simple cases, for instance when an eyelid response is conditioned to a loud click, the meaning of 'stimulus' is clear enough in physiological terms, but in more complex cases, as when a monkey learns to discriminate between a square foodbox and a round one, difficult questions arise in connection with the actual neural inputs and outputs involved. Instead of a single physiological stimulus we now have a complex stimulus situation which cannot be treated as a mere aggregate of simple physiological stimuli. We are dealing now with spatial relations of which the animal has no raw sensations. Moreover, in terms of the actual image projected on the retina, even identical foodboxes never present the same aspect to the eye on separate occasions. Neither the projected image nor the location of the projection on the retina are the same. Yet the animal learns to respond correctly even though this frequently means responding to a set of retinal inputs it has never actually encountered during training. Somehow, and by mechanisms as yet unknown, the responses that develop during learning become established as responses that are faithful to the object, not to the retinal image.

In humans, we know from the study of very young infants that from the earliest stages onwards the real shape of an object is perceptually more salient than its projective shape. The infant rarely confuses a rectangle seen obliquely with a trapezoid seen square on. Retinal similarity is not a decisive factor in the development of early visual perception. Experiments of this kind indeed suggest that, rather than being the most primitive kind of perceptual ability, the ability to register separately the information in a retinal image may be a highly sophisticated attainment acquired only by learning.

On reflection this is not surprising. The organism generally tends to respond to the total dynamic stimulus situation. This includes not only the succession of retinal images as the eyes rove over the scene but also transformations of other sensory inputs, internal as well as external. The clues needed to determine the shape, distance and orientation of the objects seen lie hidden in these transformations. During learning, these clues are not necessarily factored out by the subject in the logical order in which the scientist may be inclined to analyse them. The subject learns to evaluate them jointly in learning situations in which they are jointly relevant and to abstract them individually only in learning situations in which they are individually relevant.

The nature of the mechanisms which evaluate such clues is one of the many remaining mysteries of the nervous system. Since pattern recognition and learning are two of the major ingredients of intelligence, this is a momentous problem. Modern automata studies have looked at the problem of shape recognition but with only limited success. It is comparatively easy to construct a machine which reacts to a particular pattern of light and dark falling on an array of light-sensitive cells. The problem is to enable the machine to work out that a set of quite new patterns, seconds or minutes later, belong to the same object. Yet this is what we do all the time when we recognize particular tables, chairs, flowers or fountain pens. The problem of the mechanisms that can learn to discriminate visual shapes in a manner that is invariant to their translation, rotation and scale, and that can apply the learned discriminations to retinal images not previously experienced in their particular orientation or size, has so far defied all attempts at solution.

The reason is not far to seek. Both engineers and mathematicians are predisposed to think of this as a tidy mathematical problem to which there must be a tidy analytical key, known to nature but as yet hidden from their gaze. Whereas in truth the biological faculty of shape recognition is more of the nature of a triumphant synthesis of a host of lesser faculties of the brain, some concerned with coarse discriminations, others with finer distinctions, some relying on passive reactions, others on active explorations—and all are dependent on relating present experiences to a vast store of bygone ones.

One of the fundamental misconceptions, and one of the most difficult to banish from the mind, is that the retinal image is somehow replicated on some invisible neural screen in the inner recesses of the occipital lobes, where its components are then scrutinized and dissected by various logical analysers.

Since Hubel and Wiesel's well known experiments on the visual cortex of the cat, we know that the visual cortex contains neurons which respond specifically to certain contour elements, such as illuminated lines or bars in specific orientations. Such neurons may show different degrees of generalization. Some respond only if the particular line or bar appears in a specific part of the visual field, whereas others respond if it appears anywhere in the field. These detectors are part of the innate organization of the visual cortex*.

Indeed it makes sense to assume that in the course of evolution specific networks have evolved for factoring out of the visual inputs the visual elements that have a part to play in the important task of contour analysis. In other words, there are 'wired in' detectors for the 'letters of the alphabet' in terms of which the brain spells out the 'words' and 'sentences' of the complex contours projected on the retina.

At some levels of the evolutionary scale such 'wired in' detectors may be all the equipment needed, but the primate brain must be able to learn to discriminate between very complex novel patterns and indeed between patterns that are novel in the history of the species. At the human end of the scale we can hardly expect to find innate detectors for such things as motor-cars or teleprinters. Clearly these complex powers of classification must be acquired by learning. That is to say, the later analysers must be *trainable* analysers. They are formed or modified in learning. As soon as this is admitted, one realizes that the simple idea of learning as a process of building or facilitating new pathways between the outputs of analysers and the inputs of motor centres merely cloaks the real problems.

To return to our earlier question, when a monkey has been trained to distinguish between a round foodbox and a square one, and it has learnt to select the correct one, exactly what has become associated with what? The alternative patterns of afferent nerve volleys that we lump together as the 'stimulus' presented by the foodbox have only their objective cause in common, i.e. the box. The response, we have seen, is faithful to the object, not the image. And all that unites the alternative patterns of efferent volleys that we lump together as the 'response' is but the goal towards which the resulting movements are directed. *In objective terms, therefore, the main correlation established during learning appears to be between objects and goals rather than between specific neural inputs and outputs.*

* In the cat they function from birth. But during the first six weeks they can degenerate if the eye is occluded. After this critical period no degeneration follows occlusion.

In this book I intend to spend some time on this particular issue. We shall see that to accomplish such correlations in the most effective and comprehensive manner the brain has to build some kind of internal representations or 'models' of external objects or events and of their essential properties or relations. This power also appears to be essential to the faculties of rational thought, imagination and reconstructive memory.

We shall see that these 'models' take the form of aggregates of expectations of how sensory inputs will transform in response to the organism's movements. The question therefore turns on how such aggregates of expectations can be registered in neural terms.

These studies underline one particular aspect in which the brain differs from most man-made machines: its basic data are not passively received inputs, but input transformations resulting from spontaneous movement.

These observations suggest three main topics for investigation:

   (i) the nature of goal-directed activities;
  (ii) the nature of the internal representations which the brain forms of the outer world;
 (iii) the manner in which these representations can serve as a platform for perception, language, thought and other faculties.

The first of these topics is probably the most fundamental. There are of course machines that perform objectively goal-directed activities. Most servomechanisms are of this kind. However, this does not mean that the theory of servomechanisms is bound to advance our understanding of all the brain's control functions. In fact this is a simple example of a case in which the precipitate application of concepts derived from another field of research may sometimes cloud our view. Servomechanisms are error-controlled and to this end generally employ devices for error detection, i.e. for computing the magnitude and direction of the discrepancy between the desired and the actual output. We might therefore start searching for similar devices or 'comparators' in the brain. However, we shall see in Chapter 5 that it is a fallacy to assume that the error-eliminating activities of the nervous system necessarily presuppose the prior formation of explicit error signals. (The importance of feedback loops is not diminished by this fact.)

The same applies to the notion of 'command signal'. Most cybernetic models of the movement-controlling functions of the nervous system begin with the assumption of explicit command signals which are specifically related to the goal of the movement. These may function at a single level or they may be hierarchically organized. Sometimes both explicit command signals and explicit error signals are assumed, as in the models of Johnson for human eye tracking[127]. Sometimes only explicit command signals are assumed and the evaluation of the feedback information is left open. Examples are the models of Houk[116] and the general paradigms for voluntary control proposed by MacKay[157]. At other times command signals are envisaged in conjunction with signals indicating zero error only, as in the paradigms known as TOTE units (test–operate–test–exit program segments). Any one of these models may or may not be valid in some particular application, but we shall see in Chapter 5 that there is no prior reason to assume that invariably there exists a set of explicit command signals in the brain which can be mapped on the hierarchy of goals and subgoals that can be read into any given pattern of behaviour.

The general reader will find a useful selection of elementary cybernetic models in Arbib's *The Metaphorical Brain*[11], a book that I must here note for its title. As the title confirms, cybernetic models are no more than metaphors. As such they have limitations we must not lose sight of. Once again this points to the importance of careful analysis of our concepts before we engage in any kind of synthesis.

1.2 BRAINS AND COMPUTERS

Complex systems can often be mastered by moving to higher levels of abstraction in our thinking. However, this is not always an easy or straightforward road and there are many pitfalls for the unwary.

In general to abstract means to classify, to think in terms of general categories. It means to discriminate certain features in thought from others which are meanwhile neglected. But the abstraction must be made from the concrete material under observation and it must be carefully selected to suit the problems in hand.

Confronted with the immense complexities of the brain the neurologist is sometimes tempted to rush in with abstract concepts which happen to lie available elsewhere and which may originate in quite different fields of enquiry, e.g. in automation engineering or the computer sciences. Such concepts may relate only superficially to the real problems posed by the brain. The concepts tempt us because of the degree to which their implications have been mathematically explored. They offer a dowry of well-thought-out mathematical theories, often of great elegance. But logical clarity may be sterile if it is not backed by semantic clarity. Particularly in the case of the higher brain functions the real issue is often not how one abstract concept is related to another, but how either may relate to the world of physical observables.

From the very nature of mathematics this problem is not primarily the mathematician's province, nor a task for which he may be especially qualified by virtue of his profession. The symbols of his theoretical constructs need not have any meaning at all. To create some elegant mathematical edifice and then to add 'now let x stand for a thought and y for a memory, and this is my theory of brain functions', hardly furthers the cause of brain research so long as we are unable to say what physiological events are meant by a 'thought' or a 'memory'. Undoubtedly the failure of neurology to derive solid benefits from cybernetics and systems theory must in part be blamed on the failure of many theorists to base their abstract concepts on the concrete material that forms the subject of the neurosciences.

Weisskrantz once said that every age tends to interpret the brain in terms of its current technology. In this century we have seen the brain likened first to a giant telephone exchange, then to a giant collection of servomechanisms and now it tends to be likened to whatever happens to be the last word in general purpose computers.

In our time the development of new technologies has gone hand in hand with that of new mathematical techniques. Control theory, network theory, switching theory, dynamic programming, mathematical programming, information theory, switching theory, pattern recognition theory, coding theory, Markoffian decision processes, Monte Carlo simulation and others have variously been pressed into service. And yet the actual spin-off in advancing our understanding of the functional organization of the brain has remained disappointing. Little has emerged, for example, that could now safely be incorporated in a textbook of neurology. To some extent, of course, this is due to the sheer magnitude of the problem. I believe, however, that in part it is also due to the fact that, although analogies between particular brain functions and certain machine functions may canalize our curiosity and possibly suggest fruitful hypotheses, they can be prejudicial if they are taken too literally.

Comparisons between brains and computers can mislead in a number of ways. They can mislead not only by suggesting analogies where in fact none exist, but also because in applying computer concepts to the brain we may unwittingly commit ourselves to tacit assumptions which are valid enough in engineering but have no valid foundation in biology.

The nature of memory is a simple case in point. Computer memories are separate and localized units subject to selective address. The memory functions of the brain have none of these features. Hence the use of computer jargon like 'read in', 'read out' and 'address' suggest explicit and selective switching functions in the brain which may be quite unrealistic. In fact, 'memory' in the brain can denote two entirely different effects, neither being comparable with computer memories. In the first place 'memory' may denote merely the adaptive plasticity of the nervous system, the fact that its organization undergoes subtle and diffuse changes in consequence of the experiences the animal encounters in its transactions with the environment. To the best of our knowledge these changes are individually small, sometimes only statistical in their effects, and certainly distributed over large areas of the brain. We have no evidence for the existence in the brain of localized organs specifically subserving these or other memory functions. Secondly, 'memory' may denote the faculty we possess for reconstructing in the mind more or less reduced 'images' of events or situations we have experienced in the past. This is an advanced faculty which specifically relates to the contents of our consciousness; and although it might conceivably be more narrowly regionalized than the general plasticity I have mentioned above, it differs from computer memories in all respects bar the one that it serves to bring the past to bear on the present.

Again, computers tend to operate either in the digital or analog mode. If they are hybrid, the two modes of operation are neatly separable. The operations of the brain, on the other hand, tend to have both digital and analog aspects which are often inseparably intertwined. That is to say, in many processes both the identity of the stimulated fibres and the intensity of the stimulation matters, and it is often difficult to say which is the more critical in any particular brain function.

I have already indicated another difference between brains and computers. As the living organism is engaged in ceaseless transactions with the environment one of its main concerns is to be able to predict the sensory consequences of its activities. Thus the fundamental data the brain must process are not passively received sensory stimuli but, rather, actively achieved sensory input transformations. Hence in shape recognition it is not so much the retinal image that holds the key, as the manner in which the image shifts or transforms in consequence of the movements of the eyes, head or body.

However, these are comparatively minor points. The brain differs from man-made machines also in rather more fundamental ways. Foremost is the fact that its logic did not precede its design. It has developed phylogenetically over a very long period of time in which various selective processes have acted on small genetic variations of structure or function. New functions, therefore, had to be grafted on to old ones in whatever manner proved to be feasible and consistent with the normal processes of evolution. At every stage, as it were, evolution has had to improvise with the anatomical structures and inherent plasticities that happened to be available. In consequence it is often a mistake to look for monolithic solutions in the brain for particular organizational problems. Suppose for example that known anatomical connections suggest three alternative pathways for a particular feedback function. Intuitively one might then search for evidence that would decide in favour of one of them. Yet the chances are that the brain will avail itself of all three in varying proportions depending on context.

In the manner in which automatic machines are commonly designed, the engineer begins with a logical breakdown of the desired functions. This results in a block diagram in which each block represents a logical part-function. As the design proceeds these logical blocks are given concrete realization in the form of suitably designed electronic or mechanical modules. But in the brain we cannot expect with certainty to find what appear to us as separable logical functions to be similarly identifiable with physically (i.e. anatomically) separable structures—or vice versa. We must be prepared to find single anatomical structures performing more than one function and single functions being distributed over more than one structure.

In consequence it is probably a vain hope eventually to be able to explain the 'hardware' of the brain adequately in terms of block diagrams in which structure and function coincide. The best we can hope to achieve is to explain all significant correlations or mappings between observable events. Foremost among these, of course, are the mappings of causes and effects. However, since the brain is a teleological system, the directive correlations mentioned above also rank high among the phenomena or properties to be explained. Since these directive correlations often have a complex hierarchical structure a great deal of careful analysis is required to tease them apart and achieve a precise account of their individual elements and mappings.

This difference between brains and machines has another consequence. The engineer builds up his machine using concepts of proven determinacy and applicability. The neuroscientist, on the other hand, is confronted with the analysis of an exceedingly complex system about whose activities Man has speculated for generations in terms of concepts and ideas which, if they were all listed, would truly amount to an encyclopaedia of philosophy. Despite these efforts we are still left with the problem of finding the best concepts to use. We are only beginning to realize that these concepts must not only match the nature of the material but also the critical standards of scientific exactitude. The type of conceptual analysis to which parts of this book are devoted is thus largely irrelevant to the engineer in his own profession. For example, the concept of 'directive correlation', which I shall use in the formal analysis of goal-directed activities, will not be found in engineering textbooks, not even in those concerned with the design of goal-seeking machines. It is a concept forged to help us in the analysis of what we find—not in the synthesis of what we may wish to design.

It is sometimes said that despite all the shortcomings of technological models the insights from technology are valuable for the biologist because they can tell him the necessary conditions for any conceivable systems that can do what the brain does. The flaw in this argument is that we often do not know yet how to say in precise terms what exactly the brain does. Another flaw is that what is conceivable to the technologist depends on the tacit assumptions of his craft and these are rooted in his methods as well as in the accepted body of scientific knowledge on which he draws in his calculations and designs.

In the eyes of the public, of course, computers and brain appear to be comparable because when they are put to certain uses the net results of their performance are comparable. Both brains and computers can be used to solve logical or mathematical problems. However, net results provide no profitable basis for comparison when we are dealing with questions of functional organization. The net results of the hydraulic systems used in mechanical shovels are strictly comparable with the net results of the muscles that move our limbs. Nevertheless, it is hardly a comparison that profits our physiological studies of the musculature.

Turing's discussion of artificial intelligence is suggestively misleading for the same reason. By concentrating the argument on the question whether machines can copy the intellectual capabilities of man, and thus on the question of net results, Turing evades all questions about the actual processes of thought and about the meaning of 'thinking' in the first place. The overt results of the brain's activities are not the only aspect of the matter to be considered. There are also the subjective aspects: our subjective experiences, the nature of our mental life and consciousness.

A few years ago Putman[203] suggested that there is an analogy between logical states of a Turing machine and mental states of a human being, on the one hand, and structural states of a Turing machine and physical states of a human being on the other. This is an interesting analogy and in Chapter 3 we shall see in what indirect sense it is a valid one. However, it cannot bridge the fundamental dichotomy between mental and physical states. Mental processes, in so far as they are conscious, presuppose an element of self-awareness which is totally lacking in machines. And this is so even when the self is not an object of conscious attention. For this reason, too, no known machine, however sophisticated, engages in processes that can be likened to our conscious thoughts and feelings except in a very remote metaphorical sense.

In the next chapter I propose to go into the three main problem areas on which we shall concentrate in this volume. In the final section of that chapter we shall return to the question of net results versus intrinsic organization.

CHAPTER 2

Selected Brain Functions

Any book on as comprehensive a subject as the higher brain functions must be selective in its approach. In this chapter I intend to plunge straight into the three crucial problem areas which were singled out in the last chapter: the nature of goal-directed activities, the nature of the internal representations or 'models' the brain forms of the physical world and the manner in which these representations can serve as a platform for language and rational thought.

At a first reading these topics may seem a strangely mixed bag. Their particular significance will become apparent only as we go along and our analysis unfolds. The particular points I have selected within each of these topics may also at first seem a mixed lot. This is partly because I shall use the opportunities afforded by this chapter to clarify a number of concepts we shall need presently and partly because I shall also use the chapter to outline some results of later arguments which are relevant to topics I have to discuss before I can deploy the arguments. Although in general one would prefer a linear progression in which each subject is treated adequately as soon as it is introduced, in the present case some subjects are so closely interrelated that it is impossible to discuss any one of them without anticipating the results of discussing another.

2.1 THE NATURE OF GOAL-DIRECTED ACTIVITY

All animal behaviour is permeated by goal-seeking activity of one kind or another. There are proximate goals like pouncing on the prey, jumping a hurdle, running to a visible target. There are more remote goals like building a nest or finding the foodbox in a complex maze. And, of course, there are the ultimate goals of survival and preservation of the species.

Goal-seeking in this sense is not something extraneous that gets into the organism and makes it go. It is an objective system-property which is implicit in the very nature of biological organization. It is a phenomenon in which flexible strategies and adaptive changes contrast with the randomness and blind mechanical reactions of the inorganic world. But since we automatically tend to compare all goal-directed activities with the consciously purposed

16

activities of rational agents and with the ideation that these presuppose, the subject of goal-seeking behaviour has caused a great deal of confused thinking in the history of biology.

Any complex pattern of animal behaviour can generally be broken down into a hierarchy of goals and subgoals. Nest building, for example, includes such goal-directed part-activities as picking up moss, flying back to the nest, placing the moss on the rim, etc. One of the questions we shall be examining at a later stage is whether the hierarchy of goals and subgoals in a given behaviour pattern does or does not presuppose a correlated hierarchy in the structure of the neural organization controlling the pattern.

It is essential to realize that goal-directedness is an objective system-property which is based on a distinct set of formal relationships in space and time and that to describe biological activities in terms of their goals is not just a convenient way of classifying them according to their end results. Muscular fatigue is the invariable end result of strenuous physical activity, but one could hardly say that fatigue was the invariable goal of physical exercise.

To rule out from the start the danger of sliding into anthropomorphism it is best to begin with a machine example. When a guided missile is programmed to pursue a moving target, we have before us a machine engaged in goal-directed behaviour, in a perfectly objective sense of the phrase in which there is no suggestion that the machine has a 'mind' engaged in the pursuit of conscious purposes. The distinctive feature of the machine as it homes on the target is that it 'matches' or 'adapts' its outputs to the prevailing conditions and to the requirements arising out of the nature of the goal. Thus the course held by the missile is matched to the current direction, speed and distance of the target. Contingent disturbances are compensated for by control activities which, again, are matched to the particular circumstances concerned. And all the 'matching' relates to one final event: a hit on the target. This matching quality or adaptation represents an objective system-property of the machine which is characterized by correlations which require for their definition a reference to (a) an ensemble of alternative possibilities regarding direction and distance of target, windspeed, etc., and (b) the goal-event in question.

To assert, for example, that at a given instant the direction of the missile is 'adapted' to the position or movement of the target does not just mean that at this instant the missile happens to follow the appropriate flight path. It means in addition that the system-properties of the moving missile are such that if at that juncture the target had followed a different course, the missile, too, would have followed a different (and appropriately modified) course. It has a contingent readiness to meet certain events in certain ways. The terms 'matched' or 'adapted' here therefore imply

(i) the idea of alternative possibilities as regards the behaviour of the target,

   (ii) a comparison of these hypothetical variations with the modified outputs the missile would have produced in each case,

  (iii) the belief that each of these outputs would have been appropriate under
the circumstances despite the fact that (so far as the observer knows)
inappropriate outputs are physically open to the system.

To take another example. The intrinsic difference between a clockwork
bird pecking at a grain which happens to lie at the right position (a non-
adaptive activity) and a live bird pecking at a grain (an adaptive activity) is
not perceptible on a film taken of a single instance of either activity. Single
instances of both activities may look exactly alike. The real difference
lies in the fact that we know in the first case that if the grain had been
in a different position, the beak of the clockwork bird would have missed
it, whereas in the case of the live bird the movements of the beak would have
undergone appropriate modifications so that once again it would have hit
the target (and this despite the fact that (so far as the observer knows) false
moves are physically open to the bird). So once again the 'adaptiveness' of
the action, seen as an objective system-property, refers to a correlation which
is definable only in terms of alternative possibilities, i.e. of hypothetically
varied conditions.

The essence of goal-seeking activities (in this objective sense) lies in the
fact that they consist of movements or decisions which are matched to the
existing circumstances in this particular sort of way and in respect of the
particular end results which we call the 'goal' of the activity.

We shall look at all this in more detail in Chapter 4 and we shall then see
that the objective system properties implied by notions like 'matched',
'adapted', 'coordinated', 'goal-directed' etc. can be given precise formulations in terms of particular mappings between spatiotemporal variables and
that the essential characteristics of goal-directedness can be expressed in
terms of particular mathematical equations. This more than anything shows
that we are dealing here with objective system-properties and not with
anthropomorphic projections or similar fictions. It is essential to understand
the true nature of these system-properties if we are to tackle the neural
organization of the brain as a problem *sui generis* and without having to rely
on metaphors (including engineering metaphors). However, for the present
it suffices to know that the property of goal-directedness is objectively definable in terms of ensembles of alternative possibilities, i.e. in terms of not only
what happens in the actual circumstances but also what would have happened
in alternative circumstances. This is nothing unusual in science. A typical
example is the physical concept of 'stable equilibrium'. To say that a system
is in a state of stable equilibrium is to say that it is in a state in which possible
displacements would produce restorative forces. In concepts like these we
are really categorizing what is actual in terms of what is possible or conceivable.

In fact, superficially the concept of 'equilibrium' bears some resemblance to that of 'goal-seeking'. There are biologists whose search for objective definitions has led them to equate 'goal-seeking' with 'equilibrium-seeking'. On this view the movement of a boulder rolling down a hill, the pursuit of a magnet by a steel ball or the movement of a 'missile' drawn to its target by a thin, invisible wire would all qualify as goal-seeking activities. However, we shall see in Chapter 4 that an accurate analysis of the spatiotemporal and causal relationships involved allows us to draw a line which clearly separates these activities from hunting prey, building a house, picking up a pencil and from the action of servomechanisms and freely homing missiles. We shall also see that the goal-directed activities segregated in this manner share general properties which have important implications for the required mechanisms. Some of these implications the engineer would recognize as a need to employ special feedback circuits.

Since the directiveness of their activities is the most conspicuous characteristic of biological organizations, it is no exaggeration to say that the biologist who approaches this subject without a clear conception of the formal relationships involved in goal-directed activities is no better equipped for his task than were the pre-Newtonian scientists in their approach to mechanical problems. The superficial reductionism which may be typified by '*A* means nothing more than *B*' sometimes finds expression in such beliefs as that 'mind' means nothing more than 'brain', that 'learning means nothing more than forming new S–R associations', and that 'goal-directed' means nothing more than 'having certain end results'. Invariably this leaves something out of account which may be crucial to the issues at stake. Reductionism is the besetting sin of those whose vocational interests are so narrowly focused on the parts of a whole that they lose sight of some of the particular relationships between the parts that determine the characteristics of the whole.

The critical degree to which the outcome of a scientific investigation may depend on the prior clarification of the concepts used in the description and analysis of the data is not always fully appreciated. This particularly concerns our description of the most general characteristics of the higher brain functions. In many contexts it may be clear enough to say that the overt activities of organisms are 'regulated', 'coordinated', 'integrated', 'goal-directed' etc. However, when we are up against the difficult problem of unravelling the functional organization of the brain, we have to decide what exactly these predicates mean in terms of spatiotemporal and causal relations between observable variables if our thinking is to reach the levels of precision that a problem of this magnitude demands. We are confronted here with intricate problems of neural organization. But organization means order and order here means temporal as well as spatial relationships. To be able to translate our common descriptions of the overt manifestations of the brain's activities and faculties into this kind of language calls for painstaking analysis of many of the common concepts used. To some extent, of course, this is a semantic problem which calls for an accurate analysis of meanings. This is not here a question of pursuing a finicky perfection in our terminology (that goal is probably unattainable and may even be undesirable in a fluid medium of research). It is the plain business of analysing what type of system (deterministic, probabilistic etc.) our notions imply, what elements they take to be variable and what correlations between these variables are asserted in any particular case.

There are those who interpret teleological terms like 'purposive', 'goal-seeking' and 'goal-directed' exclusively in a subjective sense in which they can strictly be applied only to activities of rational agents in pursuit of consciously conceived aims and intentions. In this sense goal-directedness presupposes ideation. Indeed, some writers, Feigl[64] for example, have made purposiveness a defining characteristic of mental phenomena. In this sense only human beings can be goal-directed and any ascription of goal-directedness to infrahuman species must be an anthropomorphism.

But if teleological terms are restricted in this way we lose the means to discuss in non-metaphorical terms a wide range of characteristic organic phenomena and organizational relationships which belong to the very essence of life. Thus, despite the misgivings of these philosophers, many biologists have continued to insist that teleological descriptions of organic processes are objective and that they express something important which is lost when teleological language is eliminated from such descriptions. As we shall see, that 'something' is perfectly compatible with mechanical explanations of the processes involved.

The situation is still very confused. Thus, whereas D. Hull[120] recently pronounced 'evolutionary theory did away with teleology and that is that', MacLeod[154] only a few years earlier asserted 'what is most challenging about Darwin is his reintroduction of purpose into the natural world'. Obviously the two authors mean different things. In what precise sense we can say that there is an element of directiveness in evolution we shall see in Chapter 4, although we are far more immediately concerned with the directiveness of ontogenetic changes the organism undergoes during learning of the behaviour it shows in consequence.

Anyone who is aware of the philosophical muddles in which brain theory has in the past become entangled, will appreciate that these questions are of a sort which must be mastered before we can hope to be sufficiently equipped to deal with the question of the higher brain functions effectively. We still have a long way to go in this respect. We loosely describe animal activities as 'adaptive' without having a clear conception of exactly what objective relationships in time and space this term denotes. We often describe the almost universal goal-directedness of animal activities in terms of analogies with consciously purposed human behaviour, even when we wish to impute no consciousness to the organism; or we say that the animal 'aims' at this or 'tries' that, without analysing the objective features of the situation that invite such comparisons. Sometimes we say that the brain reacts according to the measure to which the sensory inputs meet its 'expectations'—again without having a clear conception of the objective system-properties this term denotes in this context. We compare the functions of the brain with those of feedback controlled servomechanisms, homeostats and other automata—again often without careful analysis of the exact system-properties that invite the comparison. All these are omissions which must be made good if we are to reach out for higher levels of accuracy in our thinking. The mathematical concept of 'directive correlation' (Chapter 4) provides the main instrument through which these levels may be reached.

It may be objected at this point that engineers and scientists frequently use similar vague and anthropomorphic terms when they talk about their machines and that they appear to do so with impunity. Indeed, some of their arguments are the clearer for it. But this is an entirely different matter. There is nothing wrong with figures of speech, metaphors, similes etc., *provided we recognize them for what they are* and do not, for example, use them as premisses for logical inferences.

In order to give a sufficient account of what brains do we have to give a sufficient account of behaviour and that means also to give sufficient account of the goal-directedness of behaviour, its most distinctive quality. Conventional biological theory has been unable to do this because until the arrival of such concepts as 'directive correlation' it lacked a theoretical framework that could cope with the abstract characteristics of this particular aspect of vital organization. This concerns all the biological sciences, not only neurobiology. The living organism is a uniquely organized system in which all the most distinctive activities and developments appear to be directed towards the realization of particular goals. This in fact is how the uniqueness of its organization is brought to our attention.

This directiveness is mainly apparent at three distinct levels:

   (i) at the *phylogenetic* level, in the processes of evolution;
  (ii) at the *ontogenetic* level, in the processes of growth and development;
 (iii) at what I shall call the *executive* level, i.e. in the adaptive flexibility of
        the overt execution of innate or acquired behaviour patterns (as in the
        pecking bird, for example).

At the phylogenetic level the directive quality lies in the progressive adaptation of structure or function to the changing requirements that arise out of the demands made by the environment or by the mode of life of the species. As in the examples analysed above the correlations that mark the 'adaptive' character of these processes relate not only to what has actually taken place in any particular instance but also to what would have happened under alternative circumstances. We call the protective colouration of an insect an 'adaptation' only because we believe it to be the outcome of a process which would have produced an appropriately modified colouration in a different environment, i.e. because we believe it to be due to causes other than chance-coincidence. A caterpillar which happened to have fallen into the right kind of paintpot would not afterwards be said to have undergone a process of ontogenetic adaptation.

One of the main advantages bestowed upon the higher organisms by the processes of evolution lies in the adaptive plasticity of their development and maturation. This ontogenetic plasticity enables the species to adapt to faster environmental changes than the slow processes of natural selection could keep pace with and it enables the individual member of the species to adapt to individual circumstances. At the behavioural level the most important manifestation of ontogenetic plasticity is the power to learn from experience. From a biological viewpoint learning changes are directive to the extent to which they produce capabilities that match the demands made upon the organism.

The third important type of directiveness is to be found in the practical execution of innate or acquired behaviour patterns, i.e. in the adaptive flexibility of the actual activities through which the behaviour patterns are implemented. In pouncing on the prey the predator knows how to adapt its movements instantly to those of the prey. It is clear that in the exercise of an acquired skill the executive adaptiveness is often the end product of an ontogenetic adaptiveness which in turn is the product of the phylogenetic adaptiveness built into the processes of evolution. The correlations implied in all these three types of directiveness relate to quite different sets of variables. These must be carefully separated if we are not to be confused by the simultaneous presence of all three types of directiveness in the same patterns of behaviour.

To give a concrete example: it is now widely accepted that the pecking movements of newly hatched chicks are innate in the sense that the neural coordinations which render them possible are fully organized by the time of the first peck. The existence of this organization at that stage constitutes one of the phylogenetic elements in pecking behaviour. An innate degree of executive adaptability also exists already at that stage for although the pecking is almost indiscriminate the chick is still pecking *at* something. As pecking continues the built-in ontogenetic adaptability shows itself in the gradual development, through learning, of visual discriminations which in due course enable it to distinguish visually between edible and inedible objects. During the early pecks the distinction is only known to the swallowing reflex. The pecking accuracy, too, improves with learning.

In the past this close intermixture of different categories of directive processes (each relating to different variables, different time-spans etc.) has caused a great deal of confusion, particularly in the discussion of instinct.

But this is not the main reason why the directiveness of organic activities has at times caused such violent controversies. The main reason has always been a failure to realize that this directiveness is an objective (though abstract) system-property which can be formulated in terms of accurately definable correlations between particular variables and which does not as such imply ideation or foresight.

The origin of these misconceptions lies far back in the history of Western thought. The problem of the peculiar purposiveness found in living nature has really been outstanding ever since Aristotle. It remained unsolved because until recently it could not even be stated clearly. Until recently, therefore, it was possible to deny the very existence or objective reality of this phenomenon. And such is the lack of communication between disciplines that even today some scientists, when they sally forth from their own special disciplines and are tempted to extrapolate their special concepts on a cosmic scale, startle us with philosophies in which the objective reality of the most distinctive characteristics of living organisms is either categorically denied or wholly misconceived. I am thinking, for example, of recent publications by Monod[171] and Skinner[225].

An examination of the mathematical formulae in which the purposiveness of organic activity can be expressed (Chapter 4) shows that they are entirely compatible with the axioms of modern science and that the alleged antithesis between manifestations of purposiveness in nature and causal determinism, is wholly illusory. Since we have been able to show that directive correlation is an objective system-property it has become perfectly legitimate to interpret organic activities in terms of their goals. Monod's insistence, for example, that true knowledge cannot be gained in this way is entirely mistaken. Nor can his radical division of cultures into 'objective' and 'vitalist–animist' be accepted as valid now that we have learnt to express in objective terms those aspects of living nature which the 'vitalist–animist' cultures tended to emphasize.

The same remarks apply to the attempts of Skinner and other extreme behaviourists to banish the concept of goal-directedness from all scientific descriptions of organic and even human behaviour. Although these attempts were made with the laudable object of placing psychology on a sounder scientific footing—indeed Skinner claims that his approach is the only truly scientific one—they have produced no more than a mere semblance of scientific objectivity. By ignoring what accurate scientific analysis can reveal about the exact spatiotemporal relationships manifested in goal-seeking behaviour (and the objective system-properties these relationships reveal), they have failed to live up to the very concepts and principles of the exact sciences whose virtues they have so consistently acclaimed.

The existence of directive correlations as objective system-properties of living organisms is now as incontrovertible as the existence of physical properties like stability, elasticity etc. To generalize about the abstract characteristics of living systems without awareness of this system-property is like generalizing about planetary motion of celestial bodies without awareness of the abstract geometrical relations which are covered by the concepts of the ellipse, parabola or hyperbola.

In the Greek concept of nature the directive, teleological aspects of living organisms were embraced by the concept of the 'soul'. The soul (*psukhé*) was the incorporeal, i.e. abstract, form or principle of life. To be ensouled or animate is what makes things alive. The soul is the form of the material body having life potentially within it. It is inseparable from the body. Aristotle here distinguishes sharply between 'soul' and 'mind'. Mind is the power to think. As such it is something implanted within the soul and less intimately bound up with the body; and it is possessed by only a small minority of living beings. Its objects are timeless.

In Aristotelian philosophy, therefore, teleology and the presence of 'soul' were one and the same and they were tied to material substance. They were abstract characteristics of particular material organizations. Only 'mind' as the principle of ratiocination was not so tied.

When in later thinking, especially in Christian theology, both 'soul' and 'mind' became separated from the body, teleology took on a new character. It became a testimony for the intelligence of something other than nature, of the divine creator and ruler of nature. After the final separation, effected by Descartes, minds and rational souls became one and the same thing. Like God they were of a substance which is nowhere and unextended. Teleology often remained only as evidence for mind and God. Those who today still decry the detached and objective study of the abstract teleological aspects of living nature are not always aware how deeply rooted their prejudices are in the particular traditions of Christian theology.

The fifth argument for the existence of God given by Aquinas[14] ran as follows:

> The fifth way begins from the guidedness of things. For we observe that some things which lack knowledge, such as natural bodies, work towards an end. This is apparent from the fact that they always or most usually work in the same way and move towards what is best. From which it is clear that they reach their end not by chance but by intention. For those things which do not have knowledge do not tend to an end, except under the direction of someone who knows and understands: the arrow, for example, is shot by the archer. There is therefore an intelligent personal being by whom everything in nature is ordered to this end, and this we call God.
>
> (St. Thomas Aquinas, *Summa Theologica*, edited by Fr. Thomas Gilby. Reproduced by permission of McGraw-Hill Book Company.)

After reading Chapter 4 the reader will have no difficulty in seeing where the non sequiturs creep in after the word 'chance'. This is not to say that some valid concept of God might not be derived from the objective reality of teleological phenomena in living nature. However, in this day and age the derivation will have to satisfy higher standards of analysis and precision than have been brought to the problem in the past.

2.2   INTERNAL REPRESENTATIONS OF THE OUTSIDE WORLD

Any outline I can give at this stage of the main problems the functional organization of the brain has to solve, in order to deal with the outer world in the way it does, is bound to be sketchy and oversimplified. Even so it is expedient first to define some basic terms and to remove possible equivocations in some of the terms I intend to use. This concerns, in particular, certain types of elementary functional relationships between physical variables and also the particular sense in which environmental variables may come to be 'represented' in the internal processes of the brain.

Figure 2.1 shows a function $y = f(x)$ over the interval AB. This interval is known as the *domain* of the function, whereas the values y may take on in

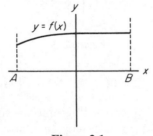

Figure 2.1

consequence of the function are known as the *range* of y. The function shown is a *single-valued* function of x, for each point on the x-axis determines only one point on the y-axis. For brevity I shall use the alternative expression *unique* function. In Figure 2.2, on the other hand, y is not a unique function of

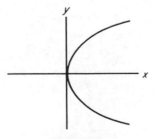

Figure 2.2

x because to each value of *x* corresponds more than one value of *y*. The function shown in Figure 2.3 is biunique in the sense that each value of *x* determines only one value of *y* and, conversely, each value of *y* determines only one value of *x*. The function represents a *one–one correspondence* between points of the *x*-axis and points of the *y*-axis.

If the elements of a set *A* can be mapped on the elements of a set *B* the two sets are said to be *isomorphic*. If each element of *A* determines a unique element of *B* and each element of *B* is the correspondent of at least one (but possibly more than one) element of *A*, the relationship is merely *homomorphic*.

Given any two sets, *X* and *Y*, the set of all elements which belong at least to *X* or to *Y* is known as the *logical sum* of *X* and *Y*. The set of all elements which belong to both *X* and *Y* is the *logical product* of *X* and *Y*.

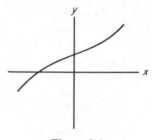

Figure 2.3

These basic concepts are applicable to biological systems despite the statistical nature of many biological phenomena. In many biological cases functional relationships are obscured by random deviations. This may have a variety of causes. The system itself may be a 'noisy' system; the conditions in which we conduct our experiments may not be perfectly controllable etc. In consequence the underlying functional relationship between two variables, *x* and *y* say, tends to be blurred. But if *x* and *y* are plotted on a dot diagram as in Figure 2.4 the relationship will manifest itself by the greater density of the dots along a certain locus. This latent curve or functional relationship

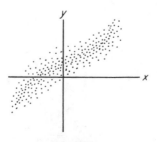

Figure 2.4

$y = F(x)$ is called the *regression* of y on x. At several stages of our analysis we shall take these facts for granted and take it to be understood, therefore, that if some variable y is asserted to be a unique function of x, the operational content of the assertion is that the observed values of y cluster around a unique function of x.

Another simplification one sometimes has to resort to in the interest of lucidity concerns the relation between discrete responses (for instance, verbal responses) and stimuli which may vary over a continuous domain. The colour spectrum is a typical example of a stimulus continuum. If several subjects are presented with a comprehensive colour chart and asked to assign a region on the chart to the word 'red' there will be some regions to which they will point with confidence and unanimously, and other regions which will cause doubt and disagreement. From a statistical sample of the results one can plot the probability distribution of the response 'red' as a function of the stimulus continuum. If the same is done for 'orange' the two probability distributions will generally be found to overlap. It is therefore an over-simplification to assume that the common colour names partition the colour continuum into a determinate set of discrete intervals. But there are many theoretical contexts in which this oversimplification is innocuous.

The image projected on the retina by an external object may be called a *representation* on the retina of the shape of that object in the elementary sense that the image is what it is partly because the shape of the object is what it is. Since the image is a two-dimensional projection of a three-dimensional shape the projection is many-to-one. It is a homomorphic representation, not an isomorphic one. Nor is the representation unique. The same object can yield different retinal images, depending on the orientation of the object, the line of vision etc.

However, it has now come to be widely accepted that the brain has the power to construct neural representations of features of the outside world which are *unique* representations of those features. We now believe that there must be processes in the brain that stand for or symbolize objective features of the outside world in a unique and relatively constant manner. The problem is to discover the nature of these processes and the neural correlates of these internal 'models'.

The concept of unique internal representations or 'models' of significant features of the environment has thus come to occupy a key position in brain theory.

The goal-directed activities of the organism call for sequences of movements which are matched to the particular circumstances in which they occur, and to achieve this the living organism must react not to the momentary stimulus qualities but to particular objects (food, implements, possessions), to the location of these objects and to their properties or relations. The activities of the organism must be matched to the objective features of the environment rather than to the subjective features of the stimuli that impinge on the senses (i.e. the sensory effects that depend on the state of the subject).

If the activities have to be learnt, then the mere question of learning economy calls for the synthesis in the brain of *unique* representations of these external variables from the non-unique representations that exist at the sensory periphery. If no unique representation can be created in the brain, so that the brain has only a multiplicity of alternating representations of the same external variable to draw upon, the correct response has to be learnt separately in respect of each of these alternative representations as and when it arises. For example, to learn to respond differentially to triangles and squares, the brain would have to learn the appropriate response to each individual projection of a triangle and square on the retina (excepting only the response generalizations which result from lack of accurate discrimination). As a mere matter of learning economy, and to facilitate the positive transfer of training, therefore, the brain needs capabilities for factoring out the elements that are common to particular classes of objects, events or situations, and for forming unique representations of the properties that distinguish these classes. The faculty of shape recognition is only a special case in point, although one of the most challenging. This problem is closely linked with the general problem of how the organism can factor out of the fleeting sensory inputs the enduring constants of a situation to which it must match its actions and adapt its visceral and other slow variables.

We know, of course, from introspection that the human brain can form unique central representations of external realities. Having surveyed a room and the layout of its furniture I can move about the room with confidence and even with my eyes closed. I can recall and describe the room after I have left it. I can imagine a rearrangement of its furniture. I can *think* about the room.

From a scientific point of view introspection is not satisfactory evidence, but even from a behavioural point of view it is evident that as I surveyed the room some neural organization must have formed in the brain which later on enables the brain to generate behaviour which is a unique function of the spatial relations I surveyed and which in some sense represents those relations.

There is ample evidence to show that similar neural organizations form also in the brains of infrahuman species. Throughout the higher orders of the animal kingdom we find a capacity to learn not only how to do something but also that something is the case. A particular example is place learning. Tolman's famous studies of place learning in rats are a case in point[251, 253]. If I walk down the High Street and notice a new phone box on my right then if on my way back I want to make a phone call I know that I shall find a phone box on my left. Tolman and his colleagues have shown that a rat has similar capabilities. They used a maze shaped like a cross and taught the animal that if it started from the south arm of the cross it should turn left to find food. If a rat was then started from the north arm it would turn right, as it should, to get to the same place, even though turning right had never been rewarded during training. Some of this work was inspired by the work of Krechevsky[142] who argued convincingly that in maze learning the naive rat does not make truly random choices but acts on primitive 'hypotheses' which are subsequently modified and refined by experience.

In another experiment Tolman used a maze in which there were three ways of getting to the goal: one short and direct path, one of medium length and one very long and roundabout. The short path joined the intermediate path a little before the goal. After the rat had been familiarized with the maze and learnt the shortest route, a block was inserted beyond the point where the short path joined the medium path. When the rat meets the block it returns to the start of the maze and should now be expected to try the medium path as in the past this had been rewarded more rapidly than the long path. In fact the animal chooses the long path. It 'knows', as it were, that the medium path is also blocked. It is hard to explain such facts on any assumption other than that a pattern of events has formed in the brain that parallels the structure of the maze. The rat has formed some kind of 'map' of the maze in the head. Beritoff[17] has noted how 'a blindfolded dog in a familiar situation comes out of its cage in response to a food signal and goes straight towards a definite foodbox, puts its forepaws on it, pushes its head through a hole and eats a given amount of food. Then it turns around and goes back into the cage. It runs to and from the foodbox by the shortest route, even in the absence of a food signal, that is to say, spontaneously, when the foodbox was closed. Moreover, the blindfolded dog may go to the place where the box is from any point of the given familiar room and then return to the cage or go to another place where food is.'

A different kind of evidence comes from the phenomena of insight. Köhler's studies on the insight of apes have become acknowledged classics[140]. In 'insightful' behaviour the animal is confronted with a novel situation to which its previous training provides no ready answer. Something other than past rewards must make the correct response appear. In a typical case a banana is suspended from the ceiling of the cage, too high for the ape to reach. But boxes are provided which the ape can move under the banana and pile up if necessary. The abruptness with which the correct solution then appears to be suddenly found and the 'pondering' that precedes the sudden insight are hard to explain except on the assumption that some reorganization or trial-and-error processes take place in the brain during the 'pondering' stage in which the whole arrangement, cage, banana, boxes and all are represented by patterns of events in the brain.

Now it is clear that to have a map in the head of a cage, a room, or a house cannot mean that in any literal sense the brain has built a little three-dimensional replica of these objects. In what sense, then, are we to understand a 'map in the head'? How are we to conceive of a neural organization which amounts to a unique internal representation of surrounding objects, their properties or relations?

The *general* answer to this question is not difficult to find, but the details of the mechanisms concerned pose exceptionally difficult problems. To see the general answer we must look at the brain in the light of the general biological functions it has to perform.

I have said that the activities of the organism must be matched to the objective features of the environment rather than to the subjective qualities of the stimuli impinging on the senses. The efficiency with which the organism can effect this control depends on the degree to which it can anticipate the outcomes of its actions and can build up expectations regarding the manner in which the sensory inputs transform as a function of time or, more importantly, as a function of its own activities. Metaphorically speaking, the effective power of the brain therefore hinges on its knowledge of what depends on what in what sort of way at any one time.

It follows that what the organism requires by way of a 'map in the head' of the surroundings at any one time is a set of neural processes or events which are representative of the way in which the scene will transform as the organism moves the eyes, head, body or limbs of the objects it will encounter as it advances in one direction or another, and possibly also of what will happen if it interferes with these objects in one way or another.

The position I shall maintain in this volume is that the primate brain does indeed form internal models of the outer world in this sense and that

(i) these models consist in the main of aggregates of expectations of how the sensory inputs will transform (a) in consequence of the movements of the eyes, head or body, and (b) in consequence of the subject's active interference with or manipulation of the objects of the outer world;

(ii) these aggregates of expectations are registered in neural terms by patterns of neural excitability (the latent form) or neural excitation (the activated form) which have two dimensions: one relating to the movements or interfering actions and the other to the resulting sensory transformations;

(iii) the overdetermination which this method of representation permits is offset by a lack of resolution in the individual expectations registered, thus keeping the demands made on the storage capacity of the brain within practicable bounds.

Thus the internal representation of a particular solid object would comprise not only a representation of the aspect the object presents to the viewer at the time but also representations of alternative aspects or perspectives, each 'tagged' according to the movements (e.g. walking around the object) or interfering actions (e.g. rotating the object) that would produce it. These expectations would be supplemented by expectations relating to other properties, e.g. to the resistance that would be experienced if one tried to move the object, compress it etc.

These expectations develop as the result of experiences which date right back to the early developmental stages of our perceptive faculties. They are encoded in terms of lasting changes in the responsiveness of particular neurons to particular input channels, thus resulting in the formation of particular cell organizations which are triggered *en bloc* when the object is perceived and in turn elicit the categorizing reactions that make us aware of the object as being one of a particular kind. Similarly when we imagine or remember an object (or event) we are dealing in physiological terms with the activation of particular cell organizations. (The difference between perceiving, imagining and remembering is not one that can be summarized in a few words in this preliminary outline. We shall come to this point when we deal with the matter in greater detail in Chapters 7, 9 and 11.)

It is evident that in this view perception is essentially action-oriented and the internal models are essentially predictive. Since the main function of the brain is to guide the activities of the organism we can hardly expect it to be otherwise. The consistent context in which the faculty of perception develops is one in which the organism is prepared to interact with the environment and the most significant information the organism can extract from the environment is the information that is relevant to its interaction with the environment.

Some philosophers have been worried by the concept of 'internal representations' because they have interpreted 'internal representations' as neural states that have structural correspondence with objects in the outer world and are 'interpreted' by the brain as signs for the external objects. This 'interpretation' would then seem to require that the representations themselves are first identified and if identification is only possible through comparison one finds oneself involved in an infinite regress. But these difficulties do not arise in the theory outlined above. Here the internal models are seen as aggregates of expectations. The activation of the expectations is part of the act of perception. Our reactions to the external world are formed physiologically as reactions to the activated models. There is no internal 'act' of comparing the models with reality and no 'act' of 'identifying' the model as a sign of the outer reality. There may indeed be discrepancies between the models and the real world: expectations may fail to be confirmed by the consequences of our actions and the brain reacts to such failures in particular ways. There may be short-term reactions (e.g. surprise reactions) and long-term reactions (e.g. modification or refinement of the expectations). But there is no separate act in which sign and significate are jointly held up for inspection and comparison.

As regards the way in which expectations about the sensory consequences of particular activities can be registered in neural terms, a few general indications may be given at this early stage of our enquiry.

The common denominator of the required neural representations is that they are all representations of how some variable (or set of variables) depends on some other variable (or set of variables). For example, they might be representations of how a particular class of sensory stimuli transform in consequence of particular self-induced movements of the eyes, head or body.

Now, to say that they must be representations of how some variable depends on some other variable is to say that they must be representations of the type of relationship that in a mathematical notation would be symbolized by expressions like $y = f(x)$, and in the sequel I shall use this notation to signify just that type of relationship. Thus x might stand for a movement of the organism and y for a stimulus input dependent on that movement; $f(x)$ then denotes how the latter depends on the former. Depending on the nature of the case, x and y in this expression may stand either for one-dimensional (scalar) variables or for multi-dimensional (vector) variables. Again, they may be either continuous or discrete variables.

Thus the basic question is: How can the brain form explicit neural representations of the manner in which some given variable depends on another, i.e. of functions of the type $y = f(x)$? To see how this may be done we must begin by realizing that the concept of how one variable depends on another, i.e. $y = f(x)$, really denotes a *set of ordered pairs of elements*, each pair here consisting of a value of x coupled with the associated value of y. *Ideally, therefore, a unique neural representation of a function $y = f(x)$ would consist of a set of simultaneous neural events which can be uniquely mapped on the complete set of ordered pairs of elements denoted by $y = f(x)$ over the domain of x. This condition can be met if there exists a set of possible and mutually exclusive neural events which can be mapped on the set of all possible combinations of x and y over the relevant domain of x, and if the brain activates simultaneously those members of this set of neural events that correspond to the particular combinations of x and y denoted by the function $y = f(x)$.* This, therefore, is the sort of thing we may have to look out for when we search for neural correlates of the internal models the brain forms of objects in the outside world.

In practice, of course, these conditions cannot be literally fulfilled unless x is a discrete variable and the domain of x is limited to a finite number of discrete values. If x is a continuous variable the internal models would have to be built up on a finite set of representative sample values of x.

In general, therefore, we must assume that the brain can form an internal representation of a function only by means of a set of simultaneous neural events which can be mapped on no more than a *sample* of the ordered pairs of elements denoted by the function. This does not matter provided each sample is sufficiently characteristic of the function concerned to prevent confusion with other significant functions. This in turn depends on discriminations expected of the organism in the practical circumstances in which it has to act.

A very simple example will suffice to show how the internal representation of a functional relationship may be conceived in neural terms. Suppose that in circumstances A an event B' would be followed by an event C', B'' by C'' and B''' by C'''. In other words, there exists a single-valued function $C = f_A(B)$ over the domain $B = B'$, B'', B'''. Suppose also that there exists a neural organization in the brain capable of producing nine different (but not mutually exclusive) neural events and that these can be mapped on the combinations $B'C'$, $B'C''$, $B'C'''$, ..., $B'''C'''$ respectively. At the simplest level we might picture these events as discharges of a set of neurons each of which is selectively responsive to the occurrence of one particular combination of B and C. Finally suppose that, during learning, the organization develops in a way which subsequently causes the perception of A to elicit simultaneously the three neural events corresponding to $B'C'$, $B''C''$ and $B'''C'''$ respectively and none of the other six. We can then say that A elicits an internal representation of the *function* $C = f_A(B)$ over the domain stated. Since C follows B in time we may also call this a neural representation of the *expectation* of how C depends on B, provided we can assume that, during learning, the responses prompted by this internal representation come to match the fact that C follows B in time.

The question of internal representations of functional relationships arises in many different spheres of activity. We shall see later that the 'stable image' of a scene, which the brain forms from the stream of images that cross the retina as the eyes move in their sockets, may be interpreted as a stable set of expectations (in the above sense) of how the retinal projections transform (translate) as the eyes move in their sockets. The 'maps in the head' of our surroundings—our 'cognitive maps', as they are sometimes called—may in turn be interpreted as sets of expectancies of how the stable scenes transform in response to head- and body-movements.

The brain forms unique internal representations not only of spatial relations. The human brain at any rate appears to be able to form internal representations of non-spatial relations, of physical properties of objects, of temporal sequences of events running their course (with or without interference by the perceiving subject), of the uses to which objects can be put and of many other features that prove significant in the subject's transactions with the surrounding world. In addition the brain can form internal representations of the posture and movements of the body itself and of the relation of the subject to the objects that surround it.

From what has gone before it is obvious that we understand by the internal representation of a physical property not merely some kind of detector system in the brain that flashes a light, so to speak, when an object having that property is perceived, imagined, or recalled in the memory. Such a light would be a *sign* of the property, not a *representation* as we understand the term here. To represent a property, in the full sense of the term as we understand it, the brain must form a neural organization which can register the nature of the property in the sense in which this affects the transactions of the organism with its environment. Any significant neural representation of the inertia of an object, for example, must contain some reference to the forces required to impart different accelerations. All this eventually reduces to a question of neural organizations capable of representing functional relationship between two (or more) variables or sets of variables in the manner explained above. Typically one set of variable relates to a class of self-induced movements and the other set to the sensory transformations resulting from these movements.

One element must be added to this preliminary account of internal representations of external properties or relations. In addition to internal representations of the way objects behave or respond in particular circumstances the notion implies that the subject derives from these representations a *categorization* of the objects concerned. By this we mean internal reactions which partition the representations in certain ways (but not always in constant or determinate ways).

For example, according to the degree of deformation produced when we apply particular forces to a set of objects we may come to divide this set into 'elastic' and 'inelastic' objects. We say that this categorization is *imposed* upon the objects. But it is *derived* from reactions to internal representations in which the shapes of object are registered as a function at the applied forces. In general these partitioning reactions develop in the course of experience and learning, as do most of the internal representations and expectations on which they are based.

By the recognition of a property we mean the activation of the respective internal representations and categorizing reactions. This activation does not necessarily presuppose the physical presence of objects manifesting the property. It can occur in consequence of the processes underlying the free play of the imagination or memory recall. The nature of these processes will occupy us at a later stage.

Behaviourists are notoriously averse to any postulate suggesting the existence of internal mediating processes or, more specifically, of unique internal representations of the outside world. Some, like Watson[270], have denied their existence outright. Others, like Ryle[212], lean over backwards to avoid them. Although Ryle, for example, allows for some internal mediating processes such as the 'silent soliloquies' he substitutes for 'thought', he generally denies the very existence of what we would normally understand in the human case by internal representations of external objects. 'True', he says, 'a person picturing his nursery is, in a certain way, like that person seeing his nursery, but the similarity does not consist in his really looking at a real likeness of his nursery but in his really seeming to see his nursery itself, when he is not really seeing it. He is not being a spectator of a resemblance of his nursery, but he is resembling a spectator of his nursery.' (Gilbert Ryle, *The Concept of Mind*. Reproduced by permission of Hutchinson Publishing Group Ltd.) Ryle is right in stressing that when we visualize a nursery or (to take one of his later examples) the smile on a doll's face, we are not 'seeing' in the ordinary sense. This would be generally acknowledged. A picture I see in the imagination is not, as snapshots are, in front of my face. It is not, therefore, in a physical space but in a space of another kind. This non-physical space Ryle cannot find. So of a child who imagines her wax doll smiling he says: 'The pictured smile is not then a physical phenomenon; nor is it yet a non-physical phenomenon observed by the child taking place in a field quite detached from her perambulator and her nursery. There is no smile at all, and *there is no effigy of a smile either*. There is only a child fancying that she sees her doll smiling' (my italics). (Gilbert Ryle, *The Concept of Mind*. Reproduced by permission of Hutchinson Publishing Group Ltd.) Nevertheless, in a very important (although metaphorical) sense there *is* an effigy and the non-physical space in which this exists is not difficult to find: it is a mathematical space relating to neural processes. It is a multi-dimensional space formed by sets of coordinates relating to patterns or distributions of neural excitations of the representational type I have adumbrated above. On Ryle's own account the child who fancies her doll smiling acts or reacts as if she were perceiving a smiling doll, just as the man who pictures his nursery acts or reacts as if he were seeing his nursery. As we shall see, either instance may imply a condition of the brain in which behaviour is controlled by representational patterns of neural excitation (or other neural functions) representing relations which are homomorphic with those characterizing the wax doll's smile or the man's nursery. There is nothing wrong in calling these homomorphic structures 'effigies'. An effigy is nothing if not a structure which is homomorphic with the object of which it is an effigy. 'Effigy' is not a term we use in this volume. 'Model' or 'unique internal representation' are preferable because they have less powerful visual connotations. That is merely a question of terminology.

It is one of the most important properties of the internal processes concerned in thinking that they have object reference in the sense of being conducted in terms of internal representation of objects (or their parts, properties or relations) rather than in terms of particulate stimuli impinging on the senses. They are true to the objects themselves (or their parts, properties or relations) not to the ephemeral projections of the objects on the peripheral sensors. Another important property is that these internal representations can be activated in the sensory absence of the objects to which they relate. This, of course, is where memory recall and imagination differ from perception.

Behaviourists do not deny that organisms regularly produce responses which are unique functions of objective features of their environment, but their dogmatic denial that, metaphorically speaking, there exists an internal platform on which external events can be reproduced or acted out, compels them to assume that the uniqueness of the representation is established at the motor periphery rather than centrally. Thus Ryle was driven to assume that thought is silent speech.

To test the assumption that thought is silent speech Thorson in 1925 used an elaborate apparatus to magnify and record tongue movements and searched for positive correlation in tongue movements when subjects first spoke test words softly and then merely thought about them. No observable correlation was found. Jacobson[124] on the other hand obtained positive correlations between records of motor potentials in the biceps and the subject imagining lifting a heavy load. Again, when subjects imagined looking up to the Eiffel Tower from base to tip recordings of eye muscles yielded results correlating with those recorded when actually moving the eyes upwards. But it does not follow that these implicit motor activities form part of the actual internal representations that compose our imaginings. The imagination is concerned with the internal acting out of external dramas, often by way of exploring alternative possibilities before we resort to overt actions. That this internal acting out should sometimes overflow into incipient motor activities can hardly be surprising on any theory. In fact Jacobson's results may be interpreted as evidence for the powerful role of expectations in the central mechanisms of the brain—the very element we stressed in connection with the formation of unique internal representations.

Throughout this section I have concentrated on a very sophisticated level of brain functions, viz. the organization of internal representations of the way in which things depend on each other and on the actions of the perceiving subject. I have adumbrated some of the general conditions the central organization of the brain must satisfy in order to factor out significant features of the physical world of which we have no raw sensation. At a later stage we shall attempt to arrive at a clearer picture of the neural mechanisms that appear to be involved in these transactions. Meanwhile we must not overlook the fact that a certain amount of this factoring out already begins at relatively low levels of perception.

The degree to which the nervous system already achieves object reference at an elementary perceptual level can be studied in the phenomena of 'constancy'. Familiar examples in this field are brightness constancies, colour constancies, size-and-shape constancies. By 'constancy phenomena' the psychologist means the tendency to see a familiar object as of its actual brightness, colour, size or shape, regardless of the conditions under which it is seen (distance, illumination etc.).

If a black disc is moved from a dark corner of a room into the bright sunlight at the window, it still appears black even though the light reflected from it now exceeds the intensity of the light that would be emitted from a white disc in the dark part of the room. Somewhere in the nervous system a constant reaction is maintained to the optical quality of the disc despite the different intensities of the light reflected from it in different parts of the room. The nervous system can only achieve this brightness constancy by taking into account extraneous clues about the different conditions of illumination to which the disc is exposed in the different locations. Experiments show that it derives these clues from the brightness of the surroundings and if the system is deprived of these clues the mechanism fails. For instance, if the black disc is illuminated by a powerful concealed spotlight whose beam strikes the disc only and none of its surroundings, the disc appears white. The nervous system now lacks sufficient clues about the conditions of observation. The same applies to colour constancies. When a blue paper is placed in yellow light it still appears blue, but if it is viewed through a reduction screen which shields the eye from all rays except those emitted by the paper, it appears grey (as would be predicted from the laws of colour mixture). Evidently, the effective internal representation of blueness is a very much more sophisticated affair than a mere set of volleys derived by convergence from particular brands of colour-sensitive receptors.

Elementary constancies of this kind are found in lower forms of life too. Chickens trained to select white grains but reject those stained yellow, choose the white grains also under strong yellow light.

The elementary constancies are not always (or even usually) perfect. Asked to say which of a number of rods of different lengths suspended at a distance of (say) ten yards, appears equal in length to a standard rod suspended at five yards, the average subject is unlikely to achieve perfect object reference and size constancy, i.e. perfect compensation for the different visual angles the near and distant rods subtend; and he is unlikely to judge the size correctly. What is perceived, therefore, sometimes represents something of a compromise between subjective sensory data and perfect object reference. Nor does the brain always achieve perfect separation of what the physicist would regard as separate physical dimensions. An audible note of 495 cycles per second received at an intensity of 55 decibels may be perceived as identical in pitch to a note of 510 cycles per second received at an intensity of 65 decibels. Similarly, monochromatic light of a wavelength of 550 millimicrons and intensity of 10 photons per second may be experienced as having the same hue as light of 525 millimicrons at an intensity of 1000 photons per second.

However, these are not very stark deviations from perfect object reference and, for the purpose of the very broad theoretical considerations that concern us in this chapter, they may safely be ignored.

What matters as a starting point is that the mature brain does in fact already achieve a considerable degree of object reference at an elementary perceptual level as well as at the higher levels of perception. It has come to be the prevailing view in experimental psychology that nearly all perception is perception of objects, that constancies pervade perception on all levels, from the most elementary to the most complex, and that the brain achieves this object reference by taking into account the clues that are available to it in the total flux of sensory inputs. By integrating these clues in the appropriate manner it can synthesize patterns of neural reactions which are specific to classes of objects exhibiting particular qualities or relations.

Sometimes the necessary clues are contained in the momentary totality of the sensory inputs, as in brightness or colour constancies. In other cases they can only be extracted from temporal sequences of sensory inputs and self-induced movements, as when we discover the shape of an object in the dark by tactile exploration.

2.3   LANGUAGE

Broadly speaking, we think in images and words. Yet, the nature of language is supremely important for our present enterprise not only because language is part of the medium in which thoughts are formed, but also because, in a sense to be explained in Chapter 3, the nature of language occupies a key position in the analysis of what separates the 'mental' from the 'physical'.

One could wish that something as important as language would be less complex and intricate, and more obviously lawful in structure and composition. As it is I must try and distil from the complexity of the natural languages those abstract features that have a particular bearing on our enterprise and that can give us at any rate a broad idea of the kind of organizational problems the brain has to solve in connection with speech and rational thought. Since what is relevant must depend on the context, it is perhaps not surprising that these abstract features are not characteristics that can be readily culled from textbooks on linguistics.

I shall also try to elucidate some of the main features that distinguish the linguistic transmission of information from other forms of information transfer and I shall discuss a number of concepts that arise in the discussion of verbal communications and their contents. All this is relevant if we are to come to grips with the fundamentals of the higher brain functions without being caught up in philosophical and semantic confusions.

In turning to the discussion of verbal communications the scientist passes from the discussion of physical events to the discussion of messages and meanings. First of all, therefore, it is important to be clear about the proper context in which we can speak of certain physical events (sounds, electrical pulses, action potentials in nerve fibres etc.) as *signals* or *messages* and attribute to them a particular *message content*.*

* In the following pages I shall avoid the expression 'information content' since this phrase is now frequently reserved for the quantitative measure information theory attaches to message contents.

Consider an electronically controlled thermostat designed to maintain an object Q at a constant temperature t'. To perform this function the device has to monitor the current temperature of Q. Assume therefore that the thermostat is linked to Q by a transmission cable T and that the thermal transducers in Q are such that the amplitude A of the current in T corresponds to the temperature of Q. Then it is obvious that to describe this current as one signalling the temperature of Q or (more elaborately) as one conveying a message to the effect that Q has a certain temperature, makes sense only in a *functional context*, i.e. in a context in which structures, states or events in the overall system are *functionally* categorized or individuated. By this I mean that they are categorized or individuated according to the *logical role they perform in the production of appropriate outputs*. In particular we can say that the current in T 'signifies', 'informs about' or 'reports' the temperature of Q only by virtue of the fact that in this machine the intervention of the current in T enables the temperature of Q to become an appropriate determinant of the thermostat's outputs. By 'appropriate outputs' (above) I mean outputs that are related to the circumstances in which they occur in a manner conducive to the attainment of a particular goal, in this case the constancy of the temperature of Q. Thus the vocabulary of 'signals', 'messages', 'information', 'message contents' etc. belongs to a language or context of discussion which explicitly or implicitly relates to the appropriateness of structures, states, processes etc., in respect of some particular goal. This goal may be explicitly mentioned or merely tacitly understood. Moreover the goal need not be one *pursued* by the machine. It may be one merely *served* by the machine, i.e. a goal *pursued* by those who designed or employed the machine.

Thus the ascription of *contents* or *meanings* to physical events in a transmission system (electrical, physiological or otherwise) can be given a rationale only by pointing out the actual or potential contribution the events make to the production of appropriate outputs, i.e. of outputs that in a normal working of the system are related to the circumstances in which they occur in a manner that is conducive to the attainment of a particular goal.

These results underline the important fact that statements asserting contents are intensional rather than extensional. The statement that our signals in T carry a message to the effect that Q has a temperature t'', does not imply that Q in fact has the temperature t'', nor indeed that Q exists or that anything exists having the temperature t''. Q may have vanished through some mishap or the temperature sensors may have broken down. This in turn is the rationale for distinguishing between *true* and *false* message contents.

When in Chapter 3 we come to consider the nature of mental as distinct from physical events, this dependence of content or meaning on a functional or organizational context will prove to be particularly important. This aspect of 'meaning' has been increasingly appreciated in recent times. MacKay[156], for example, points out that 'when a man speaks to another man, the meaning of what he says is defined by a spectrum over the elementary acts of internal response which can be evoked in the hearer'.

It follows from the above that different types of signals can have the same content. We say in that case that there are different expressions of the same messages or that they are expressions using a different *code*. Hence we can characterize a message content by paraphrasing it in a different code. Non-linguistic messages, in particular, may be paraphrased linguistically. This is commonly done in the propositional form as in 'a signal to the effect that Q has the temperature t'.

The time has come to pass from the general subject of messages and their content to the rather more specific subject of linguistic messages. Naturally, in a short space I cannot deal with the vast complexity of linguistic communication even if I were competent to do so. I can only single out certain central features which are particularly relevant to our main topics.

To make the transition to linguistic communication consider first a more sophisticated thermal control system which is designed independently to control the temperatures of two objects P and Q to which, however, it is connected only by a single transmission cable. Assume that it is informed about the current temperature of P and Q by means of pairs of pulses in the cable, the amplitude of the first pulse in each pair indicating the object and that of the second pulse its temperature. We would then have signals which resemble human speech in one important respect, viz. in that they consist of 'statements' which essentially have a subject–predicate structure and which have a 'syntax' in the sense that the significance of each term depends on its serial position within the 'statements'. This use of signals specifically relating to or 'naming' an object, in juxtaposition with signals specifically relating to or 'naming' an attribute, i.e. class, is significant because the most distinctive features of the natural languages arise from the manner in which these languages have surmounted the limitations inherent in the type of simple two-term messages we have just considered. The complexities of the natural languages are best understood if they are seen in this light.

Every consistent response by an organism to the objects that occur in its environment amounts to a *categorization* of these objects. It divides the class of all possible objects into two subclasses, viz. the objects that elicit the given response and those that do not.

Categorization in this sense is to be found throughout the animal kingdom. But, as we have seen, the observation that a particular overt response generalizes over a particular class of objects does not necessarily imply that the brain has formed an internal representation of the common denominator of these objects.

When objects are assigned to a particular class or category (I use these terms interchangeably) according to a set of criteria of which the brain has formed an internal representation, we say that we have formed a *concept* of the class concerned. Such criteria may relate to the appearance or physical properties of the objects or to a variety of other things. They may relate to the purposes for which an object may be used, to the emotions it arouses, to the dangers it presents, to its edibility etc. Concepts, therefore, are not just collections of physical properties.

For some classes we have names, for others we have not. Words may label particular objects ('John', 'Mary') but, in the main, words label realms of concepts rather than physical things. The names we find in a dictionary relate to classes and not single individuals. In general these classes are *open classes*, i.e. classes determined by a set of criteria. The category 'chair' is not determined by enumerating all objects that are given that name. It is determined by the special purpose for which the objects were designed or to which they lend themselves.

Although in some cases language may introduce a biasing factor in the formation of concepts, a number of investigations show that this is not a major influence[147]. In general we are justified in treating naming as a consequence of categorization rather than a cause. Whereas namability frequently tends to be coupled with cognitive salience, no major constraint of words upon our cognitive faculties has been conclusively demonstrated. Speakers tend to use words to label conceptualizations which develop unrestricted by the dictionary meanings of the words they use.

With Popper we may distinguish four main functions of language:

  (i) expressive or symptomatic functions (exclamations etc.);
 (ii) stimulative or signal functions (e.g. commands);
(iii) descriptive functions (information about the environment etc.);
(iv) argumentative functions (reasoned discourse).

The last two are of paramount interest in the present context. I shall take the descriptive function first.

Simple descriptive propositions ('John is tall', 'the car is red') commonly serve to convey that a particular object, event or situation is of a particular kind, i.e. belongs to a particular class of objects, events or situations. The class membership may be asserted for the present, the past or the future (the water 'is' cold, 'was' cold, 'will be' cold). For a start, however, we shall ignore this time reference and merely look at what is involved in conveying the information that a particular object is a member of a particular class.

If the vocabulary of our language were large enough to contain a separate name for each individual object, event or situation about which we wish to communicate and, equally, a separate name for each class to which we should wish to assign them, the structure of our language would be simple indeed. Apart from the time reference (tense), it could discharge its descriptive function in the form of simple two-word sentences in which the name of the object, event or situation is coupled with that of the appropriate class. 'Water cold', 'kettle hot' would be typical examples.

To serve any useful purpose the vocabulary of such a language would have to be absurdly large. A solution had to be found by which the communication of information could transcend the limitations imposed by a restricted vocabulary and simple binary word combinations. The solution found in the natural languages is basically simple and logically obvious: if the vocabulary does not provide a name for the class to which a particular object is to be assigned in a verbal message, the obvious solution is to demarcate the class in terms of the logical product of classes for which the vocabulary does provide a name.

In practice this is seen to take the form of either an explicit logical product ('Smith is tall, dark and handsome') or of the type of logical product that is implied when a species is indicated in terms of its genus and differentia. Thus in the statement 'John throws a blue ball' the constituent 'throws' assigns John to a particular class of ordered pairs, viz. the class of all subjects throwing when paired with objects thrown. This class is the genus. The differentia is provided by specifying the object thrown (blue ball), this specification, in turn, relating to a genus (ball) and differentia (blue).

The technique, therefore, is to express the class for which we have no name in the vocabulary as the logical product of classes for which we have a name in the vocabulary. In the sequel I shall call classes for which we have a single word, i.e. a name in the vocabulary, *namable classes*, and classes for which we have *no* name in the vocabulary *unnamable classes*. Using these shorthand terms, therefore, we can say that the general technique employed in linguistic communication is to express unnamable classes as the logical product of (in the last instance) namable classes. This logical process is crucial to our understanding of the deep structure of the natural languages. In the sequel I shall call this logical step the *cognitive resolution* of the unnamable class in terms of namable classes.

Relations between classes may be illustrated by Venn diagrams (Figure 2.5(a)). The members of a class are here represented by the points in the plane of the paper which lie inside the oval designating the class.

A *relation* between pairs of elements may be thought of as a class of ordered pairs. The relation 'father of', for example, may be thought of as the class of all father–offspring pairs of beings. In the idiom of Venn diagrams a relation may be represented by a family of arrows linking the respective pairs of points in the plane (Figure 2.5(b)). The cognitive resolution applied in our example of 'John throws a blue ball' may therefore be represented graphically as in Figure 2.6.

I have said that descriptive sentences typically convey the information that some particular object is a member of a particular class. In the above example we assumed that the subject of the sentence ('John') was namable

but the class was not. When the subject is not namable the same technique
of cognitive resolution must be used to specify it in terms of classes that are
namable. In the sentence, 'that strong man threw a blue ball', for example, the

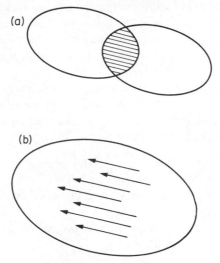

Figure 2.5. Venn diagrams

subject is indicated in a way which may be broadly rendered as 'the object to
which I am attending and which is strong and which is a man'. The cognitive
resolution which this presupposes calls for no further comment. The reader
will note that, if a cognitive resolution is analysed as a system of formal steps,
this system will have a hierarchical structure.

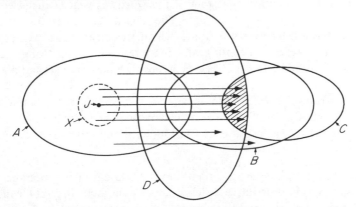

Figure 2.6. Venn diagram of cognitive resolution of the unnamable class in terms
of namable classes in 'John throws a blue ball'. *A*, beings capable of throwing;
B, throwable objects; *C*, balls; *D*, blue objects; arrows: relation of thrower to
object thrown; *J*, John; *X*, unnamable class to which John is assigned (here
defined by the roots of the arrows whose heads lie in the shaded area)

To perform these feats the brain must have the ability to see the unnamable object or class as the logical product of namable classes (in the special sense in which these terms are used here). This may be likened to our visual ability to see a perceptual figure as a composite of more elementary figures in respect of which the brain has special competences of recognition or reproduction. A possible comparison is with the action of a child which reorganizes the picture of, say, an animal in terms of the elementary shapes which it knows how to draw: ovals, circles, sticks etc.

The main complexities and differences of the natural languages arise from the code they use for expressing the resolution which has been used for specifying the unnamable objects or classes in terms of namable classes. This code avails itself of three main instruments:

(i) the order in which the names of the objects or classes (the *content* words) appear in the sentence;

(ii) the use of a standard range (closed class) of word-modifiers, mainly endings (*-ly*, *-ment*, *-s*, *-ing* etc.);

(iii) the use of a standard range of *grammatical* or *functional* words (*the, in, we, any, that, who, after* etc.).

In addition the objects or classes that occur in the cognitive resolution are themselves categorized according to certain criteria, for instance according to whether they relate to objects, properties or actions, whether the objects are single or plural, male, female etc. These *lexical* divisions generate a variety of word classes (nouns, adjectives, verbs etc.) which the code of the natural languages also takes into account in determining the final structure of the sentence. They may affect the order of the words as well as the selection of functional words or word-endings. The lexical categorization may, for example, distinguish between attributes which are constant to a class of objects and those that are merely contingent. Compare for instance, 'John is a brute' with 'John is brutal'. The first case generates a 'noun', the second an 'adjective'.

We see from this brief (and inevitably oversimplified) account that if descriptive verbal utterances are examined in the light of the ultimate information they serve to convey, at least four different cognitive processes must be distinguished:

1. The first cognitive process relates to the content of the message. In the case of simple descriptive sentences this means factoring out the information that a particular object (event, situation) is a member of a particular class.

2. The second process consists of the cognitive resolution which is required in all cases in which either the object or the class (or both) are unnamable. The unnamable object and class each now comes to be appre-

hended as the intersection of a number of namable classes sufficient to prevent confusion with other objects or classes. This stage calls for internal representations of the namable classes and of the relations in which they occur in the resolution. The structure of this resolution forms the *abstract underlying structure* on which the *overt* or *superficial structure* of the final sentence is based.

3. The third process consists of 'lexical' categorizations of the namable objects or classes highlighted at the second stage.
4. Finally, the sentence structure depends on factoring out the time reference (past, present or future) of the message.

Since our aim is to achieve a deeper insight into the mechanisms of the higher brain functions, it is worth noting at this stage some of the demands our linguistic competences make on those mechanisms.

First, we have seen earlier that language and thought call for internal representations of 'models' of the objects or events to which our descriptive utterances relate. In Section 2.2 we arrived at a general idea of what this implies in terms of pattern of neural excitations. We saw that these internal models consist of particular sets of expectations and we noted the general manner in which such expectations can be represented in neural terms. (More detailed realizations will be considered in Chapter 7.) Next, to accomplish steps 1 and 2 the brain must be able to form an appropriate set of generalized reactions to these representations, viz. reactions which are specific to the relevant attributes of the object to be described. Furthermore it must be able selectively to activate, or render effective, particular sets of these reactions. The brain must also be able to form internal representations of the fact that the attributes concerned belong to the object being described. For, although the respective categorizing reactions are implicitly associated with the object in the sense that they are elicited by the internal representation of the object, the fact of association needs an explicit internal representation as a precondition of the speaker's ability to express it explicitly. In Chapter 11 we shall see that this fact of association may itself be internally represented by a particular set of expectations. This, therefore, does not call for anything essentially new.

To accomplish 3 above the brain must be able to form an appropriate set of even more general reactions to the reactions listed above, viz. the reactions which give us the appropriate lexical categorizations. As regards the reactions required to accomplish 4 we must assume that the internal representations of the brain extend over temporal associations to which, in a given context, appropriate reactions can be formed.

The question of the role these various reactions play in the processes of speech production touches on the difficult question of the rules that govern the structure of our verbal utterances. This is the realm of linguistics.

Chomsky[41] and others[164] have initiated research in this area whose most important implication (from our point of view) is that the control of linguistic behaviour must be hierarchically rather than serially organized[176]. This means here that the reactions we have listed must exercise a joint control over the whole sentence which precedes and directs the production of its parts. Since according to our analysis the role of each class name ('content word') in the sentence is determined by the function it fulfils in the cognitive resolution that precedes the sentence production and since this role is indicated in the surface structure of the sentence by the position of the name in conjunction with the word-modifiers that may be applied and the functional words that may be added, Chomsky confirms a conclusion that follows directly from the above analysis.

So far we have only thought of the surface structure of the sentence and factors determining it. The surface structure in turn determines the string of verbal utterances through which the sentence is expressed. In linguistic analysis the smallest unit of language said to contribute to the meaning of a sentence is the *morpheme*. Morphemes, as it were, are the atomic units of the surface structure. The word 'uninterrupted', for example, may be represented as the three morphemes un–interrupt–ed.

In the vocal production of a sentence each morpheme finds acoustic expression in a string of *phonemes*. Thus the morpheme 'man' yields the phonemic string, m æ n. Each phoneme in turn may be thought of as an organized set of instructions to the muscles involved in speech production (but see Chapter 11).

2.4 RATIONAL THOUGHT

Many of those who ponder about the functions of the human brain find it impossible to conceive even dimly of any kind of bridge between the 'mechanical' functions of neural systems on the one hand and the rational or logical character of the outputs of the thinking process on the other. The neural mechanisms of reasoning seem beyond comprehension.

The difficult question of the nature of 'mental' events, such as thought, memories, imaginings and feelings, and their relation to physical events in the brain will occupy us in Sections 3.3 and 3.4. However, so as not to misdirect our efforts, it is important to stress at this early stage that what makes thoughts rational is not so much the nature of the internal events that are associated with them as the final results of those events, e.g. the interrelation of the statements they produce and of the beliefs these may express. Thus the logical order of a syllogism like

> All men are mortal
> Socrates is a man
> Socrates is mortal

need not reflect a serial order of events in the brain.

We are now concerned with the *argumentative* use of language and, as the example shows, even at the simplest level this involved *general propositions* in addition to the simple descriptive propositions we considered in the last section.

General propositions are of the type 'all A is B', 'some A is not B' and 'no A is B'. These propositions express relations between classes. The logical relations between propositions are based on class-relationships of this type.

Without general propositions the argumentative use of language would be impossible. The most fundamental class relation which enters into reasoned discourse is that of class inclusion. It entitles us to infer 'A is C' from 'A is B' and 'all B is C'. However, general propositions have a functional value in their own right, quite apart from reasoned discourse. For, functionally, the general proposition 'all X is Y' amounts to a licence to react to any X as to any Y. This function also suggests what kind of internal representations we can associate with general propositions. Obviously these representations cannot be of the same type as the internal representation (i.e. aggregate of expectations) associated with simple descriptive propositions like 'John is sleeping'. Rather, we must think of the internal representation of 'all X is Y' as a readiness of the brain to attach to any X the expectations attached to Y, i.e. as a generalization of expectations.

In practice, general propositions thus amount to a licence to extend or transform the internal representations of external situations or of elements of external situations along specific lines. In this way they may enter many fundamental processes of problem solving. By 'problem solving' we mean a process of acquiring an appropriate response or set of responses to a new situation.

Consider the case of a man who is lost on a country ramble and now reasons as follows: 'I am facing the sun. At midday the sun is in the south. It is midday. Therefore I am facing south. I want to go west. Therefore I must now turn to the right.' In terms of internal representation this example of problem solving has taken the form of a tentative exploration of internal representation of elements of the problem situation, and of transformations permitted by accepted general propositions, until a set of internal representations of elements of the situation ('I am facing the sun', 'it is midday') is found which an accepted general proposition ('at midday the sun is in the south') allows to be transformed into some internal representations to which he knows how to respond: ('I am facing south while wanting to go west'). I have illustrated the process in verbal terms but, if the descriptive and general propositions concerned are based on internal representations, it is perfectly conceivable that this type of process may run its course without the accompaniment of either 'loud' or 'silent' speech.

This example typifies much of the rational problem solving that we use as we go about our daily business. It has taken us right into the realm of rational

thought processes. Frequently, of course, we solve our problems at a perceptual rather than conceptual level. If I have to fit a carpet to a room I will
probably begin by acting out in the imagination the consequences of manipulating the carpet in one way or another until I have found a way that I
recognize as a solution. This is again a process of 'licensed' transformations of
internal representations. But in this case the representations are complex
visual representations of an entire scene and the transformations are licensed
not by verbal formulae but quite simply by the past experiences I have had in
the manipulation of objects and shapes. However, if we look a little closer
at the actual activities the brain appears to be engaged in when we think,
we come to realize that any undue occupation with the formal properties of
the end products of our thinking, the formal structure of a reasoned argument
or theory, may cloud our view of the internal processes that produce them.

To explain what I mean it is expedient to look at the exercise of some of
our lesser skills, such as playing tennis or golf. The perfection of these skills
with practice depends on the learning mechanisms that control our skeletal
movements and the coordination of our muscles. The function of these
mechanisms is to correlate and integrate the information supplied by the
senses in a way that produces the appropriate movements of body and limbs.
They achieve this function by learning to activate the correct combinations
of efferent outputs in response to all relevant combinations of afferent inputs.
Eventually the player knows how to perform movements which correctly
match the position or flight of the ball. These correct movements may have
certain formal properties. For the sake of argument let us assume that the
perfect golf stroke is a circular movement of the club and the perfect tennis
stroke a rectilinear motion of the racket. It is clear from this that these formal
properties of the appropriate actions are irrelevant when it comes to explaining the physiological processes involved in learning these actions. The learning
mechanisms have simply learnt by trial and error to produce particular outputs
in response to particular inputs. Whether the resulting outputs satisfy
$y = ax + b$ or $y^2 + x^2 = r^2$ is of no concern to them. Their only concern
is that the movements should be successful.

The situation changes only when the player begins to reflect on the formal
properties of the stroke and tests its correctness, not by watching the ball in
flight, but, for example, by watching his practice shots in a mirror. It may
then become supremely important for him to know that the perfect stroke
should be circular in the one case and rectilinear in the other and he must be
able to recognize a circular or rectilinear movement when he sees one.

The example underlines what I said at the beginning, viz. that in the study
of thought processes we must be careful to distinguish between the work and
the result of the work. The formal, logical structure of reasoned arguments
and theories may be compared with the formal relationships that characterize
the perfect stroke at golf or tennis. They may be equally irrelevant when it

comes to understanding the neural mechanisms that produce our thoughts or the neural learning changes that take place as our rational faculties develop. They become supremely important when we check (or recommend to others) the result of the work.

During learning the brain adapts to the way things are and this automatically includes adapting to the way things logically are. In learning formal reasoning the brain has to adapt to the fact that the free transformation of propositions only leads to successful outcomes if it proceeds subject to particular restraints, i.e. if it restricts itself to the 'licensed' transformations I talked about earlier on. This adaptation is not unlike the lessons the nervous system has to learn when it discovers the restraints that the forces of gravity and the laws of balance impose on the free movements of body and limbs if these movements are to be successful. To account for the faculty of reasoning, therefore, we need not assume that some radically new type of neural learning mechanisms had to develop in the brain. The restraints implied in the notion of 'licensed' transformations initially may take the form merely of inhibitions learnt in much the same way as other inhibitions the nervous system has to learn if its responses are to meet with success.

Nor must we forget that a great deal of thinking is conducted in terms of visual images rather than linguistic symbols. The activity of thinking often appears as a vague search for images as well as for words, as an acting out of internal dramas as well as the silent rehearsing of speeches and arguments. Both image- and word-formations appear among the structures that precipitate in the stream of consciousness when we are engaged in thinking, sometimes in coherent sequences, at other times in a kind of internal trial and error process in which we persist until, at last, a structure crystallizes which appears to us as a solution to our problem. Suddenly insight has occurred; the elements of the task fall into place and, in a decisive act of acquisition, the product of our thinking is accepted as a platform for action. The process as a whole is a dynamic process in time, but 'thoughts' in the sense of what is acquired as the result of these events is a new and non-episodic state of awareness, self-preparation or programme acceptance, which functions as a unitary factor in the subsequent determination of our course of action. There are no partial thoughts in this sense.

Although this is a somewhat metaphorical account of thinking, it serves to emphasize some of the ambiguities we must guard against in our use of such terms as 'thoughts' or 'thinking'. Some of these arise because we are apt to use the same terms indiscriminately for

> (i) the end product of the internal activities I have sketched, i.e. for the content of what is acquired in the course of our mental activity: 'I was thinking', John said, 'that if we attach the lever at this point we should get a greater purchase';

(ii) for the act of acquisition: 'the thought suddenly struck me', Peter replied, 'that . . .' etc.;

(iii) for the exploratory processes that precede the act: 'What are you doing, John?' 'I am thinking', John replies. But a moment later, as he jumps up and attaches the lever, he may exclaim: 'I have got it.' This time there were no verbal symbols, only a sequence of visual images and an action programme released by the end product of the sequence.

CHAPTER 3

Mind, Brain and Behaviour

3.1 SEMANTIC DIVISIONS

In the last chapter I gave an outline of rational thought processes in which I deliberately steered clear of concepts derived from introspection. Rational thought was presented as a transformation of internal representations which is confined to particular channels, viz. those licensed by the intrinsic properties of classes. And 'internal representations' were defined in purely functional terms.

All the same, the neuroscientist cannot ignore the subject of mental events in the sense in which they are revealed to us by introspection and it is important therefore to realize the methodological status of mental concepts and the particular problems this creates for the neurosciences.

The neurosciences are faced with the unique problem that many of the phenomena they are expected to explain are studied by investigators working in different disciplines, accustomed to different languages and often operating at quite different levels of thought. At one end of the scale we have the data compiled by the physiologist and anatomist. At this level we are dealing with precise descriptions of anatomical structures and accurate observations of physical and chemical events. All variables here are definable in the language of the exact sciences: electrical potentials, discharge frequencies, skeletal movements, chemical changes etc. We observe accurately definable electrical, chemical or mechanical responses to accurately definable stimuli.

Our next set of data comes from the behavioural sciences which deal with the integral results of nervous activity as they are revealed in the observable behaviour of the living organism. At this level experimental psychology furnishes a wealth of data on the overt behaviour patterns of the living organism, on the goals they pursue in different circumstances, on their powers of discrimination, learning, motor control etc.

Finally, at the other end of the scale, we have the ramified studies of human psychology, of the interplay of emotions, volitions and cognitions, of the stream of consciousness and the mental states which we ascertain introspectively or claim to infer from our observations of the behaviour of others.

The fundamental predicament is that the languages of the mental and behavioural sciences cover the things we most want to know about, but they often lack the clarity and precision of the physical sciences, whereas the language of physiology has the scientific precision required but deals only with isolated part-events in which the integral, holistic aspects of the nervous system are lost from sight. Our ultimate aspiration must be to achieve the scope of the one field of enquiry without sacrificing the standards of precision which are the virtues of the other.

There are those who gloss over this predicament by assuring us that the gap will automatically close in time as our experimental techniques improve in quality and penetration. Why not therefore forget about the 'mental' aspects of brain function and about the holistic aspects of behaviour and concentrate on finding physiological explanations of physiological observations? As fact uncovers fact, a model of the brain's functional organization will eventually crystallize of its own accord and with it a picture of the person as a single sentient and rational entity. But in practice this is not a tenable position even at the behavioural level, i.e. even if we think of a person as no more than a physical object manifesting certain types of observable behaviour. The neuroscientist must work with hypotheses and, where relations between the microscopic and the macroscopic are involved, these hypotheses must take account of behaviour. In order to be able to evaluate a hypothesis about the synaptic changes that may occur in learning, the neurologist must be able to predict the 'molar' consequences of the predicted 'molecular' events. His hypothesis must be tested against the observation of 'molar' behaviour. This means that he must make at least some assumptions about the functional organization of the nervous system, about its relevant connectivities and their effects as revealed in overt behaviour.

Even before this stage is reached he needs some sort of model to guide him in his search and to suggest the kind of things to look for. One cannot just measure everything that is measurable. In a laboratory experiment we may condition an animal to a particular response. By reversing the training procedure the response may subsequently again be extinguished. Does this reversibility mean that the synaptic changes involved in learning must themselves consist of reversible processes? And should the physiologist therefore limit his search to that class of possible physiological processes? These are questions you cannot answer without some kind of organizational model of the brain as a whole and of its relation to observed behaviour. To take another example, the researcher may play with the hypothesis that during learning the synapses undergo lasting changes simply as result of use. It would then be essential for him to know whether this hypothesis would be sufficient to explain the learning phenomena observed by the experimental psychologist and this in turn presupposes assumptions about the general organization of the learning mechanisms. There is really no part of the brain about which one can think without at some point coming up against questions concerning the organization of the whole. There is no piece of the jigsaw puzzle which can be moved with profit without the eyes roaming over the whole puzzle.

This search for comprehensive models of the functional organization and operational principles of the brain cannot be left to the end. It must run *pari passu* with the work of those whose researches lie closer to the grass-roots. We are reminded of the cautionary tale of the spy who was so obsessed with the details of his work that he tried to trace the telephone cables of the Pentagon in order to uncover the seat of the U.S. High Command—and came to locate it in the Pentagon's telephone exchange!

The experimental psychologist, in turn, cannot pursue the study of human behaviour without being drawn into discussions about the subject's mental life and data derived from introspection. In whatever experimental situation a human subject is placed, the outcome of the experiment may be critically influenced by the subject's own ideas of what is happening and the meaning he attaches himself to the experimental and environmental conditions. An extreme example is the therapeutic effect of placebos. It is well known that this depends on the beliefs which the patient derives from suggestions implicit in the experimental situation and which are only partly under the control of the experimenter.

To try to avoid the problem of mental states by substituting physiological criteria whenever this seems feasible may yield no more than a spurious objectivity. Basowitz *et al.*[15] have described an experiment in which a number of patients received small doses of adrenaline intravenously. One subject showed alarming changes in blood pressure and pulse rates although he himself did not feel particularly anxious. The same group contained another subject who complained of great anxiety and seemed to approach a state of panic although his circulatory responses showed no significant change.

To achieve objectivity must always be the scientist's aim. Coupled with this goes the demand that the results of his experiments must be capable of verification. Data derived from introspection pose exceptionally difficult problems in this respect.

Carnap[39] has defended the acceptability of introspective evidence. 'Psychological concepts', he says, 'are properties, relations or quantitative magnitudes ascribed to certain space-time regions (usually human organisms or classes of such). Therefore, they belong to the same logical types as concepts of physics . . .' and later; 'Although many of the alleged results of introspection were indeed questionable, a person's awareness of his own state of imagining, feeling etc., must be recognized as a kind of observation, in principle not different from external observation, and therefore as a legitimate source of knowledge. . . .' However, although 'in principle' observation based on introspection may not differ from external observations, in practice there is a crucial, indeed critical, difference. This is that the subject's reports based on introspection are bound to use words or phrases which may mean different things to different people and there is no operational way of defining them which could guarantee uniform and consistent usage. Since introspective concepts relate to private experiences, there is no way in which we can make sure that two people mean exactly the same thing by the statement 'I feel anxious', for example. Indeed the concept of 'meaning the same thing' may not even be applicable in this type of situation.

Special experimental methods have been designed to minimize the short-comings of data derived from introspection. Self-observation can be given a comparatively high degree of objectivity, for example, by structuring it through questionnaires which have been validated statistically against clini-cally established 'criteria groups'. However, the selection of these representa-tive groups requires subjective judgements by the clinician which in turn detract from perfect objectivity.

Many of the confusions caused by the problems I have mentioned can be forestalled if from the start we draw a sharp distinction between three languages in which we can talk about the things that go on inside our head or the overt behaviour that springs from them. For brevity we may label these three languages as 'brain talk', 'behaviour talk' and 'mind talk'. In rather more explicit terms they are:

(I) The language of the physical sciences. This includes the language of anatomy, physiology, biochemistry, biophysics etc.

(II) The language of goal-directed behaviour. In this language the reac-tions of the organism are classified not in terms of discrete physical or physiological outputs, but in terms of the goals towards which they are directed. This is the common language of experimental psychology. As has been said the vast majority of the animal responses which the experimental psychologist studies consists of families of movements which are defined in terms of the immediate goals they seek: 'building a nest', 'pressing a lever', 'approaching a foodbox', 'jumping a hurdle', 'reaching for a banana' etc. We have seen in Section 2.1 in what sense the goal-directedness of behaviour reflects a particular class of objec-tive system properties. In Chapter 4 we shall see how language II can be translated into language I through the concept of *directive cor-relation*.

(III) The language of mental states and mental events. In a strictly literal sense this language can be applied to human beings only, as it origin-ates in self-awareness and in the analysis of our own stream of con-sciousness. To this language belong terms like 'feeling', 'emotion', 'volition', 'cognition', 'remembering', 'imagining', 'expecting' and qualified feelings like 'pain', 'hunger', 'thirst', 'pleasure', 'sorrow' etc. We shall see in the next section that, contrary to beliefs fashionable today, the concepts of language III cannot be translated into language II without a change of meaning.

It is often profitable to re-define these class III concepts in class II terms, but serious confusions result if this is not done explicitly and the resulting change of meaning is allowed to go unnoticed.

The most common causes of muddled thinking spring from

(i) the use of concepts of class III for the explanation of phenomena described in terms of language II without the prior re-definition mentioned above;

(ii) the use of class II concepts for the explanation of phenomena described in language I without prior re-definition;

(iii) the rejection of language II and/or III altogether on account of their semantic indeterminacy (Watson's behaviourism being an extreme example). In our present state of knowledge this attitude is excusable as regards language III but (since the development of the concept of directive correlation) no longer as regards language II.

3.2   SCIENCE AND PURPOSIVE BEHAVIOUR

We have a great deal of commonsense knowledge about animal behaviour and our own behavioural tendencies and mental functions. But the language in which commonsense knowledge is formulated is notoriously vague. The classes of things designated by our commonsense notions may not be sharply and clearly demarcated from each other, or they may lack the specificity required to bring out important differences between the things denoted by a single concept. We can see in any dictionary of the English language that there are few terms which do not have more than one meaning. In ordinary conversation inexactitudes do not usually matter. For ordinary purposes it is not always necessary to know what exactly is asserted, particularly as there is a great deal of what information theory calls 'redundancy' built into our language. That is to say, we use far more words or signs than would strictly be required to transmit a given amount of information. In consequence what is missed out by the wrong use or the vagueness of a term may be supplemented by the context in which it occurs. But science must aim at uniqueness of reference because scientific formulae must be able to stand on their own feet without having to rely on contextual support.

The efficacy of all verbal communication ultimately depends on the listener attaching the same meaning to the terms used as the speaker. Scientific theory requires that the meaning must be definite and firmly anchored in experience. It must not be one that can change from proposition to proposition. It is well known from logic that if our concepts are ambiguous a reasoned argument can take us from any set of valid premisses to any set of false conclusions. Not every ambiguity in the use of a word, of course, amounts to a fallacy. A fallacy results from ambiguity only when one asserts that certain premisses necessitate a given conclusion and the claim is false because the use of the word in different meanings has suggested a connection which does not in fact exist. The converse is sometimes even more pertinent: when a word is used in a vague sense, covering a spectrum of possible meanings, we may fail to discern connections that become apparent only when one or more of the meanings have been isolated and separately defined. In due course we shall meet several instances of this.

Seen in this light the power of the language of the exact sciences—our language I—can be largely attributed to the scientist's insistence on publicly definable concepts. For, the only ultimate way in which we can circumscribe and firmly anchor the meaning of a concept is to define it operationally in terms of publicly witnessable objects or operations—or indirectly, in terms of concepts which can be publicly defined. It does not matter in this context whether the public operations are the laboratory operations of the experimenter or the paper-and-pencil operations of the mathematician. One of the keystones of the Relativity theory is the recognition that the notion of 'time' remains essentially ambiguous until it is operationally defined in terms of specified clocks and the state of motion of the observer is specified as well.

Inclusion of paper-and-pencil operations, in this case mathematical operations, is important. The stipulation that scientific concepts must be operationally definable is sometimes misinterpreted and taken to mean that electrons, for example, can only be defined in terms of oscilloscope traces, X-ray diffraction patterns and such like. This is not the case. They are legitimately definable in terms of particle inertia, energy quanta, electrical charges etc., so long as these in turn can be defined in terms of mathematical relations between variables (forces, displacements, time intervals) which in the last resort are definable in terms of laboratory operations and observations. Again, it must not be thought that science advances systematically by first defining variables operationally and then constructing theories about their behaviour and relations. As Popper has shown, measurement itself presupposes theories. Rather, science progresses through processes in which concepts and theories develop *pari passu*. Now a theory is modified using existing concepts, now a concept is modified using existing theories. This is not a circular process but a steady process of reciprocal refinement.

Insistence on definitions which directly or indirectly link the meaning of scientific concepts to publicly witnessable operations, does not of course reflect on the aim of the natural sciences to penetrate beyond what is directly observable. On the contrary, it makes this goal ultimately attainable. Only because our concepts and inferences are reliable can we penetrate to those deeper aspects of nature where the senses no longer provide an immediate check on our conclusions. It is sometimes said that physics has only become exact because it restricted itself to simpler phenomena, steering clear of such complex systems as the living organism. But the converse is nearer the truth: it had to restrict itself to simpler phenomena because it had learnt the importance of being exact.

It might be thought on logical grounds that any insistence on operational definitions involves us in an infinite regress. For how are the operations in turn to be defined? But this is not the case. In specifying the relevant operations we can generally avail ourselves of a highly redundant language and so rely on contextual support for our meanings. In consequence the operational definition of a concept can yield a higher level of determinacy than the level of determinacy of the concepts used in defining the operations.

In many contexts, of course, broad and metaphorical descriptions may have a useful part to play in organizing our thoughts. But there are theoretical contexts in which the precise meaning of our terms becomes critical. This particularly concerns the use of anthropomorphisms in connection with the purposive aspects of animal behaviour as when we say that a rat is 'trying' to escape from a certain noxious situation or that the 'purpose' of the bird's actions is to complete the nest. This is not poetry. There is obviously something special about the animal's activities that invites this kind of language, this use of language III. But, until these factors have been resolved, metaphors of this kind are apt to cause perplexities. Some of these are illustrated by the following passage in which Walter[265] comments on the meaning of 'learning'.

> Practice makes perfect in a great diversity of circumstances. The essential here is that the response to a stimulus 'alters when it alteration finds', as a result of previous experience with the stimulus. But we must go warily here. The bed of a river is the result of such varied responses to floodwaters; hillside and valley each year alter their responses to the torrent as a consequence of previous responses. Do earth and water between them 'learn' adaptation to gravity? Has an old billiard table with nice easy pockets 'learnt' adaptation to the balls? Is the car engine that is being run in 'learning' to do better by repetition?

This quotation from one of our leading neurologists illustrates one of the many semantic issues that must be cleared up before the biologist can handle with confidence all the main concepts on which a description of the characteristics of living organisms has to rely.

There are many other examples. I have heard leading ornithologists debate whether bird song is intentional behaviour. It was a sterile discussion because, as happens with so many discussions of this type, for most of the time the adversaries were arguing at cross-purposes as they could not make their concepts sufficiently definite. We shall see later that all these concepts derived from analogies with human behaviour can be made perfectly definite and precise provided one starts at the right level of conceptual analysis.

We need not repudiate altogether the significance of metaphorical terms like 'trying' or 'aiming' or 'purposing'. Metaphors are comparisons of one object with another in circumstances in which we feel that the objects compared have some features in common but are unable to say what exactly these features are. Every metaphor should really be prefaced mentally by 'it is as if'. The widespread use of metaphors in the description of life testifies to our inclination to search out resemblances between new experiences and familiar facts so that we can subsume what is novel under established distinctions. But when in this manner familiar notions are extended to novel subject matters on the basis of unanalysed similarities, serious errors may result if we forget that the similarities are unanalysed or if we fail to pay attention to the limits within which such felt resemblances are valid. This applies not only to familiar notions taken from everyday life but also when the biologist turns to notions that have become familiar in, say, servo-engineering or the computer sciences. In either case the answer is obvious: the unanalysed similarities must be analysed and the results of the analysis used to replace indeterminate metaphors by more determinate statements.

To some extent, of course, this means refashioning the language we use in the description of animal behaviour. But this is nothing new. In their quest for systematic explanations the sciences have always had to mitigate the indeterminacy of ordinary language by refashioning it to some extent.

A good example of the way in which old and vague concepts can be replaced by new and precise ones, and one that has made some impact on brain research, is the concept of *information*. In ordinary usage the meaning of 'information' seems definite enough: information is something we gain by observing the world around us, by reading or listening. A message is informative if it tells us something we did not know already and so reduces or removes uncertainty. However, only when, in 1948, Shannon and Weaver[218] undertook to define this function with mathematical precision did 'information' become available as an exact scientific concept—with profound effects on communication engineering. An outline of the basic concepts of information theory is given in Appendix A.

3.3   THE DICHOTOMY BETWEEN MENTAL AND PHYSICAL EVENTS

The language of goal-directed behaviour can be translated into the language of the physical sciences through the concept of directive correlation. But the language in which we describe our mental states or activities poses special problems which cannot be resolved in this way. There is a dichotomy between concepts relating to physical and mental events respectively which profoundly concerns the neurosciences and which cannot be spirited away simply by boldly denying that it exists. Even scientists of the highest repute have been known to question whether there is a real distinction between mind and brain. Yet the fact remains that you cannot seriously substitute 'weighing the mind' or 'dissecting the mind' for 'weighing the brain' or 'dissecting the brain' or cite physiological criteria for the many different categories of mental activity we are wont to distinguish.

Fifty years ago Bertrand Russell said that few things were more firmly established in popular philosophy than the difference between 'mind' and 'matter'. Today it is still true that there are some kinds of items, such as rocks, water, human bodies, trees etc., which we would unhesitatingly call 'physical' or 'material' and other items such as thoughts, feelings, emotions, desires, memories and perceptions which we would call 'mental' or 'psychical'. Whether these two kinds of items can be said to relate to different kinds of existence is another matter.

The view that the physical and the mental have radically different kinds of existence is nowhere more forcibly and comprehensively stated than in the writings of Descartes. 'Mental' is all that is given in subjective experience. Mind is the incorporeal subject of experience, contrasting with the corporeal substance that constitutes the physical universe and whose essential nature is to be extended in space. It follows that the mental and the physical are mutually exclusive of each other. The mental is conscious and the physical is in space, while the mental is not in space and the physical is not conscious. Despite this essential disparity Descartes postulated that these two types of existence were capable of mutual interaction, a postulate so productive of contradictions that to all intents and purposes it has been accepted as a *reductio ad absurdum* of dualism.

To find a way out of this impasse many avenues have been explored. Spinoza's *psycho-physical parallelism* abandoned interaction and postulated instead merely a formal correspondence between mental and physical events. Hobbes' *epiphenomenalism* substituted one-way for two-way inter-action: mental events, it was asserted, are always effects and never causes of physical events. Berkeley's idealism escaped the duality by conceding mind but eliminating matter. The physical world was presented as a logical con-struct of mental entities, viz. sense data. By contrast Watson's radical *behaviourism* and Ryle's logical behaviourism conceded matter and elimin-ated mind. Others, like Russell, represented mind and matter as double aspects of a third term.

Not unnaturally scientists have tended to favour the primacy of matter. Hence the popularity of the *identity thesis*. According to this thesis having a subjective experience is just being in a particular physiological condition and mental activities are just the activities of the brain.

None of these views has been able to escape fatal objections and contra-dictions [12, 16, 226]. Today we are in a better position to understand the reason, for modern analysis has made it increasingly clear that by the very nature of their specification and individuation 'mental' and 'physical' items belong to two logical categories of which interaction, parallelism, identity etc. just cannot sensibly be predicated. In this section, therefore, we must take a closer look at the dichotomy between concepts relating to 'physical' and 'mental' events.

The basic dichotomy arises from the way in which we are accustomed to characterize the *state* of a person at any particular point of time. It is a dichotomy which every scientist tacitly acknowledges when he compares evidence based on observation with evidence based on introspection.

1. Some of the states we attribute to individual human subjects relate to observable behaviour or other observable criteria, for instance to their physical or physiological condition. Thus we may say that an individual is in a state of motion or in a state of rest, that he is breathing, perspiring, running a temperature etc.
2. Other states are not of this kind and their relation to observable factors is a contingent rather than a logical one. People are said to be happy or unhappy, to be jealous or angry, to be thinking, remembering, imagining, perceiving, to be in pain or to be suffering from hallucinations. In the most fundamental sense *mental* states belong to this category.

Sometimes we use mental attributes in a sense in which they denote internal activities or conditions which we define in terms of observable effects and overt behaviour (or behaviour tendencies and dispositions). Indeed the scientist often feels restrained to define them in these terms in order to arrive at determinate and scientifically acceptable concepts.

However, there is a more fundamental sense in which these attributes signify, not internal activities or conditions defined in terms of overt effects, but internal *experiences* which we distinguish on private and introspective grounds. When used in this sense the relation of 'mental state' to overt behaviour is a contingent and not a logical one.

We cannot ignore this sense. It is the more fundamental sense, and it is largely in this sense that terms like 'pain', 'happiness', 'love' are used in our everyday lives.

In the sequel I shall use 'mental state' in this fundamental sense. It is only in this sense that mental states create special problems for the scientist and prove to be the source of all manner of philosophical confusions. To come to grips with some of these problems we must begin by taking a look at the notion of 'state' as such.

Common sense distinguishes between objects and their states. Broadly speaking every object denotes a certain invariable conjunction or association of properties which is different from other conjunctions and which determines the identity of the object. A car is a self-propelled vehicle driven by an internal combustion engine. In addition there are properties and attributes which are not essential to the identity of the object and which may change in time without the object, therefore, losing its identity. A car may be clean, dirty, noisy, silent, stationary, moving etc. The object persists through these changes. The current value of any set of these variables is what we call the current *state* of the object. It is important to note in this connection that *in classifying the state of an object we are in effect classifying the object.* In specifying the speed of a car we are assigning the car to a subclass of cars, viz. the subclass of all members of the class 'cars' which have that particular speed.

Depending on the set of variables chosen for consideration, we may talk about the 'mechanical' state of an object, its 'electrical' state or 'chemical' state etc. It should, therefore, be noted that these particular predicates in this particular application do not classify the object but classify the context of the discussion, i.e. the set of variables under review.

The same applies to the phrase 'mental states'. The predicate 'mental' here relates again to a particular set of variables or types of classification selected for discussion. The universe of discourse of these classifications is the class of all living human organisms—in other words, people. The types of classification concerned are those which we make when we describe people as happy or unhappy, as hungry or thirsty, as desiring this or loathing that, as seeing A, knowing B, remembering C, imagining D, believing E etc.

Depending on the context we can specify the state of a person in many different ways. We may take his temperature, note his blood-pressure, rate of breathing etc. and so give an account of his physical state. We may observe his postures and discuss his state of motion. And, of course, the subject may classify himself in the same sort of way. From the semantic point of view the advantage of these particular physical criteria is that they are publicly observable. Hence it is possible to define them demonstratively or operationally and we can achieve a uniform and consistent use of the classificatory concepts concerned. We can make sure that people uniformly and consistently distinguish between different temperatures because we can point at thermometers and publicly demonstrate their use. We can ensure that people use terms like 'fat', 'tall', 'dirty' etc. in the same sense because we can point at fat, tall or dirty people. And when we cannot demonstrate classifications of this kind we may still be able to define them verbally in terms of classifications which we are able to demonstrate publicly. But when it comes to mental states the picture changes. For now we are meeting a classification of people in which

(i) the only ultimate arbiter whether an individual does or does not belong to a given class, e.g. the class of happy people or the class of thirsty people, is the individual himself;

(ii) the criteria on which he makes his classification are private.

More precisely, the classification is solely based on 'internal' events or conditions, in the sense that the individual does not go by his observation of external events or conditions in deciding whether he does or does not belong to a given class. When declaring 'I am happy' or 'I am thirsty' or 'I have a toothache' the individual does not base his declarations on the observation of his publicly witnessable behaviour or on an analysis of his overt behaviour dispositions (i.e. on an analysis of the probabilities that he will behave in certain contexts in certain ways). Anyone can notice the onset of nausea without having to use his exteroceptors.

As these criteria are directly accessible only to the subject concerned, others can judge his mental state only by inference from his behaviour, i.e. from the publicly witnessable symptoms or behaviour dispositions which the particular mental state is commonly taken to elicit. But these inferences have an irreducible penumbra of uncertainty.

In ourselves we recognize pain directly but in others only by such public indicators as squirming, withdrawal responses, agitation, crying out etc. However, the behaviour disposition or syndrome commonly associated with any particular mental state is important not only because (within limits) it enables us to infer the mental states of other people, but also because of the part it plays in our learning the use of the respective mental state terms in the first place. We learn the use of the word 'pain', for example, mainly in two complementary ways:

  (i) by being referred to publicly observable *causes* of pain;
  (ii) by being referred to publicly observable *effects* of pain.

When a child pricks his finger he is asked if his finger is hurting and when his little brother cries he is told that the boy cries because he has a tummy-ache. The child assimilates the conventional usage of 'pain' from a variety of such situations by a process not unlike extrapolation. But note that we are never taught that 'pain' *is* to behave in certain ways. We are taught that pain is the *cause* of the behaviour. Just as we are taught that 'wind' is the *cause* of swaying trees and branches. We are not taught that 'wind' *means* the swaying of trees and branches.

There is no compelling reason why a sensation word like 'pain' should absorb into its meaning only those features of what it stands for which are causally related with something external and observable. The connection between mental states and overt behaviour is only a general one.

A child may learn the use of the phrase 'mental depression' in terms of observable behaviour syndromes long before it has personal experience of the collapse of vitality and purpose that the phrase commonly denotes. But only after he has had that experience can he say that he now really knows what the phrase means. As a matter of principle the quality and richness of internal experiences is not comparable between one individual and another. And in this case there is no telling what the child absorbs into the meaning of 'mental depression' as a result of his experience—bar the constraint that the meaning must remain generally consistent with certain observable behaviour dispositions.

Although, therefore, from the nature of the case the relation between a mental state and the associated behaviour dispositions is a close one, it is not a logical one. In consequence it is logically possible to be in pain and not show it and, conversely, to show pain behaviour and not to be in pain. In other words, it is possible to pretend.

Again, after leucotomy a patient may report that his chronic pain did not subside but he was less alarmed by it. So, although his behaviour disposition has changed, the pain is asserted to be unchanged. If 'pain' just meant the behaviour syndrome, this assertion would be a contradiction in terms.

The same applies to other mental state concepts. Sometimes we learn the use of a mental state concept mainly in terms of the commonly associated behaviour dispositions (as in the case of hunger or thirst), at other times in terms of publicly witnessable causes (as in the case of sensation words like 'hearing', 'smelling', 'seeing'). Of course, it is also possible to learn the use of a mental concept by seeing it defined in terms of concepts with which we are already familiar. Thus we can learn the meaning of 'hallucination' without having to experience one or witnessing the effect of hallucinations in others.

I have laboured this point because of the deplorable mistake of Behaviourists of interpreting the meaning of all mental state concepts as synonyms with the respective behaviour dispositions. This interpretation is often expedient but it is not a true analysis of what we commonly mean. By the very manner in which we are taught the meaning of mental concepts (and subsequently see it confirmed in our daily use of these concepts) the relation between a mental state and the associated behaviour disposition is impressed on us as a contingent one. There is no doubt that this is the way these concepts are used in common parlance and we can ignore this fact only at the risk of courting confusion.

Nor would it be a good thing if it were otherwise; just because mental state classifications are directly linked to internal events and not prompted by external observations, when an individual asserts that he is in a particular state of mind his statement carries information value over and above the information we can derive from observation of his behaviour dispositions. Although this information may not remove uncertainties about observables it does remove uncertainties, for example, about what it might be like to be in the subject's place.

Two important consequences follow from this particular character of mental state classifications:

(i) since they are based on introspection the mental concepts we use in our daily thinking apply in a strictly literal sense only to humans;

(ii) since their meaning is not definable in terms of public events or operations, or definable in terms of concepts which are so definable, they
cannot attain the uniqueness of reference which is indispensable for
concepts used in scientific theories. Their meaning is indeterminate—
bar the general constraints imposed on it by the manner in which we are
taught their use (and the manner in which we have seen their usage
confirmed on many occasions since).

The obvious way out for the scientist, of course, is to take the bold step
of breaking away from the common meaning of these mental concepts and
re-define each (so far as this is possible) in terms of the associated behaviour
dispositions. Such a procedure is perfectly legitimate provided it is adopted
explicitly and the reader is warned that the respective mental concepts are
now used in a new, behavioural sense which must not be confused with the
sense in which they occur in ordinary speech. Such a step has the profitable
consequence that we arrive at a set of concepts which can now legitimately
be applied also to infrahuman species. From a scientific viewpoint the profit-
ability of this step is beyond question, but it cannot be stressed enough that

(i) we are now no longer talking about the original (introspective)
attributes, but only about attributes contingently related to them;
(ii) the re-definition in behavioural terms should be given explicitly;
(iii) the fact that the new meaning differs from the old and that, therefore,
we are changing to a new language, should be emphasized.

Much unnecessary confusion could be avoided if these precepts were observed.
Only too often one sees a question asked in one language and answered in
another. If the answers are startling the reason may well lie in this very
discrepancy. For instance, many of the 'startling' answers the layman tends
to receive nowadays when he asks about the nature of the mind (mostly to
the effect that there is no difference between mind and brain) belong to this
category.

The main blame for these confusions must be laid at the door of Behaviourism. In modern times the most influential attempt to interpret mental
state concepts in essentially behavioural terms was probably Ryle's *The
Concept of Mind*[212]. All mental state classifications are here interpreted in
terms of people's dispositions to act in certain ways or say certain things in
certain circumstances. 'Dispositions' here include tendencies, propensities,
liabilities, inclinations, capacities etc. Feelings, moods, desires are treated as
dispositions to act in certain ways: a man is not angry if he is not at least
inclined to raise his voice and shake his fist; imagining a scene is acting as if
the scene took place; remembering is conning of something learnt. 'To
know' is taken to be a 'capacity verb' signifying that the person described can
bring things off, or get them right; 'to believe', on the other hand, is a 'ten-

dency verb', signifying a tendency to act in certain ways, make certain declarations, acquiesce in some statements while objecting to others; thought is silent soliloquy etc. The whole endeavour is a fascinating and elegant exercise—and very profitable for anyone looking for behavioural re-definitions of mental state concepts.

We must quarrel with Ryle only in so far as he fails to realize that he is substituting new meanings for old, that he is breaking away from the common meaning of mental state concepts and what people want to talk about when they use 'mind' in the sense inner experience or stream of consciousness. And he is certainly wrong when he tries to persuade us that this is what we have meant all along by the various mental state concepts concerned. In contrast to Watson's even more radical behaviourism, Ryle allows us to say that we think and feel, but all we supposedly mean by this, 'though we may not know it', is that we are disposed to behave in certain ways. The answer, of course, is that we don't know it for the simple reason that it is not true.

Watson's even more radical Behaviourism was a protest against a psychology based on introspection and his object was to make psychology a natural science by confining its propositions to those which are publicly verifiable. The goal was laudable enough. But as he was unable to forge a bridge between what we have called 'behaviour talk' and 'brain talk' respectively, he came to demand restrictions which at one stage reached a pinnacle of absurdity. The reality of subjective experience was denied along with any kind of thought, ideation or imagery. Teleologically tainted concepts, like purpose or insight, were ruled out of court.

Within the framework of this volume, I do not wish to become committed to any particular metaphysical position. There is no need to. As far as the 'reality' of mental states is concerned, for the scientific observer they are certainly real in the sense that we do make mental state classifications: individuals can (and often do) classify themselves on grounds which are not directly dependent on their observation of their own overt behaviour. The states so classified we have called the 'mental states', and I do not think that this strays from the common meaning of the phrase.

As we have seen, however, insofar as mental concepts are based on private experience and introspection, their meaning has a fundamental *indeterminacy*. This is limited only by the general *constraints* imposed on it through the manner in which we learn and maintain their conventional usage by referring to publicly witnessable effects or causes.

This is important when the question is raised whether it will ever be possible to relate mental states to particular patterns of nervous activity in the brain. The answer must be: Only within the limits imposed by the indeterminacy of the mental concepts. This means in effect that we can hope to make determinate, unequivocal identifications only if we first re-define the mental concepts in behavioural terms. All we shall ever be able to say is that such and such nervous processes are identifiable with such and such behaviours or behaviour dispositions and that neural events belonging to some particular broad category were *probably* happening in your brain when you claimed to have had a particular 'inner experience'.

There are many who, like Eccles for example, see themselves as uniquely experiencing beings and who feel that the ultimate goal of our scientific endeavours must be to explain the nature of our inner experience. But, insofar as 'explanation' is a process conducted in terms of verbal propositions, we cannot explain inner experiences unless we can first name or describe them. And to name or describe means to classify. Thus the description of inner experience presupposes the subjective classifications we discussed above. It follows from what was said in the last paragraph that in searching for scientific explanations of our inner experience we are really searching for the impossible.

As regards the generic nature of 'the mind' one fact has plainly emerged from the discussion: 'the mind' is *not* the entity of which pain, thirst, happiness, remembering, thinking etc. are distinctive states. As we have seen, all these attributes belong to a breed which denotes states of *persons*, albeit a particular class of states which, in accordance with the particular variables concerned and the private manner in which their values are decided, we have called 'mental' states. Although from the nature of the case the classification of individual persons according to their mental state has some measure of indeterminacy, there is no doubt about the universe of discourse which is partitioned by these classifications. This universe of discourse is *people* and not a class of nebulous entities called 'minds'. It is always '*I* am happy', '*he* is thinking', '*she* is thirsty' in the same sense of the personal pronoun as in 'I am tall', 'he was hit by a brick' etc. Whatever may be the philosophical ramifications of this, there is no doubt that for psychology and psychiatry the concept of person is primary and the generic meaning of 'mind' really rather irrelevant.*

For this reason I am inclined to use 'mental state' (in the fundamental sense) as the basic concept and 'mind' merely for the totality of the possible mental states of an individual. In this sense one might think of the 'state of mind' of a subject symbolically as a vector variable moving in a multidimensional abstract space representing the totality of his possible mental states. That the movement of this vector (the 'stream of consciousness', if you like) shows a special kind of lawfulness or (as some might prefer to say) lawlessness, need not as such perplex us. So long as we cannot link the constraints on its movements to known physical or physiological conditions, there is no good reason why we should expect it to be otherwise.

---

* The reader will find a stimulating philosophical discussion of this point in Strawson's *Individuals*[239].

3.4 INTERNAL REPRESENTATIONS AND CONSCIOUSNESS*

The critical characteristic of mental states, as we have seen, is their privacy. In the last analysis the distinctions between different mental states are based on subjective self-categorizations and we have no direct access to the mental state of another individual except through his introspective utterances.

Since introspective utterances are the ultimate overt criteria for different mental states, they are in a sense irrefutable. We can draw upon no other type of evidence to check them against. This is the core of introspective certainty.

There is another important quality of mental-state characterizations that must be mentioned, although it concerns the working scientist less directly and really only insofar as he is interested in the philosophical aspects of the mind/matter problem and in the nature of consciousness. However, as Eugen Wigner, Nobel laureate in physics, has said: 'our inability to describe our consciousness adequately, to give a satisfactory picture of it, is the greatest obstacle to our acquiring a rounded picture of the world.' And many scientists would agree with this.

This second quality is that the verbal characterizations of mental pheno-mena belong to the same logical type as the characterization of electrical signals when they are described not in terms of their physical constitution but in terms of the messages they convey, i.e. according to their *content* in the sense in which that term was introduced in Section 2.3. The distinction between different mental states or events is a distinction according to content in the sense that in the last analysis it is a distinction relating to functional significance within the wider framework of a goal-directed system. The reader will also recall from Section 2.3 that to say that an electrical signal conveys the message that object Q has a temperature t is not to imply that Q exists or that anything exists having the temperature t. The specification of mental states is similarly dependent on non-extensional statements which may or may not contain names or descriptions of observables, but if they do, imply nothing about the existence of the objects named or described. The occur-rence of observables in mental state descriptions, as in 'I am thinking of Spain', does not therefore diminish their subjectivity.

The situation is not quite as clear-cut as this very sketchy outline may sug-gest. In view of the complex organic nature of the natural languages, of course, this is hardly surprising. There are terms, for example, which have aptly been called 'mongrel' terms—terms like 'know' in 'John knows that it rains'. 'John *knows* that it rains' implies that it rains. By contrast 'John *believes* that it rains' does not imply this. The latter is purely a statement about John's mental state whereas the former also tells us something about the relation of John's mental state to the outer world. It is a 'mongrel' statement

* This section may be omitted at a first reading.

and one which in the present case may be interpreted as a fusion of 'John believes that it rains' and 'John's belief is true'. There are many other points of detail that have to be dealt with. The reader will find a number of these discussed in Dennett's penetrating *Content and Consciousness*[50], a monograph to which I am indebted even though my analysis of awareness and consciousness differs substantially from the author's.

Despite these complexities it seems to me that this line of analysis (which dates from the writings of Brentano[27]) offers a more convincing resolution of the mind/matter problem than any other approach to date.* For it shows that mental events can no more be said to be identical with or interact with physical events than the messages passing through a wire can be said to be identical with or interact with the electric currents. This is not to say, of course, that mental states or processes are of the nature of messages, i.e. essential links in some process of communication. All it means is that the distinctions between different mental states or processes logically are of the nature of distinctions of *content* in that they relate to functional significance within the wider framework of an ultimately goal-directed system.

These considerations also have an important bearing on the meaning of *consciousness*. To reach this concept it is expedient first to deal with the nature of *awareness*.

Although awareness is an essential ingredient of consciousness, the two concepts are not coextensive. There are indeed those who would assert (with Dennett) that 'I am conscious of . . .' is synonymous with 'I am aware of . . .', but the reader will probably agree that when some radar-controlled, anti-aircraft device first picks up and locks upon an approaching aircraft, it seems more natural to say that the device becomes 'aware' of the approaching aircraft than that it becomes 'conscious' of the object and that 'conscious' implies an element of self-awareness which is absent in the machine. Since self-awareness is a species of awareness the paramount importance of the nature of awareness is evident.

Consider the occurrence of an event A and assume that the event is witnessed by a subject S and recorded in the brain of S in the form of an internal representation A'. Now the mere fact that A has been registered thus by S does not mean that S is 'aware' of A in the ordinary sense of the term. S may forget all about the event and only remember it again the next day. When he does remember it he will be able to do a number of things he could not do in the interim period. He will be able to take the occurrence of A explicitly into account in his behaviour, for example in his linguistic behaviour. He can tell others that A occurred. What then is the effective change that took place when S remembered the occurrence A? Surely it is a change which enabled the content of the internal representation A' to assume effective control over

---

* For a modern exposition of Brentano's distinctions the reader may be referred to Findlay's *Values and Intentions*[66] and Chisholm's *Perceiving*[40].

the current behaviour of *S*. In particular it enabled *S* to express the content of *A'* in a variety of verbal utterances. (Note my emphasis on the *content* of *A'*. The verbal utterances express the *content* of *A'*, not *A'* itself, for *A'* is merely a set of neural conditions or processes. By saying that the content of *A'* must assume effective control over behaviour, I mean that *A'* must enter as a neural codeterminant of behaviour in a manner that accords with its functional significance. The behavioural reactions to *A'* must be context-dependent reactions, the context extending both over the origins of *A'* and the goals in the service of which the reactions occur. Compare the way in which the outputs of the electronic thermostat must depend on the content of the signals reporting the current temperature of the object.) I would therefore render 'awareness' thus: *S is aware of an object or occurrence X if and only if there exists an appropriate representation X' of X in the brain of S and the content of X' enters as an effective determinant into the control of the current behaviour of S.**

One might define awareness in a wider sense by saying that *S* is aware of *X* if the internal state of *S* is such that *X* enters as an effective determinant into the control of the current behaviour of *S*, or simply if *X* produces stimuli to which *S* responds. This is roughly the sense in which the anti-aircraft device might be said to be 'aware' of an approaching aircraft. But I am sure that this is too broad an interpretation and that the emphasis on appropriate internal representations is crucial—even though this means that we can now attribute awareness to the anti-aircraft device only in a metaphorical sense. In the first place, the broader interpretation would not cover awareness of events that occurred in the past. Secondly, it seems to me that stimuli make us aware of the objects or events that caused them only to the extent that they elicit internal representations of those events or occurrences. Thus the piano notes I hear make me aware of the piano or the player, not of the piano strings that actually produce the sound. The light that I see makes me aware of the table lamp, not of the electric current that produces the glow. The knock on the door makes me aware of the man beyond, not of vibrating panels of wood. (Once again we note that it is the *content* that matters: stimuli make us aware of what they signify.)

To return to the question of consciousness. I have suggested that consciousness implies an element of self-awareness. Indeed, *I shall tentatively define consciousness as awareness of the self (in a sense to be explained) coupled with awareness of the objects around one and of one's relations to them.* According to our definition of 'awareness' this implies that consciousness presupposes internal representations not only of the objects around one but also of the self and its relations to those objects.

* 'Control of current behaviour' is here to be understood in the broad sense in which it includes the subject's conditional readiness in certain circumstances to react in certain ways. Not everything one is aware of necessarily has a noticeable effect on the actual behaviour shown at the given time and place.

This interpretation of consciousness accords with the notion that the stream of consciousness is the stream of our mental events. For, as we have seen, mental events are distinguished on the basis of subjective self-categorizations and these obviously presuppose self-awareness, as shown by the use of the personal pronoun in the introspective statements through which we may express them. The primacy of the Ego in consciousness has been asserted by many writers, among them Sherrington and Adrian.

Awareness of the self may be interpreted in a narrow sense as awareness of the physical self only, i.e. of the body, its shape, posture, movements, and physiological condition. However, to cover the whole spectrum of our intro-spective utterances we need a broader interpretation which extends also over the mental dimensions of the self. *We can reach this extended concept of the internally represented self if we add to the internal representations of the physical self a further hypothetical category of representations, viz. representations relating to the self-categorizing reactions that give us the 'mental' categories of the self*; in other words, if we assume that these self-categorizing reactions can be the subject of expectations which supplement, and are integrated with, the aggregate of expectations that constitute the internal representation of the physical self. The total aggregate of these expectations would then constitute an internal representation of the self which extends over its 'mental' as well as physical aspects.

These assumptions imply that the internal representations whose content is expressed in introspective statements are changed by the very occurrence of those statements and underlying self-categorizations. I do not think this presents a difficulty. In essence it means no more than that the internal representations of the self exercise a feedback in the production of appropriate self-categorizing reactions and introspective utterances.

The sense of 'consciousness' I have discussed above is the philosophical sense in which the term contrasts with 'not having consciousness'. This sense must be distinguished from the clinical or psychological sense in which being 'conscious' contrasts with being 'unconscious', as when we say that the patient 'regained consciousness' or that in falling asleep we 'lose consciousness'. However, our interpretation of the philosophical concept also suggests a simple interpretation of the clinical or psychological concept. Since we regard internal representations of the outer world and of the physical self (and by implication of the relation of the one to the other) as the essential substrate of consciousness, the suggestion lies close at hand that unconsciousness (in the psychological sense) is a state in which either the representations have broken down or they have lost their power to control behaviour. On balance I am inclined to the first alternative. But this is a subject that must be left to a later chapter.

The sense of 'unconscious' used above must be distinguished from 'the Unconscious' as the term is used, for example in Freudian psychology. We may interpret 'the Unconscious' as an umbrella term for a set of hypothetical intermediate variables which are assumed to affect our conscious experience and according to Freud have an underlying coherence and unique goal-directedness.

The interpretation of consciousness I have given above answers one question that has frequently been raised since the demise of interactionism—viz. why consciousness should exist at all. If it is not a factor that influences biological events, what is its biological value? Is it biologically redundant? The answer is now clear: the physiological aspect of consciousness resides in the complex internal representations I have specified. To the extent to which these internal representations assist in the production of appropriate behaviours, their biological value is self-evident. In addition there is the sociological value of the subjective self-categorizations which they permit and of the introspective utterances in which these are expressed. It is clear, however, that consciousness in the philosophical sense defined above can be attributed to dumb animals only to the extent to which we have reason to believe that they can form internal representations at a level of sophistication comparable to the one I have assumed above. At least the basic categories of internal representations I have mentioned would have to be present.

All this has taken us rather far afield, but if the interpretations I have suggested are accepted it has given us a picture of consciousness in which the relation of this phenomenon to the physiology of the brain becomes discernible in terms of a chain of concepts each of which can be made precise. To conclude this section let me give a brief review of this chain of concepts.

The central concept is that of *internal representations* of the outer world and of the self. In Section 2.2 we have seen in very general terms how such representations may be conceived as neural processes. Briefly, each representation may be interpreted as an *aggregate of expectations* of how some variable depends on some other variable. This is a question of which value of the one variable is associated with which value of the other; and we have seen how such an aggregate of pairings may be represented in neural terms.

The next important concept is that of the *content* of the neural representation. By this we mean a variable denoting the functional significance of the representation in the context of the overall system, including the origin of the representation and the uses to which the representation is put. Responses to the content of a neural representation are responses to the neural representation into which this functional significance enters as a determinant. This is another way of saying that they are context-dependent responses of a particular kind: given the significance of the representation they are appropriate in respect of the goals of the system.

From these concepts we derive the notion of awareness, as defined earlier in this section. This in turn gives us the concepts of *self-awareness* and of *subjective self-categorizations*, i.e. reactions in which the subject categorizes himself in a manner which has comprehensive internal determinations but is only contingently related to the outer world and overt behaviour. The next step is the concept of *mental* state: the 'mental' state of an individual is his state in so far as this is characterized by such subjective self-categorizations and the introspective statements in which these are expressed. Mental 'events' and 'processes' in turn may be defined in terms of changes of mental state.

Next we assume that there are internal representations which relate specifically to such self-categorizations and which supplement the internal representations of the physical self. This gives us an internally represented self which extends over the mental as well as physical dimensions.

Finally, *consciousness* is interpreted as awareness (in the sense defined) of surrounding objects, of the self (as extended in the above sense) and of the relations of the one to the other.

This, in essence, is the general connection between the physiology of the brain and consciousness, as I see it. A great deal of work would have to be done to fill in all the details. In this volume we can only look at some of the details. In Chapter 7, for example, we shall take up the question of the neural networks in which internal representations may be registered. First, however, I must return to a rather more fundamental subject, viz. the precise nature of goal-directed activity.

CHAPTER 4

Teleological Systems

4.1 THE CONCEPT OF DIRECTIVE CORRELATION

It is food for profound thought that the only activities in the universe which need transmission of information (in the technical sense of the term) are goal-directed activities. The nature of goal-directedness, information flow and organic order hang together in a way that can only be clearly understood at the level of abstraction I am introducing in this chapter. It is the level of abstraction at which we can isolate the common denominator of all goal-directed activities and express this in terms of a single concept, viz. the concept of directive correlation. At this level of abstraction, therefore, we become aware of the unity of the most characteristic features of biological order.

Since the human organism is essentially a complex teleological system, new insight into the nature of these relationships is bound to influence our interpretation of human nature at a very profound level. To take a simple example. Only because, as teleological systems, we depend on information do we act at certain times in certain ways. This is so obvious as to be almost a truism. But it is not a truism to suggest that because of the biological importance of the information inflow as such, advanced organisms may have become responsive to the *information profile* of the sensory inflow and that this may be the biological basis of Man's aesthetic sensibilities. Nor is it a truism to suggest that since the individual generally functions in a social context, i.e. as a member of suprapersonal teleological systems, he may have developed sensibilities which specifically relate to the spatiotemporal and informational conditions which such systems presuppose and to the degree of integration the individual has accomplished. At this very abstract level of thought, therefore, we are reaching the common biological roots (indeed cosmic roots) of such manifestations as Man's desire for beauty, friendship, love and security.

However, these are not the sort of questions that concern us here. I have mentioned them only to indicate the philosophical implications of the present undertaking and to point out the broad range of questions which call for a deeper understanding of the formal characteristics of teleological systems. Our main object in this chapter is simply to grasp the general nature of the property of goal-directedness, so that we may deal with certain aspects of

73

brain function in sufficiently accurate terms and without having to fall back on broad (and sometimes misleading) analogies with servomechanisms or other automata.

Formalization apart, the mathematical demonstration that goal-seeking is an objective system-property [230, 231] and that, therefore, it is respectable for a scientist to use this concept in the description of animal behaviour has helped to hasten the end of that extraordinary era of mechanistic biology in which the most distinctive feature of living systems was treated as unmentionable. But although this mechanistic attitude in effect meant pouring out the baby with the bathwater, the reasons are understandable. In the absence of an adequate theoretical framework, the formulation ordinarily used for teleological phenomena were largely anthropomorphic and often appeared merely to project our own conscious strivings and ideational processes into the outside world. And the theoretical concepts introduced by the Vitalists to explain teleological phenomena were totally incompatible with the canons and axioms of the exact sciences.

The mechanistic reductionism which developed largely as a defence against the pseudo-scientific outpourings of the Vitalists overlooked one crucial fact, viz. that there is something unique about many types of organic behaviour which emphatically invites comparison with the purposive behaviour of rational agents and which makes these phenomena much more susceptible to anthropomorphisms than, say, the behaviour of a falling stone. It also overlooked that this unique something was the very hallmark of biological organization and touched on the very essence of life. The concept of directive correlation now enables us to isolate this elusive property and to demonstrate that it consists of a particular, and uniquely important, system-property. In doing so it offers us not only a bridge to span the gap between 'behaviour talk' and 'brain talk' but also a means of analysing scientifically the directive characteristics of many other types of biological processes.

The concept of 'directive correlation' formalizes the exact sense in which any goal-seeking activity is characteristically matched to the environment in a manner which raises the occurrence of the goal-event above the level of chance-coincidence. But although we are dealing here with a single set of characteristic relations, the actual terms in which these relations may be formalized allow a fairly wide choice. For systems in which all relevant functions between the quantitative variables are continuous and differentiable, directive correlation can be defined in terms of differential equations; for other systems it can be defined in terms of information transfer functions or in set-theoretical terms [13, 111].

The reader can be spared many of these details. For our purposes it is more important to know that the concept is generally definable in exact terms, than to fix on any particular formalization. What matters is that we have available a mathematically definable concept which can be used to give greater precision to many of the concepts used in the description of animal behaviour and so enables us to state more clearly the nature of the brain's system-properties as they are revealed in the overt behaviour patterns of the organism.

As was shown in Chapter 2, the key to understanding the nature of goal-directed behaviour lies in realizing that it is an activity which, in a particular sense, is 'adapted' or 'matched' to the circumstances in which it takes place and in respect of some specific end-result. The first step, therefore, must be to discover exactly what formal relations this idea implies. (In daily language 'adaptation' can mean either 'the state of being adapted' or 'the process of becoming adapted'. To avoid confusion Weiss proposed that 'adaptation' should be confined to the process and 'adaptedness' used to denote the state. Where there is danger of ambiguity I shall adopt the same convention.)

To start our analysis we may revert to the simple example of a bird pecking at a grain. When we assert that the movement of the bird is 'adapted' or 'matched' to the position of the grain on the ground, we are plainly asserting that there is some kind of correlation between the action variables defining the bird's movements and the position variables defining the position of the grain. The problem is to discover the formal structure of this correlation.

Clearly we mean more than just that the circumstances are such that, as events run their course, the bird's beak happens to strike the grain. If this were all we meant by 'adapted', there would be nothing to distinguish this case from the blind action of a clockwork bird placed in the right position. Also '*A* adapted to *B*' would then be synonymous with '*B* adapted to *A*', which is manifestly untrue. In fact the 'adaptedness' of the bird's movements in relation to the grain is the very quality which rules out the term 'happens' at the beginning of this paragraph: it is the very quality which raises the successful outcome of the action above the level of chance-coincidence.

As already noted in Section 2.1, the obvious difference between the action of the real bird and that of a clockwork toy is that we know in the former case not only that the beak meets the grain but also that if the grain had been displaced a few inches in any direction the bird would have modified its movements accordingly, whereas the clockwork bird would not have done so. Here lies the crux of the matter. Clearly we are dealing here with system-properties which cannot be defined solely in terms of what happens in a specific instance but which relate also to what *would* have happened in a specific set of hypothetically varied circumstances. They imply a conditional readiness on the part of the organism to meet certain contingencies in certain appropriate ways. As has been said, the specification of properties in terms of hypothetical or 'virtual' variations is nothing unusual in the physical sciences, as instanced, for example, by the concept of 'stable equilibrium'.

If we take a closer look at this or similar examples we also note that the assertion '*A* is adapted to *B*' has a definite meaning only relative to some understood goal-event or goal-condition. In the bird example this goal-event is that the beak hits the grain. Any analysis of the case has to be related to the occurrence of this event. An action which is appropriate in respect of one outcome may be quite inappropriate in respect of another.

On this analysis the crucial facts that distinguish the case of the real bird from that of the clockwork toy are seen to be the following:

1. The bird has physically open to it not only the actually executed sequence of movements, but also a set of alternative action sequences, containing at least one to match each of a number of possible alternative grain positions.
2. The mechanisms determining the bird's movements *are* such that they *would* have produced an appropriate matching variation for each of these possible variations of the grain position.

Before we subject these preliminary results to closer scrutiny, it is expedient to clarify a few auxiliary notions and also to show how causal relations appear in the mathematical representation of deterministic systems. We begin with the notion of the *state* of a physical system. In general the state of a physical system is specified by means of a selected set of quantitative variables which may be either scalar variables or vector variables. The state of the system at any given instant is the set of numerical values which these variables have at that instant. A *line of behaviour* is defined as the succession of states through which the system passes as it runs its course. It is specified by specifying the states and the times at which they occur. A line of behaviour may be recorded, for example, by a number of traces on a multiple-pen recorder, or it may be given in tabular form. In physics a line of behaviour may also often be specified in terms of known mathematical functions. Consider, for example, a system consisting of a point-particle of mass M moving under a uniform acceleration A. The current state of this system is then given by the current position and momentum of the particle. Let t_0 be taken as the initial time and let p_0 and m_0 denote the initial position and momentum of the particle. At any subsequent time t_1 the position and momentum are then given by the equations

$$m_1 = MA(t_1 - t_0) + m_0 \tag{1}$$

$$p_1 = \frac{A}{2}(t_1 - t_2)^2 + \frac{m_0}{M}(t_1 - t_0) + p_0 \tag{2}$$

If p_0 and m_0 are given and t_1 is taken to be an independent variable, these equations jointly define a line of behaviour whose starting point is p_0, m_0 (see Figure 4.1).

However, we may also take t_1 as given and treat p_0, m_0 as independent variables. We call this a *causal reading* of the equations. The equations now present p_1 and m_1 as single-valued functions of p_0, m_0, in the sense that each p_0, m_0 pair determines one and only one p_1, m_1 pair. When interpreted in this sense, the functions given by our two equations may be called *causal functions*. Since they are single-valued functions, the system is by definition deterministic. Note that in the causal expression for p_1 the arguments (p_0 and m_0) relate to the same point of time. The concepts of causal function and determinism, of course, apply equally when the functions concerned cannot be written in the form of known mathematical equations.

In the above example p and m are independent variables and, of course, it is only because of this that we can represent their progress in the Cartesian coordinates used in Figure 4.1.

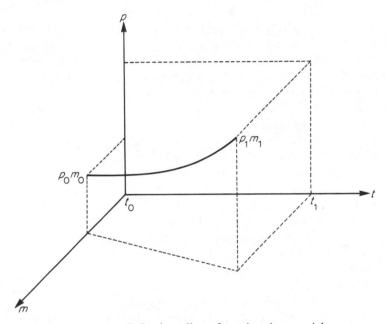

Figure 4.1. Behaviour line of accelerating particle

When we think of an event as due to joint effects of two (or more) earlier events, these events are (by implication) always taken to be independent variables.

In a closed deterministic system lines of behaviour may fuse but they can never bifurcate: different initial states of the system may lead to the same end-state, but the same initial state can never result in alternative end-states.

We may now return to the example of a bird pecking at a grain. The results of our preliminary analysis showed that the notion of a goal-directed movement implies in the first place that the bird has physically open to it not only the actions actually executed but also a set of alternative actions and that this set contains at least one to match each of a number of possible grain positions. Secondly it implies that the mechanisms determining the action are so conditioned that they would have produced an appropriately varied action for each of these variations of the grain position. There is, as I have said, a conditional readiness to meet certain contingencies in certain ways.

On closer analysis this account is seen to imply the following:

1. It implies a comparison between the actual system running its course from some arbitrarily chosen initial point of time and an ensemble of identical systems starting from initial states which differ in only one respect, viz. the position of the grain. The comparison relates to the different lines of behaviour which issue from these hypothetical variations of the initial state. (By 'system' in the above statements we mean, of course, the bird plus the relevant domain of its environment.)

2. The system is conceived as deterministic in the sense that each member of the ensemble of alternative initial states is taken to generate one and only one line of behaviour. Thus the state of the system at any point of time is conceived as a unique function of the initial state.

3. The set (A) of action variables of the bird and the set (P) of position variables of the grain are conceived as two independent sets of variables in the sense that the value of either set at any one point of time implies nothing about the value of the other set *at the same point of time* (although it may imply something about its value at a later point in time). If this were not the case we could not conceive of alternative grain position in conjunction with the same initial state of the bird and the same starting point of the bird's movements. To avoid confusion with other kinds of independence I shall in future use the term *orthogonal** for this type of independence. Thus if two variables are 'orthogonal' any arbitrary combination of their values can be conceived as an initial state of the system. This is also what I mean by saying that arbitrary combinations of the values of A and P are *physically open* to the system. It follows that any subsequent correlation between concurrent values of A and P must be a contingent one.

4. Our account implies that, given the initial time t_0 and given A_0 and p_0 as the initial values of A and P, there exists a set (S') of variations of p_0 such that the resulting behaviour lines terminate in the goal-event (G') if and only if the values of A undergo specifically correlated variations in the intervening interval. Thus the goal-event G' is really conceived as the joint effect of the behaviour of A and P after t_0 and it is implied that the variations P incurs after t_0 in consequence of the set S' of hypothetical variations of p_0 are such that G' only occurs if A is made to undergo specifically correlated compensatory variations by the brain mechanisms of the bird.

---

* In my *Analytical Biology* [230] I used the rather more cumbersome expression 'epistemic independence'.

5. The account implies that the factors determining the bird's movements are such that A in fact would have varied in the manner specified if p_0 had varied in the manner specified.

By *directive correlation* we mean this specific correlation when it is expressed as a correlation between *concurrent* values of A and P in the interval between t_0 and the terminal event.

Definition. The concurrent values X_t, Y_t of the two orthogonal variables X and Y are *directively correlated* in respect of a goal-event G' if the occurrence of G' requires that X_t and Y_t satisfy a particular condition $R(X_t, Y_t, t) = 0$ and if there exists a set (S') of possible variations in the initial state of the system such that in the resulting behaviour changes of the system, $R = 0$ remains satisfied, but only because the effect on R of the resulting changes in X_t are compensated for by the effect on R of the resulting changes in Y_t (and vice versa).

The definition may be extended to more than two correlated variables. The variables themselves may be scalar or vector variables and they may be either continuous or discrete—there is no restriction on them except that they be independent in the sense specified.

Directive correlation must be expressed as a correlation between *concurrent* values of the correlated variables because only in that case is the correlation a contingent one. That is to say, the possibility of a mismatch must not be precluded by our definition of the system. To think of 'match' or 'mismatch' in this case is to think of the goal-event G' as the *joint effect* of X and Y and this implies that we are thinking of X and Y as independent variables in the sense specified. For, if the values we think of do not relate to the same point of time there is always the possibility that the one may determine the other causally, in which case it would be misleading to speak of G' as the *joint* effect of X and Y.

Directive correlations can be given more definite mathematical formulations whenever it is possible to express $R(X_t, Y_t, t) = 0$ in more definite terms. To give a simple and illuminating example, suppose that in a practical case

(i) the condition $R(X_t, Y_t, t) = 0$ takes the form

$$F(X_t, Y_t) = 0 \quad t = t_1 \tag{3}$$

(ii) F is differentiable,
(iii) the variations of the initial state mentioned in the definition take the form of variations of a variable Z at t_0 within a domain S',
(iv) X_1 and Y_1 are differentiable functions of Z_0, then the directive correlation between X_1 and Y_1 may be expressed by the equation

$$\frac{\partial F}{\partial X_1}\frac{\partial X_1}{\partial Z_0} + \frac{\partial F}{\partial Y_1}\frac{\partial Y_1}{\partial Z_0} = 0 \tag{4}$$

coupled with the stipulation that the left-hand terms do not vanish individually (i.e. 'identically').

It is easy to see how this equation may be expanded to cover the case of more than two directively correlated variables. The equation also covers the common case when Z_0 is identical with X_0 or Y_0.

This simple mathematical model of the relations that characterize goal-directed activities shows particularly clearly what is involved and that we are here confronted with a system-property which can be expressed in perfectly orthodox terms and which as such contains nothing that would in principle be incompatible with the laws of physics or chemistry. Spelt out in detail equation (4) expresses that (a) variations in the initial value of Z entail variations of X_1, and Y_1, either of which would have affected the value of F (and thus prevented the occurrence of the goal-event) if it had occurred in isolation, (b) the effect on F of the one variation, however, compensates for the effect of the other, so that $F = 0$ remains satisfied (and the occurrence of the goal-event remains unaffected).

I have given a worked example of the application of this equation elsewhere[231]. Using equations (1) and (2) above for a particle moving under a constant acceleration the reader may verify for himself that these conditions are not satisfied, for example, by a falling stone, even though variations of the initial conditions may lead to the same end-result.

In the example of the bird pecking at the grain, of course, the system is not sufficiently specified to enable us to spell out the physical requirements for a successful outcome of the action. But that does not impair the definiteness of the concept of 'directive correlation' as such.

Directive correlation may also be expressed in statistical terms. As set out in Section 4.3 and Appendix A, for example, directive correlation, as defined above, implies in informational terms that the information transfer function

$$T_{G=G'}(X_t;\ Y_t)$$

increases from zero as t increases from t_0.

Directive correlation is an objective system-property. In simple cases the nature of this property can be readily visualized in a graphical representation. Consider a rifleman shooting at a stationary target. Let T and R be the direction of the target and rifle respectively in the horizontal plane. It is then a necessary condition for the success of the action that at the time of firing these two directions coincide. The adaptive process here consists of lining up the sights. This action may start from any initial position of the rifle. Assume that the rifleman fires as soon as his sights are aligned on the target. The directive correlation of this action may then be illustrated diagrammatically as in

Figure 4.2 (the initial position of the rifle being taken as given). It is characterized by the fact that the family of behaviour lines which is generated by hypothetical variations in the target position twists in such a manner that all lines come to intersect the sheet $T = R$ at the respective times of firing. The twisting of the sheet of behaviour lines expresses the fact that variations in target position would have elicited compensatory variations in the movement of the rifle.

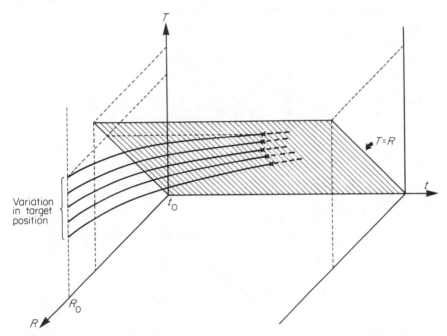

Figure 4.2. Behaviour lines showing directive correlation in system containing rifleman and stationary target

As the target is stationary each behaviour line remains in the same horizontal plane. A moving target would give us the same figure except that the lines of behaviour are no longer confined to horizontal planes of the diagram and, since the rifleman must now aim ahead of the target, the sheet F would be displaced vertically by an amount depending on the target speed. Figure 4.3 illustrates the general case of two variables, A and B, directively correlated in respect of a goal-event whose occurrence is conditional on A_t, B_t satisfying at some time t the one–one correspondence expressed by the sheet F.

It may be noted in passing that Figure 4.2 could equally be used to illustrate phylogenetic adaptation, for instance in an idealized case of cryptic colouration in which it is assumed that for maximum survival value the colour of a species must equal that of the habitat.

Adaptability is a matter of degree and this depends on the time-span considered. Phylogenetic adaptability, for example, depends on the number of generations that are taken into account. By contrast, executive adaptability depends on the number of seconds or minutes taken into account. In our original example it is clear that the nearer the bird's beak has moved towards the grain, the less it can cope with sudden disturbances in the position of the grain. In many movements, of course, the final phase is purely ballistic and devoid of adaptability. Thus during most of the action when a frog hurls itself forwards with its hindlegs to scoop up a prey with its forelegs, it can no longer see its prey.

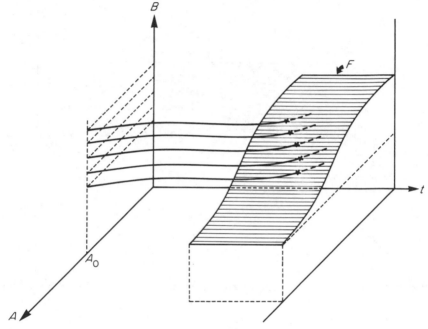

Figure 4.3. Behaviour lines showing the directive correlation between two variables, *A* and *B*, when *A* is adapted to *B* in respect of a goal-event whose occurrence presupposes the conditions expressed by the sheet *F*

The *degree* of the adaptiveness is represented by the magnitude of the set S' (see para. 4, p. 78). This in turn depends on what is taken as the initial point of time in our conception of the system running its course from some arbitrary starting point. If in the example of the pecking bird the state chosen as initial state is one in which the bird's beak is already well on its way towards the grain, the remaining adaptability is small and so is S'. If the final stages of the movement are purely ballistic then S' will be an empty set in any conceptual representation of the system which covers only this final episode. Conversely, the greater the time interval considered the greater the adaptability of the movement. If the starting point is taken sufficiently far back in time, even the hopping of the bird towards the grain enters the picture and the area over which the grain can be displaced without loss of the goal-event increases accordingly. Hence we define the *degree* of a directive correlation as the magnitude of the set S' for which the relations specified in the definition of directive correlation are satisfied.

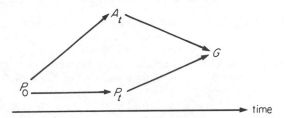

Figure 4.4. The basic categories of causal functions implied in the notion of the bird's action (A) being adapted to the position (P) of the grain in respect of some goal-event (G)

Nothing has been said in this analysis about the exact nature of the mechanisms in the bird's head which enable it to adapt its movements to the position of the grain. No mention has been made of feedback loops or error signals. This omission is deliberate. For, at present we are solely concerned with the descriptive characterization of the system-properties revealed by adaptive behaviour, regardless of the particular manner in which these properties come to be realized in nature. Only by taking this course do we arrive at a position at which we can attempt to analyse these mechanisms in terms of what they actually achieve rather than in terms of mere analogies with known goal-seeking machines such as servomechanisms and other feedback devices. It is easy to show that the outputs of such machines satisfy the conditions of directive correlation we have formulated above. But, as we shall see in Chapter 5, the mechanisms of the brain may achieve similar results in ways which have no strict analogies in servo-engineering.

The directive correlation which characterizes the adaptive nature of the bird's movement involves four causal functions (Figure 4.4). The role of the bird's brain is to establish A_t as an appropriate function of B_0, i.e. as a function which satisfies the stipulated correlation to B_t. At a first reading this may seem confusing because the reader may be accustomed to think of the action A_t as a causal function of P_{t-k}, where k is the transport lag of the neural mechanisms in the bird's head. But there is no contradiction, because in a deterministic system P_{t-k}, in turn, is a causal function of P_0 (Figure 4.5).

Adaptation is not a symmetrical relation. 'A is adapted to B' does not mean the same as 'B is adapted to A'. The two cases are illustrated in Figures 4.3 and 4.6 respectively and are compared in Figure 4.7. The difference lies in

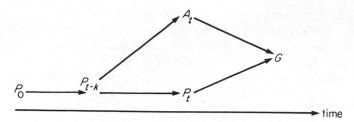

Figure 4.5. The same as in Figure 4.4, but incorporating the additional notion that the current values (A_t) of the action variables are determined by the position of the grain as perceived at time $t-k$, where k is a constant time lag. Since P_{t-k} is a causal function of P_0, A_t is a causal function of P_0 by implication. This representation, therefore, is consistent with that of Figure 4.4

the variable whose variation in the initial state of the system is assumed in the specification of the directive correlation. In *A adapted to B (but not B to A)* only variations in B_0 generate a sheet of behaviour lines satisfying the stipulated conditions. In *B adapted to A (but not A to B)* only variations in A_0 do so.

The variable whose variations at t_0 generate the sheet of behaviour lines

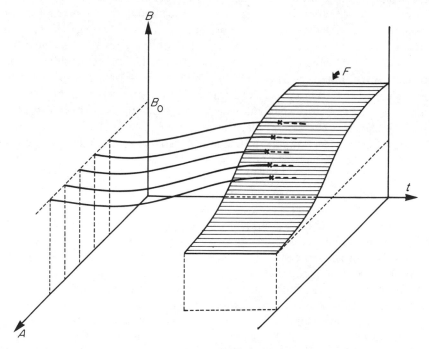

Figure 4.6. Same representation as in Figure 4.3, but for the case when *B* is adapted to *A* instead of *A* to *B*

satisfying a particular directive correlation is called the *coenetic variable* (B_0 in Figure 4.3 and A_0 in Figure 4.6). Its variations within S' represent the 'disturbances' for which the system can compensate by virtue of its adaptiveness.

As mentioned above the *degree* of a directive correlation depends on how far back in time the starting point of the behaviour lines is chosen, i.e. on the choice of the initial time t_0. In future the time-span considered, the span between t_0 and t, will be known as the *back-reference period*. The degree of a directive correlation is therefore a function of the magnitude of the back-reference period. In general it will be a monotonically increasing function of this magnitude.

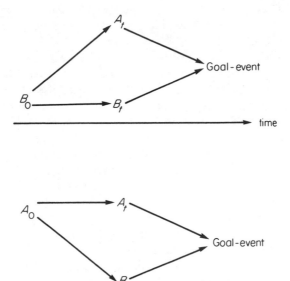

Figure 4.7. Causal functions implied in *A adapted to B* (top) compared with *B adapted to A* (bottom)

Goal-directed systems are sometimes described as *feedback systems*. This can be misleading. One of the simplest devices to illustrate the notion of 'feedback' is the thermostat. An electric heater warms the room. When the temperature reaches a certain level a bimetallic strip operates a switch which cuts off the heater. When the room cools again the bimetallic strip unbends and the heater is switched on again. The activity of the heater is here controlled by signals 'fed back' from the thermostat's field of action. These feedback signals drive the system in a way which minimizes the discrepancy between the actual state of the system and the desired state. It is easy to see the general connection between 'feedback' (when used in this sense) and directive correlation. If the action A of a given system is repetitive or continuous and has to be directively correlated to an environmental variable B, then A_t must be currently generated as an appropriate function of B_0 (or B_{t-k}). If B is influenced by A it belongs to the field of action of A and the system therefore requires that information is 'fed back' from the field of action of A to the controller of A. We must note, however, that this is a special case, albeit a common one. Not all directive correlations relate to continuous or repetitive activity and not all directive correlations are between variables which influence each other reciprocally. Thus when a boy throws a ball to a playmate there is only a single action and the question of feedback from the external field of action does not arise. (A contrasting case would be if the boy aims a continuous jet of water from the garden hose at his playmate.) It is a mistake, therefore, to equate all goal-directed activity with feedback activity, although this assertion is often found in the literature.

Directive correlation is defined as a relation between *orthogonal* variables only. This is important for here lies the difference between *goal-seeking* as defined above and *equilibrium-seeking* in the classical sense in which a physical system is said to return to a state of stable equilibrium when displaced from it. The true nature of the teleological character of organic activities slips from our grasp if we fail to see the formal difference between these two sets of phenomena. In either case a disturbance from a given state elicits forces tending to restore it, but in the case of the stable equilibrium the restoring forces and the disturbance are *not* mutually orthogonal variables whereas, when a given state is restored through goal-directed activities (the restoration being the goal), the corresponding variables are orthogonal. Thus, in contrast to goal-seeking, equilibrium-seeking requires no information flow. When a pendulum is displaced from equilibrium the restoring force is an unalterable function of the displacement. It is not an independent variable: random combinations of the two are not possible initial states of the system. No decorrelation between displacement and restoring force is physically open to the system. This is also the crucial difference between a steel ball pursuing a magnet and a cat pursuing a mouse. It would be tendentious to describe the magnet as the 'goal' of the ball. The reactions of the ball are merely 'Newtonian'. The direction of the target and the direction of the force controlling the ball are not orthogonal variables. *No feedback loop could be cut that would result in a deviation of the ball failing to produce a restoring force.*

It is a common but mistaken belief that the stability which the living organism derives from its organization within a certain range of conditions, is solely of a kind that can be accounted for in terms of potential energy minima. Closely allied to this view is the belief that the degree of organic order of a living system can be expressed adequately in terms of negative entropy. Both beliefs ignore the points brought out above. The stability of the physical and chemical part-structures on which the organization of the body depends is indeed of the type stated. But the total stability conferred on the internal environment, by homeostasis for example, additionally depends on a multitude of directively correlated processes which represent an altogether higher type of organization.

The stability of the internal environment depends on a host of coordinated processes which spring into action when deviations from the norm occur or are threatened. Thus when the athlete makes extra demands on his body his respiration and heartbeat will accelerate to increase the supply of oxygen to the muscles; extra red blood corpuscles will be released into the blood stream; arterioles will dilate and capillaries open; meanwhile the pressure of the labouring muscles, the contractions of the abdominal muscles and the pumping action of the diaphragm will increase the return flow of blood to the heart; adrenaline will be secreted to adjust muscle tonus; perspiration will reduce body temperature etc. These are but a few simple examples of the running adaptations and compensations which confer on the living organism a protective order of a kind that belongs to the very essence of life. Similar types of protective and organic order also exist on the social scale for socially integrated individuals. In one form or another they are to be found at all levels of social integration, including the most abstract level: the integration of Man with nature. Not only our physical health but also the more elusive forms of health which we sometimes describe as 'mental health', vitality, happiness etc. depend on, and relate to, conditions of organic integration and protective order which, even at this very abstract and intangible level, are yet of much the same general type. (It is my personal view that Man's religious beliefs are a cosmic projection of the protective order he experiences in these sundry ways, whose essentially directive qualities he has felt unable to interpret except in terms of an all-pervading intelligence.)

Before we proceed a word must be added about the application of the concept of directive correlation to systems which are partly or wholly described in terms of probabilistic variables. In the preceding analysis we have assumed a deterministic system, that is to say a system in which the value of any descriptive variable at any point of time is a single-valued function of the initial state of the system and the time which has elapsed since. It is evident from this analysis that the concept can also be applied to systems which are described in probabilistic variables provided these variables, in turn, fulfil the same condition. Systems in which this is the case are known as Markoff systems. In a Markoff system the initial state of the system is defined in terms of probability distributions over a basic set of physical variables and it is assumed that the probability distributions over these variables at any subsequent point of time are single-valued functions of the initial distributions and the time that has elapsed since. It is evident from our definitions that this condition is sufficient to permit the concept of directive correlation to be applied to these probability values when the circumstances warrant it.

This is relevant because during learning an organism may undergo a change of state (attitudes, reaction patterns etc.) which relates to the probability of particular stimuli occurring in particular situations. These changes of state may be adaptive. It is therefore important that we should be satisfied that we can apply the concept of directive correlation to the relation between the state of the organism and a state of the environment which is defined in terms of probabilistic variables. We conclude that this is legitimate provided that the variables which occur in the asserted correlations are elements of Markoff processes. (The reader will find a more detailed treatment of probability in my *Analytical Biology*[230].)

4.2 MAJOR TYPES OF DIRECTIVE CORRELATION

The example of the bird pecking at a grain and that of protective colouration represent two opposite extremes of adaptivity. In the first case we have the instant adaptability of what I have called 'executive' processes. We may distinguish the directive correlations that characterize this type of instant adaptability as *executive* directive correlations. We find them in the dynamic exercise of all skills and practical competences. They typify the flexibility of the actions through which the animal comes to implement the goals of the moment. At the other extreme we have the long-term and slow phylogenetic adjustments of evolution. These show directive correlations of any significant degree only if we consider back-reference periods which extend over many generations. The goal of these *phylogenetic* directive correlations is not so much a goal-event as a goal-condition, commonly the optimization of some particular condition (e.g. minimal detectability by predators).

An intermediate position between the executive adaptations and phylogenetic adaptations is occupied by the *ontogenetic* adaptations, the gradual adaptations through which the individual organism adjusts during its lifetime to the special circumstances of its existence. The rigours of cold winters may lead to reactive growth of fur; local pressure on tissue may lead to resistive toughening: the development of skeletal muscles may adjust to the degree of exercise to which they are put etc. In the context of this volume the phenomena of *learning* form the most important class of ontogenetic directive correlations.

The three classes are mainly distinguished in the magnitude of the back-reference period which must be chosen to yield significant degrees of the directive correlations concerned.

As we know, in many biological situations all three types of directive correlation are present and closely related. The executive adaptiveness shown by a predator pouncing on the prey presupposes nervous pathways formed by learning, i.e. ontogenetic adaptations. These in turn presuppose a functional organization in the brain which rests on phylogenetic adaptations. In the context of executive adaptation the ontogenetic adaptations appear as preadaptations. In the context of ontogenetic adaptations the phylogenetic ones appear as preadaptations.

Much confusion surrounding the phenomena of adaptation in their various forms can be resolved by translating the problem concerned into the precise language of 'directive correlations'. The importance of this type of analysis is brought home by the observation that two of the main variables which distinguish the different types of adaptation, viz. the coenetic variable and the back-reference period, are never explicitly mentioned in the common cases in which the term 'adaptation' is used. The goal-event, too, is often taken to be understood. These omissions in what is explicitly mentioned in statements like '*A* is adapted to *B*', together with the fact that statements of this kind relate not only to what is happening or has happened but also about what would have happened in different circumstances, account for much of the confusion that surrounds the notion of adaptation. The crux of the matter is that such statements appear to be about particular variables but in fact are statements about particular system-properties. The following assertion is a typical example of the resulting confusion: 'Animals are adapted to their environment. And all that this means is that their characterization is such that in those environments they are able to live.'* This interpretation misses the very essence of adaptation, viz. that the observed fitness to survive is the outcome of a process which would have produced appropriate modifications in different circumstances. It misses the essential system-property which 'adaptation' commonly denotes. On Woodger's interpretation we might with equal justification say that mountains and stones are adapted to their environment.

We can also at this point answer the questions Walter asked in the passage quoted in Section 2.1. We now see that, in the full sense of the term, 'learning' denotes an adaptive process which is characterized by (ontogenetic) directive correlations which are absent in the examples of the river or the billiard table.

The course of the behaviour lines shown in Figures 4.3 and 4.4 illustrates '*A* adapted to *B*' and '*B* adapted to *A*' respectively. A special case arises when *both* conditions are satisfied simultaneously: variations in either A_0 or B_0 generate compensating variations in subsequent values of the other variable. This case of *mutual* adaptation is commonly implied when we describe activities as *coordinated*. In most of these cases more than two activities are likely to be involved, but, as we have seen, the concept of directive correlation is readily extended to more than two variables. Coordinated activities of all types, from walking to playing tennis, typically show such mutual adaptation of the movements concerned. In anthropomorphic terms we might say that the central control mechanism for each limb or joint takes into account what the others are doing and adjusts its commands in the manner best suited to secure the collective goal of the combined movements. Formally this means

* J. H. Woodger, *Biological Principles*[273], p. 436.

that we are dealing with complex directive correlations between the movements of the limbs in which each of these variables may figure also as a coenetic variable.

The number of variables concerned in a directive correlation may be called the *compass* of the directive correlation, as distinct from the *degree* of the correlation as defined above. When in ordinary language we talk about different degrees of adaptiveness we may mean either measure, but the distinction is rarely critical. As we move up the scale of life the adaptiveness of the organism increases in both respects. This general increase in the manifested compass and degree of the directive correlations is probably the most meaningful sense in which we can distinguish between 'higher' and 'lower' forms of life.

It must be clear now that the concept of directive correlation enables us to define the goal-directedness of behaviour objectively and to use the term 'goal' in a sense in which it can be applied to animals as well as humans without committing an anthropomorphism or imputing any kind of 'conscious' mental activities to the animal. Defined in terms of directive correlations the objective goal-event no longer runs the risk of being confused with the idea of a subjectively thought-of purpose. Of course, in Man, the *thought* of a particular goal may be instrumental in generating a behaviour sequence which is not only subjectively goal-directed (in the sense of involving mental processes in which the thought of the goal occurs) but also objectively so (in the sense of manifesting the respective directive correlations). The one does not guarantee the other. Behaviour may be subjectively goal-directed in the mentalistic sense but fail to become objectively so. This is *one* sense in which we distinguish between *successful* and *unsuccessful* behaviour. But it is not the only sense. Biologists frequently pronounce an animal activity unsuccessful without any intention of imputing conscious thought processes to the animal. This commonly occurs when the animal shows behaviour which *within a given range of situations* is known to be directively correlated to the environment in respect of some specific goal but, owing to special circumstances, the actual situation happens to lie outside this range. Hence the goal-event may not materialize and there is a perfectly objective sense, therefore, in which we may call such behaviour unsuccessful. Thus the hawk may swoop upon the prey but the prey may be rather more nimble than usual.

When a given situation lies outside the range of situations for which the animal has directive responses available in respect of some ultimate goal, a typical effect (and one that we should expect on logical grounds) is the appearance of random factors in the choice of proximate goals the animal comes to pursue. This is characteristic, for example, in the activities we know as *searching* and *trying*. These random factors prevail until, while searching or trying, the animal chances into a situation which lies *within* the mentioned range of situations, when normal directive behaviour will be released and the searching or trying ceases. In this case, too, there is a use for 'successful' and 'unsuccessful' in an objective sense. This objective interpretation is particularly worth noting by the reader who may have wondered how our definitions of goal-directed behaviour fit the cases in which the goal is not attained.

The fact that we can show the directiveness of organic activities to be an objective system-property which is definable in terms of ordered relations in space and time, does not as such solve the more pragmatic problems of the working biologist. Its main value lies in the fact that it enables us to realize the full implications of many of the concepts biologists have to use, that it brings into the orbit of accurate scientific analysis a number of supremely important features of vital organization and that it enables the biologist to develop his own concepts in contexts in which he previously felt constrained to borrow concepts from other sciences, e.g. engineering and the computer sciences.

We shall see at a later stage how this type of analysis helps us to disentangle some of the problems surrounding the nervous system.

4.3   INFORMATION THEORY AND CYBERNETICS

I have mentioned before that the only events in the universe which require the transmission of information are goal-directed activities. Only through the transmission of information can the particular correlations be realized in which, as we have seen, the goal-directedness of a process resides.

The concept of directive correlation itself can be defined in informational terms. The definition in Section 4.1 was based on a deterministic conception of the physical system concerned. But, as was said at the time, directive correlations can also be characterized in statistical terms. The most suitable terms for this purpose are those of information theory. A brief résumé of the central concepts of this theory is given in Appendix A. For anyone versed in this theory, it is not difficult to see that the formal relationships embodied in the concept of directive correlation can be characterized in terms of information transfer functions. As already indicated, if a system S, developing from an initial state S_0 at time t_0, contains a variable A whose value at t is directively correlated to the concurrent value B_t of a variable B in respect of a goal G, the directive correlation implies that the information transfer function

$$T_{G=G'}(X_t;\ Y_t)$$

increases from zero as t increases from t_0. In statistical terms, therefore, this may be taken as a formal criterion of directive correlation. I mention this only as a matter of passing interest.

The significance of 'information' in goal-directed activities was one of the factors which motivated Wiener and his followers in the development of a branch of studies which they called *cybernetics*. The name, first introduced by Wiener in 1948, derives from the Greek for 'steersman'. Wiener and a group of scientists around Rosenblueth were aware of the essential unity of the problems centering on control and communication. It was unfortunate, therefore, that they fell short of factoring out the formal structure of the space–time relationships in which this unity resides, the formal structure of goal-directedness. In consequence cybernetics remained, as someone said, 'a unifying name in search of a unifying concept'.

Unknown to these scientists the central concept which their endeavours lacked meanwhile developed in another sphere of activity. But although the concept of directive correlation was already being advanced by the present writer in 1950, the link with cybernetics was not established until years later, mainly through the influence of Ross Ashby. By that time, not surprisingly, cybernetics had lost much of its identity. Moreover Wiener's followers had settled in a trend which looked at machines in the first instance and at the living organism only derivatively. Thus cybernetics came to increase the biologist's dependence on engineering concepts instead of diminishing it, as it might have done had it lived up to its original promise. Meanwhile, of course, control and communication engineering had developed as major disciplines. In consequence, 'cybernetics' is now often used merely as a collective name for these disciplines or, in a more restricted sense, for the study of the basic scientific principles on which they depend.

Owing to its failure to start with a unifying concept cybernetics has failed to bring about a concerted endeavour to come to grips with the common elements in all teleological processes and to develop a general theory which would cover both the form in which they occur in nature and the form in which we can achieve them in man-made machines.

Attempts to develop artefacts which imitate the performance of living organisms, and then to reason from the machine to the living prototype, have largely failed for reasons given in Chapter 1. We now have machines capable of displaying the superficial appearances of instincts, taxes and kineses, machines capable of trial-and-error learning, self-correcting and self-optimizing machines and many other 'brainlike' devices. But most of this work has remained on the level of performance imitation without shedding light on the physical or physiological organization which accounts for these capabilities in the living prototypes—just as hydraulic systems can imitate muscle performance but shed no light on muscle organization.

The gulf between organism and machine is immense. It has been said, quite wrongly, that since directive correlations can be achieved by machines (as in guided missiles) the concept of directive correlation blurs this difference. This is certainly untrue. On the contrary, it enables us to see the differences more clearly. Organic activities are not typified by discrete and unrelated sets of directive correlations, but by integral hierarchies of directive correlations in which phylogenetic, ontogenetic and executive correlations combine to produce a self-regulating, self-reproducing, self-repairing and self-maintaining, stable and yet flexible entity. No machine has as yet been designed to emulate these features of organic integration, nor are we likely to meet one in the foreseeable future.

4.4 POSTSCRIPT AND PREVIEW

The main purpose of this chapter has been to show how teleological concepts can be defined in terms of particular correlations—as typified by equation (4) —and within the framework of a causal–analytical approach. The following is a selection of concepts which can be given a precise definition in terms of these 'directive' correlations:

appropriateness	in the sense of an action or process matching ambient circumstances in a manner conducive to the attainment of a particular goal; the goal may be the occurrence of a particular event or of a special condition (such as the optimization of the value of some particular variable);
adaptation, adaptive process	in the sense of a process resulting in appropriate activities or changes of state;
adaptedness	in the sense of having become appropriate in consequence of an adaptive process;
function	in the biological sense of an organ having an inherent mode of action serving a particular goal;
coordination	in the sense of two or more activities or processes being mutually adapted in respect of a common goal;
integration	in the biological sense of two or more activities or processes being closely interrelated in a manner serving a particular goal;
organic order	in the sense of organizational relationships manifesting themselves in activities or processes directed towards a biological goal.

To be able to define these concepts in terms of specific correlations between specific variables is important to the life sciences not only because all are concepts which at one time or another have caused a great deal of confusion but also because the definitions now enable us to use these concepts with confidence and with knowledge of exactly what we are asserting when we use them. In science there can be no excuse for using terms in a vague sense when an accurate and equally pertinent sense is available. (Should anyone wish to use any of these concepts in a different sense he will be well advised to use the same analytical method for making this sense clear. We know from pure mathematics that mappings between specified sets of elements is the best conceptual tool we have available for the definition of abstract concepts.)

The reader who is unaccustomed to seeing mathematical concepts employed solely for the purpose of conceptual analysis may at first fail to grasp this point. Thus he may now expect to see the equations given in this chapter applied to the solution of some mathematical problem arising from neural functions, or used for predicting some particular sequence of neural events. In the absence of such applications he may wonder why the mathematics were necessary at all. To have these misgivings is to misunderstand what we set out to do. Briefly it was this:

1. To analyse and expose the logical and linguistic structure of the concept of adaptation and related concepts.
2. To show how a concept that makes integral use of reference to a future state may be phrased in perfectly orthodox and straightforward causal–analytical terms.

Object (2) has been fulfilled in the following successive steps:

(i) the description or specification of a 'state of affairs' by means of values attached to coordinates;
(ii) showing how the successive sets of values adopted by these coordinates in a time-sequence may be represented (a) temporally, i.e. as a function of time, given some definite initial state, (b) causally, i.e. as a function of initial state, given some definite time.

Obviously a logical prerequisite of treatment (ii) (b) is the use of the concept of

(iii) 'virtual variations'. We have to examine the consequences of the initial state having been other than in fact it was. Without using this concept one is forced to adopt the unsatisfactory position of saying that the 'adaptedness' of an organism to, e.g. the environment, merely affirms that the environment is there, the organism is there and the organism is alive in it.

Mathematical notations for these elementary concepts were introduced in the interest of precision, lucidity and ease of deductive development. It could all have been said in words, but only at a loss.

As the result of this analysis we can now tackle teleological phenomena as manifestations of objective system-properties and we can describe them without being compelled to use anthropomorphisms or possibly misleading analogies with servomechanisms or other automata. We now know that in making assertions about the goal-directedness of a process we are making assertions about a particular set of correlations, but we also know that these correlations can be defined only in terms of hypothetical variations of the circumstances in which the process occurs.

I must conclude with a few remarks about the use to which these results will be put in our analysis of brain functions. Some of this ground has already been covered when we discussed goal-directedness as an outstanding characteristic of the overt behaviour of the higher organisms and when I pointed out that the associations formed during learning appear to relate to objects and goals rather than discrete inputs and outputs of the nervous system. We also know that a single change in a stimulus situation or a single physiological event can change not only the actual responses of the organism but also its conditional readiness to react to certain circumstances in certain ways. In other words, it can change goals and cause one set of directive correlations to be succeeded by another. We can see all these phenomena in a clearer light once we interpret them in terms of specific classes of correlations.

The question 'How does the brain work?' is not as simple as it may seem. As J. Z. Young once remarked, it is not too much to say that the whole structure of our logic and language is influenced by the concepts we use to discuss this problem and to formulate the detailed questions that shelter behind it. The introduction of the concept of directive correlation has profound effects in this respect. When an engineer is asked to explain how some complicated machine works he will produce a 'block diagram' in which the installation is broken down into functional units and the relations between the units is indicated in a suitably symbolic form. He can do this because in man-made machines structures can generally be identified with functions and functions with structures. There are many neuroscientists who hope that some day we may similarly be able to produce a block diagram of this type for the brain. I believe this to be a vain hope except at a very coarse level of representation. As was pointed out in Chapter 1 the brain has not developed as the physical embodiment of a preconceived set of discrete logical functions. Thus we can hardly expect to succeed in representations of the brain which show it to be neatly divided into blocks, each designating both a discrete physical structure and a well-defined logical function. What then can we hope to achieve? Naturally the neuroanatomist can hope to arrive at ever more detailed wiring diagrams of the brain, and the neurophysiologist at ever more comprehensive causal explanations of particular neural events. Yet, neither can satisfy us completely for, in the end, we want more than a blueprint of the brain or causal explanations of contingent events: we want explanations of the brain's *accomplishments*. That means, we want explanations of how the brain comes to produce outputs that are appropriate in the circumstances in which they occur and in respect of specific goals, i.e. explanations of directive correlations of one kind or another. For a final answer to the question 'How does the brain work?', therefore, we must rely on a policy of *research programmes which tease apart the main directive correlations that account for the brain's accomplishments* and which seek to discover the processes and pathways through which these correlations are brought about. I do not believe that in the last analysis there is any other way.

As we proceed along this road we are likely to discover that one neural pathway may serve more than one correlation and that the goal of one directive correlation figures as one of the correlated variables in another and to encounter a variety of other complications which prevent what is functionally distinct from coinciding with what is structurally distinct and what is structurally distinct from coinciding with what is functionally distinct—thus destroying our prospect of finally arriving at comprehensive block diagrams of the type we may have dreamt of.

In the remainder of this volume I shall broadly follow the above policy, although within the compass of what is feasible in our present state of knowledge we can do no more than concentrate on certain basic categories of directive correlations. The main categories we shall consider are:

1. The adaptive changes which result in the brain building and storing models of the external world.
2. The adaptive changes which result in the formation and storage of particular action programmes.
3. The executive adaptations through which these models and programmes come to be used in intelligent decision making to achieve goals that are suitably related to the organism's drive state.

Two closely related questions will be given paramount attention, viz. the neural counterpart of these processes and how far what is functionally distinct in these processes may also be structurally distinct. (As already indicated in Section 2.2, the positive transfer of learning is one of the most important signposts we have available here.)

CHAPTER 5

Clarification of Some Critical Concepts and Relations

5.1 INTRODUCTION

The main value of the demonstration that goal-directedness is an objective system-property which can be expressed in accurately definable correlations is that it has delivered the biologist of the burden of semantic inhibitions which have frustrated the discussion of directive phenomena in the last hundred years.

For the particular purposes we have in mind in this chapter it is sufficient to know that the characteristic relationships of goal-directedness can be expressed in precise terms and that, in particular, the notion of 'goal' can be given a precise definition in objective terms. The question of the different ways in which these relationships can be formalized is largely irrelevant.

In this chapter I propose to deal with a select number of issues which are particularly liable to cause confusion. The first problem area concerns the implications of activities in which progress towards some ultimate goal is punctuated by a hierarchy of subgoals. The question arises, for example, to what extent such hierarchies must be reflected in the information flow in the brain and whether we can assume (as many contemporary writers do) that for every discernible goal or subgoal there must be somewhere in the brain a signal that specifically relates only to that goal or subgoal. We shall see that this assumption is unwarranted.

At a later stage we shall also see that it is unwarranted to assume that, even when there exist specific command signals relating to particular goals, the execution of the commands presupposes the use of 'comparators' in the sense of mechanisms designed to compute explicit error signals in the manner of common servomechanisms. These are typical examples of the way in which machine analogies can sometimes mislead us.

Two other problem areas will be dealt with. The first relates to the notions of instinct and drive. We shall see that if these notions are to be used without ambiguity it is important to distinguish between particular classes of directive relationships. The second problem area relates to the use of the notion of 'expectation' in the explanation of animal behaviour. We have seen that many

97

forms of behaviour suggest that the activities of an organism are often determined by the 'expectations' it has formed as the result of prior experience.
Once again, to be able to use this concept with confidence we must be able to
define it accurately and in objective terms. We must be sure that we are not
unwittingly sliding into the use of mentalistic concepts. The alternative course
is to avoid the concept altogether. Although this course has been adopted by
a number of writers, it is a stultifying one.

5.2 HIERARCHIES OF GOALS AND SUBGOALS

It is a truism to say that the coordination of the many types of movements
which the body and the limbs can perform presupposes an elaborate organization on the part of the nervous system. The crucial question is what inferences
about this organization we are entitled to draw from our observation of the
different types and degrees of coordination found in human or animal movement and from the organization of goals and subgoals which these movements
implement. It is easy to jump to conclusions here. It is easy, for example, to
think of 'open' organizations, such as that of an army division or of a large
business enterprise, and to compare the type of coordinated activities which
such an organization permits with the coordination of our body and limbs.
It would be a fallacy to assume that there exist analogies here which entitle
us to conclude that the organization of the nervous system must be based on
the hierarchical pattern that is found in armies, business organizations etc.
However, it requires a certain amount of analysis to see at what points the
analogy breaks down.

  As we are meeting hierarchical relations of one kind or another in other
contexts, too, it is expedient first to say a few words about the general nature
of such relationships. Most people have a general idea of what is meant by a
hierarchy and are familiar with some particular types of hierarchy. We are
all familiar, for example, with the hierarchical structure of the armed services,
large business organizations, the judiciary, the civil administration etc. In all
these cases we are dealing with a set of relationships which can be symbolized
by an inverted tree branching at a number of discrete levels. Thus in the mili-
tary example the stem could represent the divisional command, the first
set of branches the brigade commands, the next set the regimental commands
etc. The formal implications of the concept of hierarchy were fully analysed
by Woodger[274] in 1937. Briefly, the formal structure of a perfect hierarchy
is characterized by the fact that the elements at each level (bar the lowest)
stand in the same asymmetrical one–many relationship to the elements of the
level below as do these elements to those of the next lower level. The interlevel
relation concerned may be called the *defining relation* of the hierarchy. Thus
the descendants of Queen Victoria form a hierarchy defined by the parent–
offspring relation. In the hierarchical organization of the armed services the

principal defining relation is that each command centre computes the goals to
be pursued by each of the subordinate units of the next lower level.

An important type of hierarchical relationship we meet in the objective
description of human or animal behaviour is that between the ultimate goal
of a behaviour sequence and the various subgoals which appear to punctuate
the sequence. Many goal-directed activities appear to be plainly punctuated
by a number of easily discernible subgoals. To what extent this is objectively
true must depend of course on whether the respective directive correlations
do in fact exist in the behaviour sequence under observation. It must also be
stressed that when we speak of the 'ultimate' goal of an action this is to be
understood only in a relative sense. In any wider context the goal in question
may appear as a subgoal towards an even more distant goal. Depending on
the context we can detect in most vital activities some goals which are long-
term, some which are relatively short-term and some which are very short-
term. To take a simple example. A dog runs for a stick its master has thrown,
picks it up, returns to the master and drops it at his feet. Such a sequence of
actions may be viewed in two ways:

(i) as a single goal-directed behaviour pattern: retrieving a stick;
(ii) as a sequence of separate activities each having a specific goal and each
    of which may in turn be analysed as a sequence of actions serving
    their own proximate goals. The action of returning to the master, for in-
    stance, implies fixing the eyes on the master, running in a particular
    direction, balancing the stick while running, negotiating any obstacles
    on the way, etc.

These two ways of looking at the same events are rendered formally compatible by a theorem which follows directly from the definition of directive
correlation:

Theorem. If G_A is the goal of a directive correlation A and if the occurrence of
G_A is a necessary condition for the occurrence of the goal G_B of a directive
correlation B, then G_B is also a goal of A.

Definition. G_A is called a *subgoal* of G_B. This theorem expresses the formal
relation between goals and subgoals. It has an important logical bearing on
the kind of organizational problems with which we are here concerned.

Often the goal-event of one directive correlation may figure as one of the
correlated variables in another. In a discrimination experiment a bird may be
trained to peck at one of a set of coloured discs in order to receive a food
pellet. After training is completed and the respective directive correlations
have become established, the goal of the individual pecking movement
(bringing beak in contact with a specific disc) may itself be thought of as a
variable which has become directively correlated to the learning situation in

respect of the ulterior goal of receiving a food pellet. The proximate goal of the pecking movement then appears as a subgoal of this ulterior goal.

From such formal relations we can derive the concept of hierarchies of directive correlations, hierarchies of subgoals derived from ulterior goals.

The relation between goals and subgoals is sometimes lightly dismissed with the remark that if X is a goal and X implies Y then Y is a subgoal. But this is certainly untrue in any objective sense. If an action is directively correlated to the environment in respect of a goal-event X and the occurrence of X presupposes Y, it does not follow that the action is directively correlated to the environment (or anything else) in respect of goal Y. Y may be a constant of nature for instance. The example illustrates once again the importance of analysing in detail what exactly we mean by 'goals' and 'goal-directedness' in any given context.

To clarify certain important issues it is expedient to imagine a behaviour pattern and a sequence of events which can be broken up into discrete stages. For simplicity let us also assume that the circumstances in which the actions take place admit of a discrete set of alternatives. The argument will not be affected by these simplifications.

Consider some agent-plus-environment system and assume that the activities of the agent are directively correlated to the environment in a manner which has the occurrence of an event A as ultimate goal. It will then generally be true that A is the node of sets of behaviour lines which converge and fuse at various points of the preceding time interval. Assume, for example, that the occurrence of the goal A presupposes the occurrence of one of two alternative conditions, B_1 and B_2, at some stage t_{-1} preceding the occurrence of A. Assume also that each of these presupposes the occurrence of one of two alternative conditions at a time t_{-2}, and each of these in turn presupposes one of two alternative conditions at a time t_{-3} (Figure 5.1). If t_{-3} is taken as the initial time we are thus visualizing eight hypothetical alternatives (D_1–D_8) for the initial state of the system as preconditions for the occurrence of A.

As regards the activities of the agent in this imaginary situation we shall consider two distinct cases.

1. Assume that the system runs from C_1, C_2, C_3 or C_4 at t_{-2} to the goal-state A without requiring any intervention by the agent. But also assume that it runs from $D_1, D_2, \ldots$ or D_8 to C_1, C_2, C_3 and C_4 only if the agent performs some specific action which is uniquely related to the particular initial condition concerned. In other words in order to secure the occurrence of the goal-event A the agent has to do no more than perform the correct triggering action at t_{-3}. On this assumption, therefore, the whole left hand column of arrows (but no others) imply responses on the part of the agent which are uniquely correlated to the environmental circumstances in which they occur. If the agent is so

conditioned that he produces these responses in the respective circumstances we can discern the following hierarchy of directive correlations.

(i) The two responses elicited by D_1 and D_2 respectively may be said to
show a directive correlation which has C_1 as goal-event. A similar view
may be taken of the three remaining pairs of responses implied by the
arrows of the first column.

(ii) The set of four responses elicited by D_1, D_2, D_3 and D_4 respectively
may be said to show a directive correlation which has B_1 as goal-event.
Similarly, the responses elicited by D_5, D_6, D_7, D_8, may be seen as
arguments in a directive correlation with goal B_2.

(iii) The total set of eight responses caused by D_1, D_2...D_8 respectively
(or any subset of this) may be said to show a directive correlation which
has A as goal-event.

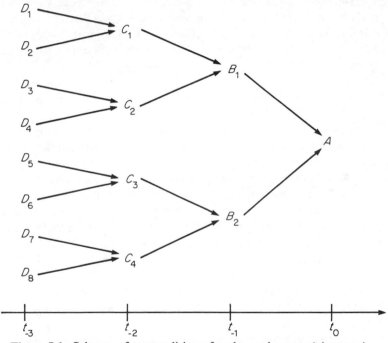

Figure 5.1. Schema of preconditions for the goal-event A (see text)

2. The second case to be considered is the one in which all the remaining
arrows of the diagram also presuppose a specific response on the part
of the agent which must occur at the appropriate moment and must be
matched to the circumstances in which it occurs. Thus instead of having
to perform only one act at t_{-3} which (if appropriate) triggers a chain of
events resulting in the occurrence of the goal-event A, the agent now has
to interfere appropriately also at the times t_{-2} and t_{-1} if A is to occur.

In a schematic way these assumptions model the common case in which we have a sequence of adaptive actions which takes us right up to the occurrence of the 'ultimate' goal or consummatory event of the behaviour pattern under consideration, as was the case in the example of the dog retrieving a stick. In this case we can distinguish all the directive correlations of the previous case plus an obvious number of additional ones relating to the responses of the agent at t_{-2} and t_{-1} respectively. In the earlier case we were dealing with a single action which triggers a set of events which run their course to the final goal-event without further intervention by the agent. This is a comparatively trivial case, but the example shows that even in such a case of a single action of this kind we can legitimately think of a *hierarchy* of directive correlations, i.e. a hierarchy of subgoals generated by a single ultimate goal, the goal-event A. And the sense in which this notion applies is exactly the same as in the second case, i.e. the case in which there was a discrete sequence of actions, except that in the latter case one can distinguish *additional* hierarchies of directive correlations, viz. those relating to the actions taken at t_{-2} and t_{-1}.

The example also shows that from the mere existence of a hierarchy of goals and subgoals no inferences can be drawn about the structure of the organization which produces the responses concerned We cannot conclude that this, too, must be hierarchical. Even in the second case considered, i.e. when all arrows in the diagram imply the performance of responses uniquely correlated to the circumstances in which they occur (and when, therefore, we have a hierarchy of directively correlated response values) there is nothing that implies the existence of a hierarchical organization in the brain mechanisms producing the agent's responses. Our assumptions require no more than that the agent is so conditioned that he reacts in the appropriate way to each of the possible conditions listed, i.e. to D_1–D_8, C_1–C_4 and B_1, B_2. For all we know the environmental conditions relating to each of the terms shown may differ in respect of one stimulus dimension only and all that is required of the agent is that each of the relevant values of this stimulus variable should elicit the appropriate action.

Goal-directed action sequences of this type are very common. They may be acquired or innate. Tinbergen's studies of innate behaviour patterns in birds give very detailed analyses of the behaviour sequences involved in nest-building, for instance. The goal of each stage of such a sequence is not a consummatory act itself, but the completion of a situation fit for the next stage to be released. The completed action stage provides specific signs which act as *releasers* for the next operation. When the bird arrives at a suitable territory a searching activity is released until an acceptable site has been found for the nest. This triggers the collection of moss, which is in turn followed by placing the moss in the fork of the branch etc. In his observations on nest-building in the longtailed tit, Tinbergen[250] has analysed eighteen releasers and fourteen distinct movements or combination of movements. To account for the action of each releaser Tinbergen postulates innate releasing mechanisms (IRMs)[249]. All the same, there is a danger here of reifying what is merely a logical relationship. There is nothing in all this to compel the conclusion that these releasing mechanisms must be discrete functional units or organizational entities. Only if we bear this in mind is it safe to use the term 'mechanism' in this particular context. We are dealing here with logically distinct sets of input–output relations and not necessarily, therefore, with anatomically distinct organizations in the brain. The upshot of all this is that from a study of the hierarchy of goals and subgoals which we may discern in the particular behaviour patterns of an organism we cannot infer that something of the nature of an isomorphic structural organization must exist in the nervous system to make such patterns of behaviour possible. We cannot infer, for example, that in respect of every goal and subgoal there must exist a feedback loop generating a correlated error signal and that the hierarchy of goals and subgoals therefore implies a correlated hierarchy of specific error detectors or 'comparators'. Additional reasons for rejecting these notions will become apparent later in this chapter.

This is not to say that the brain *may* not have developed independent or semi-autonomous mechanisms for the pursuit of frequently recurring subgoals. But if it has done so the reasons are likely to be purely pragmatic ones originating in the biological advantages (e.g. learning economy) such an arrangement might confer. Thus if the pursuit of a particular subgoal is likely to occur in a great variety of different contexts (such as the optical pursuit of visual targets) it pays to have a separate organization available for this, for it makes the skill acquired in one context immediately available in another.

5.3 INSTINCT AND DRIVE

The hierarchies of goals and subgoals that we find in all complex forms of animal behaviour are further complicated by the different admixtures of phylogenetic and ontogenetic elements that we can discern in them. The ends pursued and the means chosen may be innate and stereotyped at the one extreme or entirely flexible and modifiable by experience at the other. These elements can only be separated by a careful analysis of the directive correlations and classes of correlations concerned and by an accurate specification of the actual variables that enter these correlations. Only by an accurate analysis of this kind can we sharpen up our concepts and observations sufficiently to avoid needless confusions or pseudo-problems.

A simple example of mixed correlations is furnished by the activity of *searching.* The fact that in certain situations the animal initiates searching behaviour may be innately determined and hence an instance of *phylogenetic* correlation. Searching (for food for example) itself is goal-directed activity which yet contains random elements. But these contrary aspects can be separated. Although searching contains random elements it is not a disorganized activity. Running hither and thither in the search for food the animal executes movements which are directed towards local goals: running for this corner, looking behind that tree. These individual activities show directive correlations to the environment which are of the *executive* class (Chapter 4). But the local goals of these directive correlations are not related to the main goal of the search. This is the random element. On the other hand, the manner in which the animal evaluates the clues it picks up during the search will be related to the main goal. The experienced outcome of a search may also effect lasting changes of behaviour which are of an adaptive kind. This then is a directive correlation of the *ontogenetic* class.

We may describe behaviour as more or less *instinctive* according to the degree of prominence of the innate elements that determine its goals. This may vary according to the level of the hierarchy of the goals and subgoals that we can distinguish in the behaviour. In general the innate element increases as we ascend the hierarchy from the proximate to the ulterior goals. Tinbergen's analysis of nest-building in the longtailed tit again serves as a convenient example. The action begins with the search for a suitable site for the nest in the chosen territory. When this has been found the collecting and placing of moss begins. Once the tufts of moss have been placed in a suitable fork of the chosen tree the collecting changes to spider's silk, followed by rubbing the silk on the moss and stretching when the silk has stuck to the moss. This continues until a platform has been constructed, when the collecting changes back to moss. And so the construction continues. Fourteen different types of action appear to be executed in all, elicited at the proper stage by eighteen different releasers. Four of these consist of the four innately recognized materials: moss, spider's silk, lichen and feathers. The others consist in the recognition of the completion of different stages of construction. The relations between goals and subgoals in the sequences are the two that were given above: either the goal of the one process is a state of affairs which is essential for the next process (the moss must be picked up before it can be taken to the site), or the proximate goal is itself a variable which is directively correlated to the situation in respect of some ulterior goal (choice of moss, spider's silk, lichen or feathers, depending on the stage reached).

All these action patterns are based on phylogenetic adaptations but, although the innate elements predominate, there is some element of ontogenetic plasticity as well. The actions may improve with learning: random elements still apparent in the first performance gradually drop out upon repetition. We know from the study of newly hatched chicks that pecking accuracy improves with experience. In general, too, the choice of pecking objects is modifiable by experience and in some cases even entirely acquired by learning. In pigeons, for example, the drinking movements are innate but the bird has no concept of water as the stuff to drink and takes some time to learn this. Trial-and-error learning also improves the choice of nest material. In many birds, too, knowledge of the main landmarks of the territory is not absorbed in one complex unit, but gradually acquired through tentative exploration of the territory. Thus we can expect the flight path of the tit homing on its nest to improve with learning: whereas it may be somewhat erratic to begin with, soon some new landmark gains in associative significance and more direct paths result. The new landmark now releases an executive action it did not release before. It has become an acquired releaser in contrast with, for instance, the sight of moss, spider's silk, lichen or feathers, which are innate releasers. When the platform of the nest is completed a new type of behaviour emerges: the bird now sits on the platform and this releases the placing of the moss on the rim. But the releasing effect of a completed platform may not be entirely innate either. It is likely that the pattern constituting a completed platform sharpens with repetition and experience.

Now it is self-evident that if a particular state S_1 of the bird is defined in terms of a particular goal G, which the bird pursues while in that state (e.g. construction of platform), then the attainment of G_1 terminates S_1 and so leads to a new state, S_2 say, which will be characterized by the pursuit of different goals and subgoals. If G_1 consists of the attainment of a particular external state of affairs (e.g. completion of a platform), then one may say that the attainment of G_1 (or stimuli flowing from this) acts as external 'releaser' of S_2 and of the actions resulting from S_2. If G_1 is an innate rather than an acquired goal one may also call this fixed sequence of events an 'innate releasing mechanism' or 'IRM'. Finally, one may say that until G_1 arrived, S_2 was 'blocked'. In this terminology any hierarchy of innate goals and subgoals (in so far as they are innate) may then be represented in the manner of Tinbergen's well-known hierarchies of 'centres', IRMs and 'blocks'. But it is important to realize that this is a *formal* order of relationships which does not necessarily reflect a *structural* organization of the nervous system.

The 'appetitive' behaviour, resulting when no 'releasers' for the lower level of Tinbergen's hierarchy are realized, formally means no more than that random (i.e. non-correlated) elements appear in the behaviour when the circumstances lie partly outside the domain of the directive correlations pertaining to the goals of the given level. By the *domain* of a directive correlation I here mean the range of circumstances in which an action is elicited which is directively correlated to the circumstances in respect of the goals concerned. The appearance of these random elements does not, of course, mean totally disorganized movements, but only movements whose proximate goals are decorrelated from the ulterior goals that characterize the given pattern of behaviour.

There is no need for us to pursue these matters further. I have taken them up only to show that in behaviour patterns like the above we are dealing with complex relationships which in the long run can be clarified only if we analyse the directive correlations involved, ascertain their place in the respective hierarchies and, above all, separate carefully the three main categories of directive correlations: the executive, the ontogenetic and the phylogenetic (reserving the term 'instinctive' for the last-named).

The notion of *drive*, like the notion of 'instinct', has a chequered history in which it has taken on many different shades of meaning. Even today it is often difficult to decide whether a writer intends the term to stand for a physiological condition. The notion has oscillated between denoting, at the one extreme, a general state of tension or disequilibrium resulting in undifferentiated activity or mere restlessness and, at the other extreme, a specific state resulting in a specific directed activity—something, therefore, which can be differentiated as extensively as the goals we detect in the activities of the organism. There are those who regard 'drives' as *physiological* stimuli which are related to physiological 'needs' and others who take 'drive' to stand for the *psychological* consequences of 'needs', i.e. for the psychological incentives for action or cues for differential responses.

There are also writers who think of 'drive' as a factor which selectively strengthens certain classes of activity, whereas others think of it as a factor determining which events will strengthen the activity. Finally there are those who, like Skinner[223], define 'drive' merely in terms of a set of laboratory operations which have effect upon the rate of responding (e.g. withholding food for a certain number of hours).

This is another problem area in which the concept of 'directive correlation' can help us to think in more definite terms. In the following paragraphs I intend to do no more than illustrate a few aspects of the matter in which this is the case. I am not advancing any particular theory.

The notion of drive was originally invoked to explain the difference in behaviour when an animal is placed in the same environment and invariably it is taken to denote a variable *state* or *condition* of the individual. Sometimes we know enough about the parameters concerned to warrant the idea of drive as a physiological input. When modelling particular mechanisms of the brain this is often a convenient concept. But, although I use this concept myself in a variety of theoretical contexts, I would hesitate to assert that it is legitimate in all circumstances. Each case has to be examined on its merits.

There are two aspects of 'drives': a qualitative aspect which relates to the different behaviours, i.e. the goals pursued in particular circumstances, and a quantitative aspect. Drives may be strong or weak.

As regards the first element it is expedient to divide the goals we can discern in animal behaviour into *internal* (physiological) and *external* goals. In general this depends on the particular fragment of a behaviour sequence that we take into account. When a predator pounces on its prey and subsequently devours it we may look at only the first half of this sequence, and so have an activity with an external goal, or we may look at the second half (or the whole sequence) and see this as a behavioural unit with an internal goal, e.g. to redress the caloric balance of the organism. The first half may not invariably be tied to the second: presented with many rats in succession, cats will continue to kill prey, long after they have ceased to eat it. In other words, not all behaviours are tied to a condition of the animal which is sufficiently variable to be called a 'drive'.

The division of goals into 'internal' and 'external' enables us to establish a distinction between 'drive' and 'motivation'. This, once again is a question of expediency. Looking through the literature one notices a tendency to search for a definition of 'drive' which relates exclusively to the state of the individual regardless of external circumstances. If we accept this aim we must limit the class of goals which may be used as defining goals for 'drives' to

  (i) internal (physiological) goals;
 (ii) external goals defined at a level of abstraction at which external particulars drop out of sight.

On this interpretation building a nest would qualify as a drive-defining goal, but not 'building a particular nest on a particular site'; 'escaping from danger' would qualify but not 'diving for cover to escape the hawk'; 'aggression' would qualify but not 'hitting John'. The non-qualifying goals would then be taken to define 'motivations' rather than 'drives'.

So far we have thought in terms of goals of executive directive correlations. But if the organism is capable of learning, every frequently recurring executive directive correlation defines the goal of a potentially fruitful learning process (and so of a possible ontogenetic directive correlation), viz. to improve the organism's capacity for achieving the executive goal. In this sense any given drive defines a class of responses to be strengthened selectively if the capacity of the organism to attain its goal is to be expanded.

The above analysis gives us objective criteria for distinguishing, if we want, between different drives in terms of different directive correlations manifested in the overt behaviour of the organism. The notion of drive *strength* is more difficult to clarify in objective terms. In laboratory experiments drive levels are in practice often controlled in terms of measurable deprivations. The animal may be starved for two days or three. But it would generally be admitted that this practical procedure is not to be interpreted as a conceptual identification of drive with deprivation or need. There are deprivations which produce no drive (e.g. oxygen starvation) and drives which cannot be induced by specifiable deprivations (e.g. nest-building). Moreover, the resulting drive level is a function of all needs coexisting at the time.

The overall level of activity of the organism is often taken as an alternative index of the strength of a drive. Another possible index is the neurological state of 'arousal' produced by the drive. Both interpretations are common in the literature. But the concept of 'directive correlation' offers yet another alternative in the form of the 'domain' (as defined above) of the directive correlations associated with the defining goal of the drive. What this means in effect is that we may compare drive intensities by comparing the range of conditions to which the resulting activities are adapted in respect of the goal that characterizes the drive. The almost satiated animal performs activities appropriate to the furtherance of food intake in only a very restricted range of conditions: only when the food is immediately under its nose, for example, but not when the food is out of sight. With rising levels of food deprivation the range of circumstances expands in which actions appropriate to the procurement of food are elicited. We have here a definable criterion which appears to cover a significant aspect of what is commonly meant by the 'strength' of a drive, or drive 'level'.

If the circumstances lie outside the domain within which they elicit determinate actions directed towards the defining goal of a given drive (e.g. food intake), we must expect on *a priori* grounds

(i) less activity and/or
(ii) activities directed towards irrelevant goals (displacement activities) or
(iii) activities directed towards the same goal but showing random elements in the choice of subgoals (searching).

As already said, it does not follow from our analysis that movements must become totally disorganized or undirected, for the hypothetical circumstances we are considering only lie outside the domain of the high-level directive correlations pertaining to the high-level goal taken to characterize the drive in question (food intake, building a nest etc.)—not outside the domain of the directive correlations that characterize the pursuit of low-level goals like picking up a twig or running along an alley in a maze.

Of course, the domain of the directive correlations concerned may change with learning but, given the state of learning, we would expect it to vary according to factors commonly taken to affect the 'strength' of a drive. Whether this concept may in practice prove useful as an index of drive level, I would not like to say. The issue does not arise in this volume.

5.4   THE NATURE OF EXPECTATION

One of the main functions of the analysis given in the last chapter is to help clear a path through the clutter of concepts with vague and often misleading connotations which tend to obscure the real nature of the higher brain functions. The analysis enables us to translate descriptions of animal behaviour couched in terms like 'adaptation', 'regulation', 'coordination', 'goal-seeking', 'learning', 'drive' etc. into precise statements about particular correlations between particular variables in respect of particular end-results. In this section we shall be concerned with the exact sense in which concepts like 'expectation' and 'anticipation' can be applied to animal behaviour. However, to see the questions arising in connection with 'expectancy' in a proper context I must first give a brief outline of the general phenomena of conditioning.

Traditionally the aim of learning theory has been to interpret the plastic changes which behaviour undergoes during learning as lawful events and to discover unifying principles for these events. An important and valid part of this endeavour has been to isolate regularly occurring phenomena which can be studied under controlled laboratory conditions. The two most important categories of phenomena that have satisfied this condition are those of 'classical' and 'instrumental' conditioning. Broadly speaking, the former relates to the observation that, if a given stimulus regularly elicits a given response and if this stimulus is then repeatedly paired with a second stimulus, in due course the second stimulus comes to elicit the same response (or one grossly similar). Instrumental conditioning, on the other hand, relates to the observation that, if a given response is regularly rewarded, it tends to occur with increased frequency. Conversely if the response is punished it tends to diminish in frequency.

The systematic investigation of classical conditioning goes back to the work of Pavlov[192] in the second decade of this century. The impact made on learning theory by the work of Pavlov was largely due to the fact that from the enormous complexity of acquired behaviour patterns he managed to separate out an apparently simple and elementary phenomenon which could be studied in a pure form under laboratory conditions: the *conditioned reflex*. Pavlov showed that the animal acquires the capacity to respond to a given stimulus with the reflex action proper to another stimulus when the two stimuli are applied concurrently for a number of times. The strengthening operation for the resulting behaviour changes here, therefore, consists of the mere pairing of the stimuli. Classical conditioning, in this sense, is essentially a process resulting in a degree of stimulus equivalence. Appropriately timed pairings of a previously neutral stimulus (the 'conditioned stimulus', CS) with a second stimulus (the 'unconditioned stimulus', US) to which there is an established response (the 'unconditioned response', UR) results in a capacity of the CS to elicit a broadly similar response (the 'conditioned response', CR). Thus a mild shock (US) to the leg generally results in leg flexion (UR). If this shock is repeatedly preceded by a loud tone (CS) there comes a time when the tone will elicit leg flexion (CR) without the necessity of shock.

It is clear that when it is conceived as a simple abstract paradigm the conditioned reflex as such is a non-directive mechanism, a blind stimulus–stimulus (S–S) association which is insufficient to account for the directiveness of behavioural changes.

The directive aspect of learning changes came into focus with the isolation of a more complex phenomenon, viz. 'instrumental' or (to use Skinner's phrase) 'operant' conditioning. It was shown for a wide range of activities of higher organisms that if a particular action is regularly rewarded (e.g. with a food pellet), the action begins to occur with increasing probability; conversely if it is punished (e.g. by a mild electric shock) the probability diminishes. In other words, there exist stimuli ('rewards') which, when added to a given situation, 'reinforce' on-going activities and other stimuli ('punishments') which diminish or extinguish them. These generally valid principles were first given systematic prominence by Thorndike around the turn of the century[247, 248]. When a cat is shut in a cage with a simple latch on the door, it tends to become agitated and make various movements until it happens to knock the latch open and escape. Thorndike noticed that if this situation is repeated over and over again the cat escapes more and more quickly. He then argued that the accidental actions occurring just before the escape must somehow be boosted by the satisfying effects they produced so that they occurred with greater probability at the next occasion. This process continues until eventually the cat comes to perform the required movements as soon as it is placed in the cage.

In a well known series of experiments Skinner[224] showed that if a pigeon freely moving in a cage is regularly rewarded with a food pellet whenever it happens to raise its head above an imaginary demarcation line drawn by the experimenter, it soon comes to strut around with the head permanently erect.

Skinner has also pointed out an important operational difference between classical and instrumental conditioning. In classical conditioning we are dealing with responses which are elicited by known stimuli. By presenting the appropriate US the experimenter can summon the response at will in suitably controlled situations. In instrumental conditioning, on the other hand, we are dealing with 'spontaneous' responses, with responses elicited by no known stimuli. The experimenter has to wait until the response happens. Skinner calls the first type 'elicited' responses, the second type 'emitted' or 'operant' responses.

Thorndike's conclusions were given expression in the so called *Law of Effect*. As formulated by McGeoch[162] this law states: 'Other things being equal, acts leading to consequences which satisfy a motivating condition are selected and strengthened while those leading to consequences which do not satisfy a motivating condition are eliminated.'

In the 1930s Hull[121] suggested that the reinforcing effect of food pellets, lumps of sugar etc. is to be explained in terms of the drive reduction the food intake effects in the hungry animal. Indeed, Hull went a good deal further than this and in a monumental theoretical edifice attempted to explain all learning changes in terms of drive reductions of one kind or another.

At a superficial level of thought this offers a tempting simplicity. But when it comes to developing the hypothesis in detail the picture changes and in the event Hull's theory proved to be a *tour de force* which highlighted the immense difficulties that confront any attempt to discover unitary principles in the complex operations of the brain. By contrast, Skinner has consistently tried to avoid postulating 'intermediate variables', internal variables or mechanisms which could not be defined operationally in terms of the dimensions that he regards as the proper province of psychology.

From the standpoint of those who think of the nervous system not as a black box the psychologist is allowed to observe from the outside but not to look into but as a complex machine whose secrets we have to unravel, all attempts to find simple laws in observed learning changes must inevitably seem somewhat misplaced. We have to recognize that we are here dealing with a system which nature had to develop within a framework of what proved physiologically and phylogenetically feasible. If learning phenomena are to be fully understood we must be prepared to explore the special mechanisms which have developed within this framework for monitoring the appropriateness of behaviour and to study their effective mode of action. It is wishful thinking to expect these mechanisms in any sense to be simple ones and to assume that they operate according to a single universal principle which is merely waiting to be discovered. The nervous system has no automatic indications available for detecting the appropriateness of its responses. Nor are we entitled to assume that the reinforcement of selected connections between stimuli and overt responses is the only way in which the nervous system can (and in practice does) increase its capacity for appropriate behaviour as the result of experience.

Now it is a truism to say that if the probability of a response changes in a given situation there are likely to be events that account for the change. In instrumental conditioning we are dealing with particular instances of such probability changes in which a causative factor can be identified with the occurrence of some discrete external event occurring as the result of the organism's activities e.g. receipt of a food pellet. If the Law of Effect is understood merely as an affirmation that behaviour patterns tend to become modified by their outcomes, it becomes controversial only if this is taken to imply that in all cases of learning such identification must be possible, in other words that adaptive learning changes only happen in consequence of overt acts and their outcomes. As we know now, this is certainly untrue. As the result of past experiences and past reinforcements the brain may develop information-digesting processes which enable subsequent experiences to result in improved performances or improved capabilities even when these experiences are passive rather than active. The formation of expectancies as the result of passive observation of the external world is just one example of this category of events.

Emphasis on the importance of the development of particular 'expectations' in learning is generally associated with the name of Edward Tolman[252]. In the 1930s Tolman developed a systematic learning theory in which the main learning phenomena were seen in terms of the acquisition of expectancies or knowledge of 'what-leads-to-what' in the environment. This was essentially a cognitive theory, a 'theory of sign-learning', as it has been called, which allowed for the occurrence of adaptive learning changes also in situations involving no overt activities.

We are familiar enough with the role of expectations in our own lives. From the earliest age onwards experience teaches us to expect certain consequences from the events we observe or initiate. Already by the second week of life an infant appears to 'expect' a seen object to have certain tactile consequences. Already at that age, too, an infant will respond with a backward jerk of the head and by raising its hands when the shadow of an object is cast on a translucent screen and its size increased at an accelerating rate, thus giving the impression of an approaching object. Faced with the same display turtles pull in their heads and monkeys rush to the back of the cage. Whether the early responses of the infant or the reactions of the turtle are innate or learnt is not relevant at the moment. The point is merely that there are certain patterns of behaviour which invite the notion of 'expectation'. This is true even at very elementary levels of behaviour.

When a dog is conditioned to salivate in response to the sound of a buzzer in a series of trials in which the tone of the buzzer regularly precedes the presentation of food, it seems natural to say that the sound of the buzzer comes to create an 'expectation' of food. The animal comes to behave as if 'expecting' a definite event at a given time. This view of events is also promoted by the observation that classical conditioning works best if the CS precedes the US by a short interval (about half a second).

A monkey can choose correctly when it has seen a banana hidden underneath one of a set of containers. Moreover when, before the choice is made, the banana is secretly replaced by a lettuce leaf, the animal does not accept this upon lifting the container, but goes on looking for the banana. Again it seems natural to say that the monkey is 'expecting' a banana. Krushinsky[144] has shown that if pigeons are first familiarized with a food stimulus which moves with a constant velocity along a straight line and if a screen is then interposed behind which the stimulus temporarily disappears, they can extrapolate the place where it has to appear from behind the screen.

Expectancy in this sense is real enough also in physiological terms. EEG recordings show a sustained rise in surface electro-negativity of many regions of the frontal cortex in the period between the presentation of a conditioned stimulus and the succeeding unconditioned one. To give another example, after training to a double click when only a single click is given some cortical areas show an evoked potential response when the second click is expected. R. John[126], who is well known for his experiments in this field, goes so far as to say that the brain appears to construct a facsimile of an expected event at the expected time of occurrence.

The Principle of Expectancy, which postulates that during learning the animal builds up a 'what-leads-to-what' expectancy, became the cornerstone of Tolman's theory of learning. I have already mentioned some of the experiments from which Tolman inferred that during place learning, for example, the animal forms, as it were, a 'map in the head' of the external situation and, therefore, an 'expectancy' of what it will meet, say, around the next corner of a maze. But the concept also extends over 'expectations' of what experiences the animal *would* meet *if* it were to start on a certain course of action. The main question Tolman raised was really how far internal processes must be supposed to go on inside the animal which in some sense symbolize the actual or possible flow of events in the outer world, in other words, to what extent the brain forms internal representations of the dynamic as well as static properties of the world the organism inhabits.

The reader will recall from Section 2.2 in what sense internal representations of the way the perceived world transforms in response to our actions may be thought of in neutral terms. In Chapters 7 and 9 we shall look at the kind of neural networks that could form such representations as the result of experience. There can be little doubt that in the last analysis these internal constructs depend on being confirmed in practice. This was also Tolman's view: learning takes place by confirmation of expectancies. Since the expectancies are formed as the result of experience, a sequence of experiences which contradicts existing expectancies will tend to build up contrary expectancies and in doing so disrupt the existing ones. Tolman's Principle of Expectancy, therefore, did not contradict the Law of Effect as such, but it took this law to operate at a deeper level: rewards may act not only by reinforcing specific responses but also by reinforcing the expectancies from which the responses are derived. Since the same set of expectancies may enter into the determination of a variety of behaviours *this is the point at which you break away from simple S–R theory*. Nor did Tolman rule out the efficacy of drive reduction in certain respects. It might account, for example for the choice of goal-object, e.g. for the choice of a banana by the hungry monkey. But he rejected drive reduction as a universally valid principle for explaining adaptive learning changes.

It is clear that the mere formation of neural connectivities representing particular expectancies, and their subsequent correction in the light of progressive experiences, cannot as such furnish complete explanations of learning. One still has to explain how the organism comes to act on the expectancies in the way it does, how it comes to treat them as relevant in particular circumstances and how it comes to modify its reactions to them in the light of experience. As has often been pointed out, Tolman's theory is weak on specifying just how the expectations lead to appropriate actions. This throws us back again on the Principle of Effects. Though this principle may not suffice to explain all adaptive learning changes, no complete explanation of adaptive learning changes can do entirely without it. I shall return to this question in Section 6.5.

Much of the opposition to the Principle of Expectancy was due to the fact that, strictly speaking, 'expecting' and 'expectancy' belong to 'mind talk'. It is not surprising therefore that these concepts were alien to the behaviourist schools of animal psychology. The concepts have, as Hebb said, the smell of animism.

On a number of previous occasions I have been able to point out that one of the invaluable services of the concept of directive correlation is that it allows us to re-define apparently animistic concepts in strictly objective terms. 'Expectation' is another case in point.

We can take a first step towards removing 'expectation' from 'mind talk' by looking at the notion of 'anticipatory reaction'. This notion is easy to clarify in objective terms. To react in a way which 'anticipates' that an event A is followed by an event B, is to react in a way which is *adapted* to a situation characterized by the fact that in it A is followed by B. The notion therefore implies a directive correlation between some response variable on the one hand and some situation variable on the other. Thus when one shoots at a moving target, to anticipate where the target will be by the time the bullet reaches it is to react in a way which is adapted to the angle through which the target moves during the transit time of the bullet. And the adaptation, of course, here takes the form of aiming ahead of the target by an appropriate amount. In this rendering of the meaning of anticipation there are no concepts with mentalistic connotations.

The notion of 'expecting' an event A to be followed by an event B may go further than this in three ways:

1. It may denote an internal condition or reaction which need not necessarily be expressed in overt behaviour.
2. It may relate to probabilities. A may be expected to be followed by B with a probability of 30% and by C with a probability of 70%.
3. It may relate to hypothetical occurrences. It may be expected that *if* A is followed by B then the final outcome will be X, but *if* it is followed by C then the final outcome will be Y.

From an objective point of view 'expectancy' or 'expectation' in any of the senses illustrated here denotes what the psychologist would call a particular 'set' of the organism, i.e. a state of adjustment to the overall situation which is expressed in a conditional readiness to meet particular contingencies in a particular sort of way. The concept of directive correlation enables us to define these states of adjustment in perfectly objective terms. Thus to expect that A will be followed by B may be interpreted in objective terms as being in a state which is matched (directively correlated) to a particular property of a particular situation, viz. to the property that in this situation A is followed by B. The expectation is erroneous if the situation to which the adjustment has been made does not in fact prevail but the organism acts as if it did.

The case 3 cited above is particularly important. According to the thesis expounded in this volume the neural machinery that controls our actions operates importantly in terms of expectations concerning the possible or probable consequences of the various actions open to us at any particular juncture. It is asserted that the 'models' of the outside world which are formed in the brain consist of aggregates of expectations of how the subjective sensory inputs transform in consequence of the aggregate of self-induced movements open to us. To have a model of a room in my head is to have certain expectations of what I shall see if I cast my eyes around, or move my head or body.

An expectation of how subjective inputs transform in consequence of self-induced movements may be called a *transformation expectation*. Internal models, then, are largely composed of aggregates of transformation expectations.

Expectations relating to hypothetical events and to probabilities can be defined objectively in terms of directive correlations in the same way as before. To have an expectation that if A occurs it will be followed by B with a probability of 50% is to be in a state which is adapted (i.e. directively correlated) to a set of situation-characteristics which are such that the occurrence of A entails the occurrence of B with a probability of 50%. It was mentioned in Chapter 4 that we can treat the description of a situation in terms of probabilities as an objective scientific description. This interpretation of 'expectation' thus removes the difficulties some biologists have seen in the concept. It now enables us to use the concept in the knowledge that we can make it absolutely precise whenever doubts about its meaning or implications arise.

The problem, of course, is to discover the neural substrate of such expectations, the neural substrate of the 'set', of the state of adjustment of the organism to situation-characteristics of the type illustrated above. We shall see in due course that this problem has no unique solution. As the examples show, the expectations concerned can be of many different kinds.

The concept of 'expectation' is also sometimes used in a particular probabilistic sense in which it stands in an inverse relationship to the 'uncertainty' of information theory (see Appendix A). For example in his *Perception and Communication*[29] Broadbent has a lot to say about the 'information loading' of stimuli. By this he means a quantity which is a function of the size of the ensemble from which stimuli are 'expected' to be drawn. 'Expectation' in this sense can also be made precise in terms of directive correlations. To 'expect' that a stimulus will be drawn from a particular ensemble is to be in a state which is *adapted* to a particular set of characteristics of the experimental situation. In this case they are characteristics which limit the ensemble of probable stimuli. The 'adapted' here denotes an ontogenetic directive correlation which has come about as the result of previous experience of similar situations. The domain of this directive correlation determines a range of stimuli such that stimuli drawn from outside this range have the subjective character of novelty or surprise.

It is frequently said that the brain reacts according to the degree to which our experiences meet our expectations. The explanatory virtues of this statement are slight. Fundamentally it means no more than that the reactions of the organism to a given stimulus depend on the degree to which the organism is adjusted to the situation of which the stimulus forms a part. If the stimulus lies outside the domain of those (ontogenetic) directive correlations the reaction will be partly random, but only partly so because the occurrence of a 'surprising' or 'novel' stimulus in itself constitutes an event which the organism is innately equipped to deal with in a biologically appropriate fashion. It is an event to which the organism has become adapted phylogenetically, i.e. an event which comes within the domain of phylogenetic directive correlations. The 'orienting reactions' and general 'arousal' which novel stimuli elicits are examples of appropriate and non-random elements in the common responses to novelty and surprise.

5.5   THE QUESTION OF EXPLICIT ERROR-SIGNALS

The control of goal-directed activities in servomechanisms and other automata is commonly effected by means of error signals which inform the control units about the magnitude and direction of the discrepancy between the desired output state and the actual one. It is frequently taken for granted that this must also be the case in the motor control functions of the nervous system. In the present section I intend to show that this assumption is questionable. In so far as the overt activities of living organisms are goal-directed they may, of course, be viewed as error-reducing or error-eliminating activities. But this does not necessarily mean that their control mechanism depends on the generation of explicit error signals of one kind or another.

The bewildering complexity of the motor apparatus of the higher vertebrates makes it particularly difficult to distil the basic principles of its organization from the welter of interrelated details. This is partly due to the fact that the final motor responses are the end product of an efferent outflow of nerve impulses which originate at several distinct levels of the nervous system, and partly due to the number of degrees of freedom of the system. Each hinge-joint contributes one degree, each ball-joint two. Each degree of freedom requires at least two muscles, the agonist and antagonist. But when there are several degrees of freedom the function of the muscles may not be so neatly divided. At the ball-joints there may be a series of muscles acting in several planes. Again, many muscles act not over one but over two joints. In general, therefore, to move any part of the body, or to hold it in a determined position, requires the complex coordination and concurrent regulation of many muscles—particularly since most voluntary movements must be accompanied by appropriate adjustments of the rest of the musculature. Moreover, the task of the muscle control system is not only to establish the desired position or posture of body and limbs but also to maintain it against external disturbances or against a variation of specific metabolic parameters, as in fatigue. The coordination of so many elements requires an equally impressive flow of afferent information. As we know, each motor decision must be backed by information not only about the environment but also about the current position and state of movement of the body and limbs. Both exteroceptors and interoceptors take part in this information flow. Much of this information must have a feedback character, i.e. serve as a check whether the brain's movement decisions have been properly executed. Internally the information originates in the proprioceptors, the monitoring receptors in the muscles, tendon and joints. This information relates to both static and dynamic elements. But these elements, too, may not be neatly separated. The most important receptors monitoring the position of a joint are the Ruffini endings. Flexion, extension or rotation of the joint causes these units first to respond with a momentary overfiring or underfiring and then to settle to a new impulse frequency which is characteristic of the new position of the joint. So even this primarily static transducer function contains dynamic or 'phasic' elements in addition to the main static or 'tonic' elements. Other afferent fibres come from the tendon organs or from the muscle spindles.

Various degrees of integration and effective evaluation of the information conveyed by the proprioceptive afferents may occur at all relay stations to which they project: at the segmental levels of the spinal cord, at the dorsal nuclei of the brain stem, at the reticular formation, at localized subcortical regions and over wide areas of the cerebral and cerebellar cortices. At several different levels integration may occur in time as well as in space. Rhythmic patterns of movement, for instance, may be sustained even within the networks of the spinal cord.

Owing to the fact that each single movement may receive contributions from several levels of the brain, it is clear that one cannot think of movement as the product of a single mechanism whose secrets may some day be revealed in the form of a simple flow diagram. All the same, it is natural that any kind of goal-directed behaviour in the living organism should bring to mind the error-controlled servomechanism of modern automata such as automatic pilots, guided missiles and other robot devices. This is particularly true when we think of animal movement as modified postural control and compare this adaptive position control with the position control mechanisms used by the servo-engineer. It is therefore natural to ask whether such parallel functions imply parallel organizations.

Analysis shows that this is dangerous ground. The comparisons often seem so compelling that it is easy to jump to conclusions which may prejudice important neurological issues.

There is one aspect of servomechanisms to which these remarks apply in particular. This concerns the generation of *error-signals*. If this aspect is not properly understood the neurologist may be trapped into searching for mechanisms in the brain which do not in fact exist. To make this point it is not necessary to think in terms of very sophisticated hardware. Examples of quite simple servomechanisms suffice to show at what stage our thinking may go astray.

Servomechanisms commonly operate on an *error-control* principle in which an *error-signal generator* (ESG) computes the mismatch or error between the desired position of, say, an output shaft and its actual position. This error-signal is then fed to the *controller* or *evaluator* which computes the corrective action that must be initiated in the *motor* or *effector* system (Figure 5.2). (Error-signal generators are more commonly known as *comparators*, but as this term is open to certain ambiguities I shall avoid it for the present.) Servomechanisms are *feedback* mechanisms in the sense that they rely on a constant flow of information about the progress of the operation back to the centre which controls it.

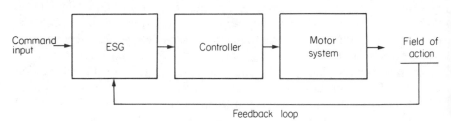

Figure 5.2. Block diagram of a simple servo

A simple example is given in Figure 5.3. The ESG here consists of the circuits containing the potentiometers P_1 and P_2. These generate an error voltage proportional to the misalignment of the output shaft. The controller consists of the amplifier and the field coils of the motor.

The steady state errors of some servomechanisms may be reduced or eliminated if functions of the input (command) signals are fed into the controller in addition to the error-signal. This is known as *feedforward*.

On the face of it one would expect systems of the same general type to be used for similar functions in the nervous system. But, as has been stressed before, it is inherently risky to transfer to a biological situation ideas which have developed in other disciplines. Tacit presuppositions valid in one field of research may not be justified in another. Close attention to the special problems the nervous system has to solve suggests that we can expect to find something analogous to these servomechanisms at the lower levels of motor control but not at the higher levels where learning takes place.

At the lowest level of motor control we in fact find a mechanism which broadly parallels that of error-controlled servos in the *gamma-efferent system* for the control of muscle stretch. We know that the actual commands to the muscles by the central nervous system (CNS) may not act directly on the muscle effector neurons, but instead adjust the 'zero point' of a stretch-sensitive receptor attached to the muscle so that its firing rate will be at a minimum when the muscle achieves the desired degree of stretch. The output of the stretch receptor is fed back to the muscle and causes it to seek out the amount of stretch that minimizes the firing rate of the receptor. These discharges, therefore, may be likened to the error-signals of a servomechanism. But, we are dealing here with a specific low-level mechanism and, for reasons I shall give presently, it would be rash to conclude that similar methods are used at the higher levels of brain function.

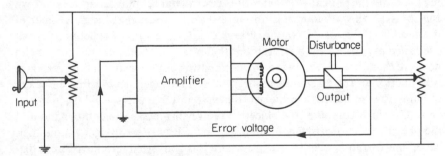

Figure 5.3. Simple positioning servo

The more intricate a scientific problem the more important it often is to look closely at the concepts we use in dealing with it. The concept of *error-signal*, for example, may have two different meanings which must be carefully distinguished:

1. It may denote a binary signal which merely indicates whether or not a discrepancy exists between the actual and the desired value of an output variable, without informing about the magnitude and direction of this discrepancy. Ordinary alarm signals are of this kind. We may call such signals *error-signals of Class I*.
2. It may denote an analog signal which informs not only about the existence of a discrepancy between actual and desired values of a variable but also about the magnitude and direction of the discrepancy. We may call this a *Class II error-signal*. Typical examples are the error voltage

of the servomechanism of Figure 5.3 and the discharges of the muscle spindles mentioned above.

Although the example of the gamma-efferent mechanisms shows that some explicit Class II error-signals are generated in parts of the nervous system, the point to be made is that we are here dealing with the lowest and most mechanical level of the motor control system where innate ESGs are possible. It must be questioned whether the same type of error-controlled servo action is compatible with the flexibility and adaptability that exists at the higher levels of the brain at which learning takes place. We shall see presently that the main advantage of using Class II error-signals and Class II ESGs is one of economy in the number of input–output associations that have to be learnt by the control mechanisms concerned. But we shall also see that the demands of plasticity and adaptability conflict with the restraints required by effective ESGs.

Strictly speaking, all we can say from observation is that the overt activities of the nervous system are *error-eliminating*. When I approach an object with my hand my movement eliminates the 'error distance' that separates the two. But to assert this, of course, is no more than to assert that the movement of my hand is *goal-directed*. On the other hand, to assert that the action is *error-controlled* may be taken to assert more than that. In a weak sense it may mean no more than that the action is error-eliminating as above, or that the response is a function of the error magnitude. But in a stronger sense it may be taken to imply that somewhere in the nervous system there is a special mechanism, an ESG, which computes the objective vector distance between my hand and the object and converts this into an explicit Class II error-signal—this then being sent to another control centre where it is converted into the efferent discharges required to correct the misalignment.

This is jumping to conclusions. Though suggested by the example of mechanical servomechanisms, the inference is not strictly warranted and it is also suspect on theoretical grounds. As we shall see, a response may be generated as a function of an error magnitude without the intervention of a mechanism which first computes the error magnitude and then converts this into an explicit error-signal. To that extent, therefore, the notion of 'error-controlled' activities in any sense other than 'error-eliminating' or 'goal-directed' may be suggestively misleading when applied to animal behaviour. It may tempt us to search for functional units in the brain which do not in fact exist.

We must draw a distinction here between ESGs which may be innate, such as the muscle stretch receptors mentioned above, and ESGs which would have to be trained for special applications as the organism learns to adapt its skills to the demands of the environment. We cannot expect to find innate ESGs for any possible goal that the human subject learns to pursue, for example. On the other hand, the obvious network complications that trainable ESGs require are such that one must question the possible biological value of trainable ESGs on purely *a priori* grounds.

For a sound approach we must describe the activities of the organisms as what they are, viz. error-eliminating or goal-directed, and take this as the starting point of any further analysis. From the very nature of the case we must expect that the methods of the nervous system differ from those employed by the servo-engineer.

Suppose X' is the actual value of an output variable, such as a shaft position in a servomechanism or the position of a limb, and X'' is the desired or commanded value. Then the response of the controller which computes the required corrective action (R_m) must be a suitable function F of the error ($X'' - X'$):

$$R_m = F(X'' - X')$$

The normal procedure for the engineer is first to design a device that generates an error-signal

$$E = X'' - X'$$

and then to design a controller which computes an appropriate function $R_m = F(E)$.

Whereas this may be the most economical solution for the engineer it is not the only possible solution. In theory it is possible to have a servomechanism which fulfils the same function without first generating an error-signal. The controller could be supplied with independent information about X' and X'' respectively and compute the corrective action required directly from these twin inputs. For instance, it could act according to a list on which all possible combinations of X' and X'' are entered against the corrective action required in each particular case.

The mathematical and engineering advantages of the standard method are obvious. But the nervous system was never engineered in the manner of a modern machine. Where the engineer uses mathematical formulae, the actions of the higher nervous centres in compounding the correct output functions are more aptly compared with the use of lists or tables. The problem confronting the nervous centres is not one of mathematical analysis but the pragmatic problem of learning to produce the correct pattern of output signals in response to two (and probably widely dispersed) sets of input signals, one set reflecting the actual position of the limbs, the other set reflecting the required position.

To the extent, therefore, to which the control of limb movements and posture is to be achieved by learning and is to be capable of adaptive modifications in the light of experience, the problem of the motor organization is to learn to associate the right sets of output signals with a double set of input signals, one set reflecting the actual state of affairs and the other the desired one. And it may well be the case that this is more expediently accomplished by learning to associate the appropriate controller responses with the respective (X', X'') pairs directly rather than by a process involving the intermediate step of first generating from these two sets of input distributions a new and distinct stream of neural signals representing the error function $E = X'' - X'$ and then learning to attach the right response to the respective value of E.

If we think for a moment only in terms of sets of discrete values of the variables concerned, one can see that the advantage of an ESG lies in the fact that the *variety* of E is bound to be considerably smaller than the variety of the possible combinations of X' and X''. In this respect, therefore, far fewer input–output associations would have to be learnt by the controller if E is computed first. But in real life this saving may be more than offset by the fact that at these higher levels of control we cannot assume any ESG to be a blindly mechanical and stereotyped system. To compensate for growth and development, injury, ablation and malfunction, and many other variants it must itself be capable of undergoing adaptive modifications and contain the necessary learning systems. Above all it would have to learn what type of error is significant in various contexts. It could not *a priori* provide for every possible comparison between every possible pair of variables or sets of circumstances. Particularly in the human case it would be absurd to assume that there exists a built-in ESG capable of computing explicit output signals reflecting the difference between the reality with which we are confronted and any goal-situation we may be striving for. Moreover every new goal which could not be compounded of variations of old goals would require a completely reorganized or new ESG. Any learning systems built into the ESG that could meet these requirements would be of the same order of complexity as the mechanism that would have to be provided if no ESG were used in the first place: both its input variety and its output variety would be of the same order of magnitude. In these circumstances the use of an ESG might well be a pointless encumbrance.

But there is an alternative way in which considerable economies may be effected and, in a broad sense, this appears to be also the basic method prevailing in the nervous system. In this method a hierarchical organization superimposes regional and subregional systems of fine control on rather more global systems of coarse control. In the nervous system a hierarchical organization, of course, has the additional advantage that it enables high level *learnt* reactions to avail themselves of low level *innate* reactions. Not all associations have to be learnt from scratch.

In view of the intricacy of the nervous system and the organic processes which have shaped its growth and development during phylogeny it is doubtful whether it will ever be possible to visualize its activities completely in terms of neat block diagrams linking tidy functional units each performing a clearly definable operation. But the urge to grasp the functional organization of the brain in terms of such conceptual models, at least in outline and at some permissible level of abstraction and simplification, is fundamental to our desire to comprehend the incomprehensible.

By rejecting the assumption that the brain must be expected to rely on Class II ESGs for producing goal-directed behaviour we are left with something of a vacuum in the search for suitable conceptual models. The various types of feedback servos envisaged by the engineer have always had a certain suggestive quality as potential building blocks for conceptual models of organic motor control systems. But without the ESG in which the feedback loop achieves a clear analytical function the block diagrams of orthodox servomechanisms are virtually disembowelled. A glance at Figure 5.2 shows how comparatively uninformative a block diagram of a servo without ESG becomes. It tells us little more than that the motor unit is actuated by a 'controller' or 'evaluator' which receives two sets of inputs, one reflecting the actual state of affairs and the other the desired one.

The inadequacy of these particular machine analogies is even more serious than this analysis suggests. Throughout this section we have tacitly assumed that error-eliminating mechanisms are controlled by explicit 'command signals', i.e. signals solely relating to the desired output state. We shall see in the next section that in neural control systems not only the notion of explicit error-signals but also that of explicit command signals can be misleading.

Throughout this section I have confined the discussion to directive correlations of the executive class. We have looked only at motor control functions involved in the pursuit of given goals and the implementation of given strategies. We have not considered the type of error-signal that is relevant in directive correlations of the ontogenetic class, i.e. in monitoring the success or failure of existing strategies and in the control of learning changes. When a particular behaviour strategy brings my hand into contact with a hot surface I know that I have made a mistake. The resulting pain is a Class I error-signal which is likely to produce a quick revision of my strategy, i.e. an ontogenetic change. I have learnt a lesson. Pain and punishment may obviously be regarded as explicit error-signals in this sense.

Once again the question arises whether all directive learning changes presuppose explicit error-signals of this type. Since we shall be looking at possible learning mechanisms later on in some detail I shall not pursue this question here, except to point out one incidental consequence of what went before. To be able to reinforce successful responses and suppress unsuccessful ones, the brain needs explicit or implicit criteria of success or failure. If the mechanisms engaged in the pursuit of a particular goal operate by means of explicit error-signals, then these signals themselves can furnish explicit criteria for success or failure. If the mechanisms operate otherwise then this source is not available and the brain has to fall back on more indirect indicators, as indeed appears to be the case.

5.6 THE QUESTION OF EXPLICIT GOAL-SIGNALS

The theoretical models one finds in the literature for particular motor control functions of the nervous system are frequently based on analogies with various types of servomechanisms or units found in servomechanisms. Often the overt responses of the system to various types of inputs are virtually all that is known. The approach is then to attempt to design a theoretical system or model which can account for all of these responses. Some of these models are quite complex and envisage a multitude of feedback or feedforward loops. The building blocks of these models are generally based on the type of functional units one finds in servomechanisms and other automata: comparators, switches, amplifiers etc. In line with these analogies it is also frequently assumed that the inputs to the system (or parts of the system) comprise goal-specific command signals, i.e. signals solely related to the goal of the control function, such as moving an arm to a particular point in space or holding it in a particular attitude, or tracking a given curve with the finger.

This assumption of goal-specific command signals calls for a closer examination. Are we entitled to assume that every goal-directed activity presupposes the prior formation in the brain of goal-specific command signals? Indeed, can we say anything definite about the nature of the goal-determining excitations in the brain?

We have seen that when an organism is engaged in a particular goal-directed behaviour it is temporarily in a state in which it has system-properties which are characterized by particular mathematical correlations between particular sets of variables. When a hungry ape reaches for a banana it is, objectively speaking, temporarily in a state in which the movement of its arm is directively correlated to the position of the banana in respect of a particular goal-event—in this case to gain possession of the fruit. One has to say 'temporarily' because, of course, an animal may seek one goal at one time and another goal a few minutes later. It may pass from a state characterized by one set of directive correlations to a state distinguished by another. As one physiological need is satisfied another may assert itself. Again, as the proximate goal of one stage of a behaviour sequence is reached the next stage is ushered in and a new proximate goal comes to be pursued.

From simplicity let us think only in terms of a few elementary drive states, such as hunger and thirst, and (although this is an oversimplification) start by assuming that these drive states are induced by explicit neural signals emanating from specific drive centres. It is clear that such basic drive determining signals need not carry any information about the details of the goal-event or goal-condition to which they relate, i.e. of the exact nature of the conditions that terminate them. For this reason it seems preferable to call these signals *demand signals* rather than *command signals*. Thirst and hunger signals, for example, carry no information about the nature and variety of liquids or solids that satisfy these demands. They are relatively non-specific, low-variety goal-determining signals. They generate specific high-variety goal-determining signals only when impacting with high-variety sensory inputs, as when the hungry monkey sees a banana and the conjunction of demand signals and sensory inputs results in an activity aimed at gaining possession of this particular object.

To illustrate at a very simple level what is implied in a system being able to pursue alternative goals arising from different 'drive' states, consider a simple learning machine capable of learning to satisfy either of two alternative 'drive states'. Let these 'drive' states' be represented by internally generated demand signals D_1 and D_2 respectively. Assume that in the circumstances in which the machine functions these demands can be met by achieving the external goals G_1 and G_2 respectively. Finally, assume that a particular set of alternative external conditions H, I, J, K (represented by sensory inputs H', I', J', K', respectively) must be matched by actions P, Q, R, S, respectively if G_1 is to occur and by actions W, X, Y, Z if G_2 is to occur. To perform correctly, therefore, the machine must learn the following input–output associations:

Inputs	Output	Result
D_1, H'	P	
D_1, I'	Q	G_1 occurs and D_1 terminates.
D_1, J'	R	
D_1, K'	S	
D_2, H'	W	
D_2, I'	X	G_2 occurs and D_2 terminates.
D_2, J'	Y	
D_2, K'	Z	

The example shows that there is no particular mystique involved in a single system producing alternative sets of directive correlations under alternative 'drive' conditions.

By way of contrast with the *demand* inputs D_1 and D_2, we may call the inputs H', I', J', K', the *contingent* inputs. The demand inputs cease (or undergo specific changes) when the goal is reached, whereas the contingent inputs may undergo continuous changes as the action runs its course. The goal of the directive correlation is determined by the demand inputs, whereas the directive correlation itself is a correlation between the actions and the external variables represented by the contingent inputs.

Now let us take the matter a step further. Consider only the demand input

D_2 and assume that in order to achieve goal G_2 the machine must first achieve a subgoal SG which consists of changing some external condition L into a different condition M. After this change has occurred G_2, we assume, can be brought about if conditions H, I, J, K are met by responses W, X, Y, Z respectively. Finally we assume that to achieve SG under condition L the appropriate responses are P, Q, R, S respectively. Then the machine must learn the following input–output associations:

Inputs	Output	Result
$D_2L'H'$	P	
$D_2L'I'$	Q	SG occurs; L changes to M
$D_2L'J'$	R	D_2L' terminates (replaced
$D_2L'K'$	S	by D_2M').
$D_2M'H'$	W	
$D_2M'I'$	X	G_2 occurs;
$D_2M'J'$	Y	D_2 terminates.
$D_2M'K'$	Z	

In this example, when learning is complete, the combination D_2L' plays the same formal part as a goal-determining input as did D_1 and D_2 in the earlier example. That is to say, the directive correlation between the action values P, Q, R, S and the environmental values H, I, J, K in respect of the goal SG is here conditional on the input D_2L'. The goal-determining input is the combination D_2L'. Despite its simplicity this example typifies the most common cases of goal-directed activity, as may be seen by comparing it with the example of the monkey grabbing the banana. We see therefore that *goal-determining inputs generally consist of specific combinations of drive inputs and sensory inputs, and typically these combinations remain constant (or continue to satisfy certain constant conditions) until the goal is reached.*

It is important to keep this simple example in mind because it illustrates an objective sense in which we can say that during learning sensory inputs can come to set up goals. When learning is complete (i.e. the machine has learnt to respond in the way specified by the table above), in the presence of D_2 the occurrence of L' produces behaviour directed towards the goal SG.

It is clear that these goal-determining combinations of drive signals and episodic sensory signals are not of a kind that one would commonly mean by 'command' signals. The essence of a 'command' signal is that it should be a goal-specific decision signal issuing from a control centre, whereas the L' component above relates to passively received sensory inputs. The above machine contains no command signals in the sense given.

It follows that *we cannot assume that the brain forms goal-specific command signals in respect of every external goal which we can discern in the overt behaviour pattern of the organism.*

If we cannot assume this for all goal-directed activities, need we assume it for any? Need we assume that to move a limb to a particular position the brain must first form an internal command signal solely related to that position? I can see no valid reason for this assumption. Nor is it supported by the evidence. Electrical stimulation of particular areas of the motor cortex may indeed result in a limb moving to a particular position, but it is also then generally found that the terminal position depends on events that went before and on the context in which the stimulation is applied[195]. Command signals *may* exist (as in the gamma-efferent mechanism mentioned in Section 5.5). But we cannot assume that they *must* exist.

To some readers the conclusion reached above may already have been evident from the analysis given in Section 5.2. I have illustrated the matter in detail because the conclusion is important and the contrary assumption is often made in the literature.

All we can say is that as the organism expands its capacity to make appropriate responses in all manner of circumstances, types of behaviour develop which manifest particular hierarchies of directive correlations and corresponding hierarchies of goals and subgoals. The neural signals that govern the type of activity that will be released in particular circumstances (and hence the goals that will be pursued) are determined by a conjunction of:

(i) action-sustaining inputs which are related to the physiological needs of the organisms and which may function in the manner of demand inputs (as defined above) in relation to ulterior physiological goals, and

(ii) 'episodic' sensory inputs which undergo particular changes, or come to satisfy new conditions, when a particular external goal or subgoal is reached.

The need detectors of the brain function as important sustainers of overt activities. In a sense they may be regarded as Class I error-signals. Some of the most important of these act through the drive centres of the hypothalamus (see Section 6.3). The feeding centre is a typical example. When bilateral lesions are made in the lateral hypothalamus the animal ceases to feed and may die of starvation unless force-fed. If, rather than being destroyed, this same region is stimulated through implanted electrodes, food intake increases strikingly. Such drive centres may be sensitive to a variety of need metering stimuli. The feeding centre may be sensitive to the hunger contractions of the stomach or duodenum as well as to blood glucose levels. The physiological details of these functions are not particularly relevant in the present context. From the organizational point of view, however, it is important to note that the centres responsible for initiating a particular drive state are generally distinct from those responsible for terminating it. Strictly speaking, therefore, it is the latter that determine the physiological goals of the resulting behaviour.

The cessation of hunger contractions does not correlate with the termination of eating.

Again, eating may cease long before digestion and absorption can redress the caloric balance. Food intake is monitored by separate systems in the mouth, pharynx oesophagus and stomach. These systems may possibly act through a special 'satiety centre' in the hypothalamus which terminated eating by inhibiting the drive centre. But, although this assumption is supported by the results of some ablation and stimulation experiments, it is not universally accepted.

The upshot of this discussion is that in the study of the control functions of the brain it may be erroneous to search for models which are controlled by explicit command signals in conjunction with explicit error signals. Rather we should concentrate on the observed directive correlations and search for explanations of how these correlations may come to pass. Our simple examples have made it clear that the changes of neural excitation which may cause the organism to pursue one goal at one moment and another at the next are unlikely to be generally confined to pathways or networks solely devoted to this function.

The preliminary conclusions we have reached in the last sections may seem somewhat negative. This is not entirely the case since it must be reckoned a positive gain to have reached a clearer insight into the true nature of the phenomena it is sought to explain. To advance further we must take a closer look at the practical problems the brain has to solve in order to achieve the required correlations, and this means looking at the general organization of the nervous system and at the functional units it has available. In short, the time has come to start looking at the actual machinery of the brain.

5.7 SUMMARY OF PART I

Before we move on it is expedient to pause and take stock.

The main premiss of our analysis is that before we speculate about the overall functional organization of the brain we need clearer ideas about the main system-properties it is sought to explain. In view of the complexity of the subject we chose three categories of phenomena as representative of the higher brain functions in general and the special faculties of the human brain in particular. These categories were: the goal-directedness of behaviour, the power of the brain to form internal models of external realities and the faculty of speech and verbal reasoning.

The keystone of our analysis was the fact that the goal-directedness of behaviour represents an objective system-property which can be formally expressed in terms of directive correlations between particular variables. This formalization enabled us to deal with a variety of conceptual and philosophical problems. In particular it enabled us to give a precise and objective meaning to a variety of concepts which relate to the directiveness of organic activities and which many biologists have so far eschewed for fear of their apparently animistic connotations. Typical examples are the concepts of 'goal', 'adaptation', 'coordination', 'organic integration', 'drive', 'expectation', 'regulation' etc.

The directive correlations we find in living nature fall into three distinct categories: the phylogenetic, the ontogenetic and the executive. The executive directive correlations express the instant adaptability with which we can match our actions to the current configurations of objects and relations in the environment. In the higher orders these directive correlations are mainly acquired through learning, e.g. through the reinforcement of appropriate responses and the extinction of inappropriate responses as the result of experience. This process in itself amounts to an ontogenetic directive correlation. The highest forms of life are mainly distinguished by the exceptional range of both their executive and ontogenetic directive correlations.

Complex behaviour sequences typically exhibit hierarchies of executive directive correlations and corresponding hierarchies of goals and subgoals. It was shown in Section 5.2 that such hierarchies do not presuppose the existence of correlated hierarchical organizations in the brain. It was also shown that the manifest pursuit of a particular goal or subgoal does not necessarily presuppose explicit and goal-specific command signals in the brain, or explicit error-signals.

We can take it that the ultimate physiological goals of our activities are in the main determined by demand signals emanating from specific need detectors. As the organism learns to respond to these demand signals and to respond appropriately in all manner of circumstances, complex behaviour patterns develop which are seen to be punctuated by a variety of external goals and subgoals. The nature of these activities and of the goals or subgoals is determined internally by the conjunction of the basic demand signals and sensory inputs representing the current external circumstances, body posture etc.

It follows that the closest approximation we can expect to find in the brain to regions in which 'goals' are represented must be regions in which neural excitations representing the physiological demand inputs can impact with neural excitations representing the relevant sensory inputs or input conditions.

All these topics pertain to infrahuman species as well as to Man. The special capabilities of the human brain arise mainly from the faculty of speech but also from more extensive faculties for forming internal 'models' of the external world.

In Chapter 2 it was argued that in the interest of learning economy we must expect the brain to synthesize patterns of nervous activity which are of the nature of unique internal representations or 'models' of external objects, events, situations and of their significant features, properties or relations in space or time. Apart from introspective knowledge, there is also abundant objective evidence to support this assumption. The quality and compass of such internal representation, of course, is likely to be a matter of degree. Even in Man the internal 'models' are often nebulous and ambiguous. It is likely that some measure of this capacity exists in all higher vertebrates, but that it expands monumentally as we reach the primates and Man.

As to the nature of these internal representations in terms of neural processes we argued as follows. The basic function of these organizations is to represent what depends on what in what sort of way. In particular the brain needs internal representations of the way sensory inputs transform in response to the organism's self-induced movements. To have an internal representation of a room means in essence to be able to predict how my sensory inputs will transform when I enter the room, glance around it or move about inside the room. At a more elementary level, to have a stable image of a scene means to be able to predict what projections will strike the retina at what locations when the eye moves in its socket.

Fundamentally this means that the brain must form neural organizations which represent functional relationships between specific variables, i.e. relationships of the type $y = f(x)$. A stable visual image, for example, needs a neural organization which can represent the retinal location of the image as a function of the position of the eye.

Functions of the type $y = f(x)$ stand for sets of ordered pairs of elements. We concluded that the neural representation of a function of this type must be expected to consist of a pattern of neural excitations which can be mapped on a representative sample of ordered pairs of elements denoted by the function. That is to say, to activate an internal representation of $y = f(x)$ means to activate an aggregate of neural excitations containing components which were formed during learning as the product of neural excitations representing sample values of x and neural excitations representing the associated values of y. It follows that to find the sites in the brain at which internal models are formed, we must look for sites at which the respective intermodal combinations can be registered. This subject will be resumed in Chapter 7.

In addition to forming internal representations of significant features or properties of the environment, of course, the brain must develop appropriate reactions to these models, depending on the circumstances (drive state etc.) in which the actions take place. This implies reactions which generalize over appropriate classes of internal representations, i.e. appropriate 'categorizing reactions' or 'discriminations'.

For purposes of linguistic communication the brain must also be able to attach specific verbal labels or 'names' to the classes of objects that are relevant in the context of an intended message, for instance in the context of a descriptive communication. Descriptive statements assign particular objects to particular classes. If our vocabulary were to contain a name for every possible object and class, the narrative use of language could be confined to strings of simple two-term utterances. Since it is impossible to acquire vocabularies that contain a name for every possible object and class of objects that might be relevant in a verbal communication, unnamable objects and classes must first be specified in terms of namable classes. This means that the relevant unnamable class or object must first be 'seen' as an intersection of namable classes. In addition to such cognitive resolutions, the code of the natural languages calls for specific categorizations of the namable classes, the 'lexical categorizations', and it calls for a factoring out of the conditional time reference of the message (past, present or future). These neural processes supply the main inputs relating to the content of the message which the speech mechanisms need in order to form the appropriate string of verbal utterances in the context in which the communication is made.

From the narrative use of language we went on to the argumentative use. Stripped of all inessential details this presupposes general propositions of the type 'All A is B'. In functional terms general propositions of this type amount to a licence to react to any A as to any B in the context in which the proposition is accepted and formulated. In neural terms we may think of this licence as a set of facilitations or disinhibitions applied to the respective internal reactions. We interpreted the process of verbal reasoning as a further instance of licensed transformations (in this case of specific propositions in conjunction with general propositions) which the brain learns as part of the process of adapting to the way things are (and so to the way things logically are).

All these, of course, are broad generalizations largely depending on a considerable degree of oversimplification. Our main concern was to interpret the structure of the natural languages and the processes of rational thought in terms of operations which can be broadly visualized in terms of neural functions—even if the outlines of these functions are still only shadowy and their details still unresolved.

PART II

CHAPTER 6

Outlines of the Nervous System

6.1 INTRODUCTION

This chapter is an interlude.

Our analysis has focused attention on two main concepts, that of directive correlation and that of internal representation. So far these have been discussed only at an abstract level. Only in very general terms, for example, have I been able to indicate how internal representations of the outer world may be thought of in neural terms. The time has come to relate our concepts more closely to the 'hardware' of the brain.

Since this volume is intended not only for the student of neurophysiology but also for the philosopher, the psychologist, the engineer and anyone else who nowadays joins the debate, I must begin with a brief outline of relevant aspects of neurology and learning theory. This is a difficult task. One has to rely on simplifications and sometimes on interpretations which may have their opponents. One cannot just give a recital of experimental results. Frequently one has to resort to generalizations which a comprehensive textbook would hedge with qualifications. One has to select what seems most relevant in the context, and there are bound to be those who will quarrel with the selection.

The reader must therefore accept the contents of this chapter with due reservations. This is the price we have to pay for bringing the 'hardware' of the brain into the picture at all. However, since my aim is not to compound a textbook, but only to develop and illustrate a line of analysis, the risks are worth taking. For a general introduction to the anatomy and physiology of the nervous system the reader may be referred to the works of Crosby, Humphrey and Lauer[48]; Thompson[246]; and Ruch et al.[211].

6.2 THE NEURON

Both the afferent and efferent flow of information in the nervous system is coded in terms of the identity of the activated nerve fibres and the frequency of the impulses transmitted in them. The amplitude of the individual impulses travelling through a fibre is approximately constant and irrelevant from the point of view of information flow. The individual impulse is an all-or-nothing event.

Although at the sense organs the frequency-coding of the information is significant, the subsequent discriminations in the sensory pathways and the choice of action in the premotor pathways appear to depend on the identity of the excited neurons or fibres rather than the frequency of the impulses. The latter seems less important further from the sense organs and muscles than 'line-labelling', i.e. the identity of excited fibres[115]. The actual information processing inside the CNS (central nervous system) thus hinges on the identity and distribution of excited fibres rather than the absolute frequencies of the impulses. But the final motor performance of the organism depends largely on the disequilibrium produced in the balance of mutually antagonistic efferent systems and at this stage, therefore, the impulse frequency again assumes special importance.

The principle that sensation depends on what fibres are excited and not how they are excited peripherally was first enunciated by Johannes Muller in 1830. This concept of specificity, as dependent on line-labelling, has since been confirmed for numerous sensory systems.

One of the most important questions concerning the plastic changes which the CNS undergoes during learning concerns the site of these changes. It follows from the paramount significance of line-labelling in the CNS that this plasticity must be expected to reside primarily in the devices by which one activated neuron may come to activate another. The main device for transmitting signals from one neuron to another is the *synapse*. It is to be expected, therefore, that learning changes take the form of (or act through) enduring changes in synaptic transmission. The question of the physiological nature of these changes is not one I shall take up. The more we learn about synapses the more we realize the complexity of these processes. When the final answer is known it is unlikely to be a simple one of synaptic growth or straightforward structural changes. The changes may not even be purely local ones. Recent research, for example, suggests that the metabolic supporting cells of the brain, the *neuroglia*, may also be involved in the synaptic changes of the neurons they support.

One of the prominent features of the peripheral receptors is that they do not commonly generate a set of signals representing the static characteristics of an applied stimulus. Many receptors are *phasic* rather than *tonic*. That is to say, the operative condition for activation is a *change* in the input variables rather than their absolute value. Frequently the impulses cease to be produced after a period of time irrespective of whether the stimulus continues to be applied, or the discharge drops to a lower level. This type of 'phasic' behaviour, really a rising of threshold with stimulus duration, is known in neurophysiology as *adaptation*. Neural thresholds (see below) may also rise with stimulus strength. This is known as *accommodation*. (Both these terms are unfortunate terminological choices and in the context of our analysis it is not a quibble to say so. In the ordinary use of the term, 'adaptation' implies usefulness in respect of some variable function or goal; in other words, it implies an element of directive correlation. This is not the case in this special physiological use of the term. This is a point to remember. The same applies to the narrow physiological use of the term 'accommodation'.)

The nerve fibres along which the messages travel through the brain are the *axons* of individual nerve cells (see Figure 6.1). The axon is a long and slender process which grows from the cell body of the neuron and continues to be nourished by it. If severed from the parent body the axon decays. Each nerve cell sprouts only one axon, but each axon may have many branches or *collaterals*. The axon carries the outgoing messages which take the form of nerve impulses consisting of brief changes in the electrical potential across the axonal membrane. These may be electrically recorded as *action potentials*, also known as *spikes*, from the way in which the impulses show up on the electrical records. They are propagated along the whole length of the axon without decrease in amplitude (about 100 mV). Each impulse is an all-or-nothing event of fixed amplitude and shape. Human nerve fibres can transmit up to about 1000 pulses per second.

Between the surface of the nerve cell and the interior there is normally an

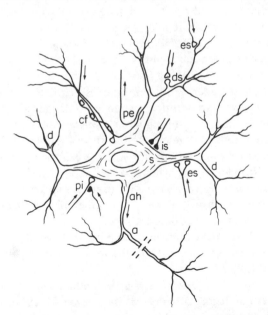

Figure 6.1. Composite representation of neuron to illustrate different types of neural elements. a, axon; ah, axon hillock; cf, climbing fibre; d, dendrite; ds, dendritic spine; es, excitatory synapse; is, inhibitory synapse; pe, presynaptic element; pi, presynaptic inhibition; s, soma

electrical potential difference of 50–100 mV (interior negative). This *resting potential* arises from asymmetries in the ion exchanges across the membrane. The nerve impulse is triggered at certain sites of the cell, e.g. the *axon hillock*, whenever the potential difference at the site drops below a certain threshold value in consequence of the stimulation the cell receives from other parts of the nervous system. But in some cells impulses may also be initiated elsewhere (Figure 6.2(a)). Stimulation comes via axons impinging on special receptive processes, the *dendrites*, or on the cell body (*soma*). These points of near-contact are the *synapses*. A central neuron may be covered with up to 50 000 synapses. As each approaching axon may have several junctions with the same cell, the number of other neurons from which a given neuron may receive afferent volleys will be less than this number, but it may still amount to many thousands. At the synapse the axonal branches have swellings, *boutons*, which approach the membrane of the receiving neuron or dendrite, leaving only a minute cleft of about a millionth of an inch. These presynaptic boutons contain the *synaptic vesicles* which probably contain quantities of a chemical transmitter substance. The rate of release of this substance is quantal and controlled by the presynaptic nerve endings. As the transmitter substance diffuses through the gap it effects permeability changes in the membrane resulting in a local depolarization which spreads electrotonically and summates with the effects of similar events at other stimulated synapses of the neuron. When the total depolarizing effect, known as the *excitatory postsynaptic potential*, or EPSP, results in a sufficient depolarization of the electrically active part of the cell membrane, the cell 'discharges', i.e. transmits an action potential or 'spike' along its axon. In the course of this discharge the remainder of the somadendritic membrane is depolarized and this in turn is followed by a hyperpolarization whose magnitude varies for different cell types. The potential changes resulting from a single stimulus to the synapses, therefore, run approximately the course shown in Figure 6.2(b).

The discharge is followed by an *absolutely refractory period* of the cell, lasting a few milliseconds during which no new spikes can be generated. This passes into the *relatively refractory period* in which spikes can be generated but only at a reduced sensitivity. In this manner the frequency of the discharges comes to reflect the overall intensity of the afferent stimulation and the excess of the EPSP over the threshold requirements of the cell. The summation of the afferent excitations has a sophisticated dependence on the extended geometry of the dendrites.

In addition to this *spatial summation* of individual synaptic transmissions there is also a certain degree of *temporal summation* which may extend over 100 milliseconds or more. Hence repetitive subliminal stimuli can summate in their effects on the cell potential and in this sense facilitate subsequent discharges.

Some synapses are *inhibitory*. Their action tends to suppress rather than

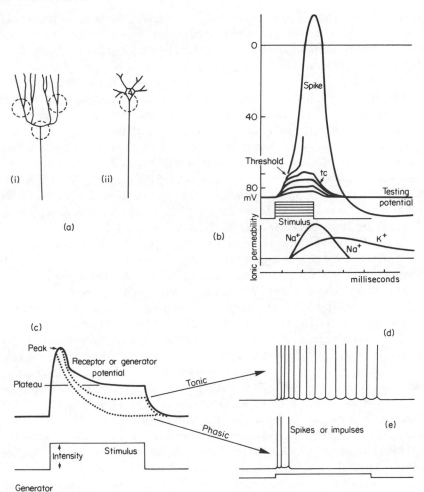

Figure 6.2. Receptor or generator potentials and spike initiation. (a) Anatomical situations in which impulses are initiated; (i) typical vertebrate motoneuron; (ii) vertebrate sensory arborizations. (b) Spike initiation. An electrical stimulus, as shown in six increasing strengths, depolarizes the membrane to increasing extents. At a certain degree of depolarization, as indicated by the threshold, the membrane resistance to sodium ions is reduced and further current begins to flow, thus causing the spike. The upward phase of the spike is caused primarily by the increase in permeability to sodium ions, shown by the Na^+ curve below, allowing sodium ions to flow in. The recovery phase of the spike is caused primarily by the increase in permeability to potassium ions (curve K^+ below), allowing potassium ions to flow out. (c) Typical relations between stimulus, receptor potential and spike activity in a receptor. The magnitude of the receptor potential can be measured either to the peak or to the plateau. (d) and (e) Adaptation of impulses can depend on the decay of depolarization in the generator region, as shown by the broken curves, or by change in sensitivity at the spike-initiating region. The resulting spike trains may be quite different (From *Interneurons, their Origin, Action, Specificity, Growth and Plasticity*[115], by G. Adrian Horridge. W. H. Freeman & Company. Copyright © 1968.)

promote a discharge. The total effect of the inhibitory influences on the cell is known as the *inhibitory postsynaptic potential*, or IPSP. The character of the synapse is generally determined by the presynaptic neuron, in the sense that the axon collaterals of any one neuron have either only excitatory or inhibitory effects on other neurons. Consistent structural differences between excitatory and inhibitory synapses have only recently come to light through the work of Gray[92]. His 'Type 1' and 'Type 2' synapses are now widely held to represent excitatory and inhibitory synapses respectively.

An important point to note is that the relative efficacy of synapses may depend on their topographical distribution on the cell or its dendrites. Somatic synapses, for example, are generally held to have the greatest relative efficacy. It is worth noting in this connection that inhibitory synapses are mostly found on the soma. Synapses are also sometimes found on the presynaptic fibres. This allows for *presynaptic* modulation (Figure 6.1).

Over and above the topographical advantages enjoyed by synapses situated on the soma of the neuron against those situated on the dendrites, some presynaptic fibres establish a dominating control over the postsynaptic cell by forming numerous collaterals which envelop the cells in a *pericellular nest*. This provides for an exceptionally large number of synaptic contacts. A similar device is the *climbing fibre* (Figure 6.1). These fibres entwine the cell body or basal dendrites like climbing plants and thus again provide opportunity for exceptional degrees of synaptic control over the postsynaptic cell.

The dendritic apparatus of a neuron can perform important integrating functions even within itself. This particularly applies to the long dendritic trees of the pyramidal neurons which dominate the cytoarchitecture of the cortex. It is now widely accepted that the summation of afferent volleys to distant dendritic branches can result in *local responses*, i.e. local action potentials within the dendrites which then propagate to the impulse firing zone of the soma or axon hillock. This provides for more effective transmission of synaptically induced depolarizations, particularly if on the way they summate with similar local responses arriving from other branches of the dendritic tree. As Andersen[10] has pointed out, since the membrane surface increases where two branches meet, it may even be the case that one such local response is held up at a nodal point until another local response arrives from the adjoining branch and summation occurs. In respect of the information flow along the dendritic tree, therefore, such a nodal point would come to act in the manner of a logical AND gate. Instances are known of inhibitory synapses being situated at such nodal points, so that from a functional point of view we then virtually have the picture of a neuron operating within a neuron. It is important therefore not to take too simple a view of the dendritic apparatus of large neurons. This particularly concerns the neurons in the cortex.

The dendrites of some neurons, of the pyramidal neurons in the cortex for example, sprout small projections or *spines* at the points of contact with a presynaptic fibre (Figure 6.1). It is significant that these spines have been observed to atrophy after prolonged stimulus deprivation[85, 210]. But there is no general agreement as yet that growth or decay of the spine apparatus can be identified with learning changes.

Our physiological concepts of neurons are far from static. New discoveries still continue to produce startling results. Recent researches, for example, have produced evidence that some cells have dendrite-like processes containing 'presynaptic elements' (Figure 6.1) which can release transmitters in the manner of axon terminals[205]. These elements were first suggested for their amacrine cells of the retina and the granule cells of the olfactory bulb, but there is now evidence that they exist also in several other areas of the central nervous system.

Looking back we note that in a sense all central neurons have a certain potential for pattern discrimination in the sense that they tend to be more responsive to one pattern of activated input fibres than to another by virtue of the physiologically active connections of its dendrites. The extent to which a stimulus is effective depends on the degree to which it approaches the optimal configuration of inputs to the neuron. But temporal as well as spatial summation must be taken into account, as well as the topography of the synaptic sites and possibly independent integrating functions in the dendritic trees.

Learning changes in the central neurons may therefore be thought of as changes in the particular pattern or distribution of inputs to which the neuron comes to be most sensitive. In detail the learning changes may be thought of as increments or decrements in what, for want of a better term, we may call their *synaptic potency*, i.e. in the efficacy of the mechanism of synaptic transmission. Unfortunately our understanding of the brief events involved in synaptic transmission, neural discharges and impulse conduction is not matched by a comparable understanding of the long-term changes that must occur at particular points of the neural network during learning. Such changes could be postsynaptic, e.g. changes affecting the sensitivity of the cell membrane; or they could be presynaptic and relate to the synthesis, storage, distribution or release of transmitter substance[56, 126]. Nor can we exclude the possibility that the ultimate learning changes take place in the deep protein metabolism of the cell, exerting their effect on the pathways followed by neural excitations in the brain only indirectly through one of the factors mentioned above. Indeed there may be different changes in succession: changes of one kind to start with, followed by more profound and lasting changes of a different kind as memories consolidate.

However, since only the effective network properties of the nervous system concern the subject of this volume, we need not look beyond the changes in synaptic transmission as such.

When we turn to the question of the organization of assemblies of neurons that might have the kind of adaptive plasticity suggested by behavioural learning changes it is important to avoid a number of mistakes from the start. Three are particularly common:

1. The attempt to explain learning in terms of neurons conceived as excessively simple logic devices, e.g. as simple switches which can learn to open or close at the right moment. The neuron is a many-input, single-output threshold device in which a large number of inputs undergo both spatial and some degree of temporal summation.
2. The attempt to reduce the learning problem to one concerning the discharge probability of single neurons as a function of present stimulation and past history, without taking into account the intimate network within which the neuron functions and which may expose it to important interactions with neighbouring cells which share some or all of its input channels.
3. To think of a natural stimulus to the nervous system as a lump of excitatory energy which then travels along various pathways. This is untrue.

In the lightly anaesthetized animal the average level of excitation in the cortex is a fairly constant quantity independent of the stimulation applied[36]. The mean frequency of discharge of cortical neurons remains broadly constant over long periods of time and is not radically altered by afferent excitation. The effect of natural stimulation, therefore, must be thought of as a redistribution of an existing flow of excitation rather than the initiation of a new one. At the level of individual neurons some of this constancy results from the complementary innervation to be discussed in Section 6.8: in some situations the absence of a particular stimulus may be just as important as is its presence in other situations. In consequence the sensory systems, right up to the level of the cortex, are often so organized that there are not only normally quiescent neurons which are excited by a stimulus, but, equally, there are normally active neurons which are inhibited by the same stimulus[174].

Just as in some circumstances the absence of a stimulus may be functionally as significant as is its presence in other circumstances, so, too, learning *not* to respond may be functionally as important as learning to respond. From a functional point of view responses may have to be extinguished either because they are relevant but detrimental, or because they are irrelevant. Responses are detrimental either because they are incompatible with useful responses or because they have detrimental external effects. In both cases the unwanted response is likely to be extinguished through *interference*: the central mechanisms are such that they inhibit the unwanted response in the course of establishing the wanted one (Section 6.8). Since, as we shall see, overt responses may generally be thought of as the result of a disequilibrium between mutually antagonistic and counter-balancing organizations, this condition is not as exacting as it may seem at a first reading. The elimination of irrelevant responses is known as *habituation*. In a sense, habituation is the simplest kind of learning and, in one form or another, is universal in animals. But habituation must be distinguished from sensory adaptation (see above). It is not a loss of sensitivity. Habituation is directive in the sense that it represents a relatively permanent waning of a superfluous response as a result of repeated stimulation which is not followed by any kind of reinforcement. It is a selective inhibition upon attention or performance which is specific to a particular stimulus situation [61, 158]. If the stimuli are changed, the extinguished response may reappear. In the cat, for example, a habituated response may return if the animal is distracted by the sight of a mouse. Again, a response habituated to a particular tone may reappear if there is a change in the frequency, duration or strength of the tone. Habituation thus differs essentially from the extinction of a response through fatigue or punishment.

6.3   THE CENTRAL ORGANIZATION OF THE NERVOUS SYSTEM

Throughout this volume we are mainly concerned with the *somatic* nervous system as distinct from the *visceral* system. In a narrow sense 'somatic' means having to do with structures related to the somites, such as muscles, tendons and bones. In the wider sense used here the concept includes all sensations that deal with the outer world and that are aroused by our own muscular responses to it—pain, touch, temperature and also the special senses of sight, hearing and balance. By visceral functions we mean functions having to do with the viscera, for example the respiratory, circulatory and digestive functions, but also the smooth muscle, cardiac muscle and the endocrine glands. The visceral efferent system is known as the *autonomic* system. Under

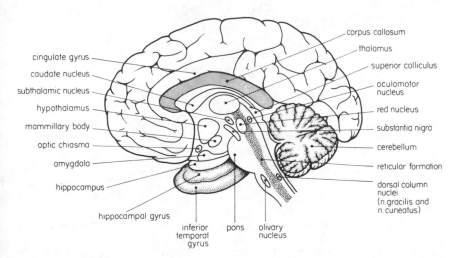

Figure 6.3. Schematic cross-section of the human brain

control of its central nervous connections the regulatory functions of the autonomic system aid in adapting the behaviour of the individual to the environment while yet maintaining the constancy of essential physiological variables (*homeostasis*).

In broad outline the central nervous system, CNS for short, is seen as a highly organized network of interconnected pathways in which the afferent information derived from the receptors is transmitted to the highest level, the cerebral cortex, along a variety of ascending pathways. None of these are uninterrupted. Even the most direct pathways typically contain at least two relay stages. At each of these intervening stations signals may depart for other regions, ultimately affecting the descending, efferent signals which carry instructions to effector organs such as the skeletal muscles. Conversely each relay stage (as well as the receptors themselves) may receive signals from other regions which can establish a certain degree of gating control.

Some of the ascending flow of information is *specific* in the sense that the signals are specific both to the modality of the peripheral stimulus and to the exact location at which it is applied—although the former may not always be a definitely definable relationship and the latter is commonly subject to some degree of regional diffusion. But in other ascending pathways the information flow is *non-specific* and relates to more than one modality and to extended peripheral regions.

The vast convoluted sheet of the *cerebral cortex* (Figures 6.3 to 6.5) harbours the extensive laminated networks which are indispensable for all the higher functions of the brain. The two hemispheres are conventionally

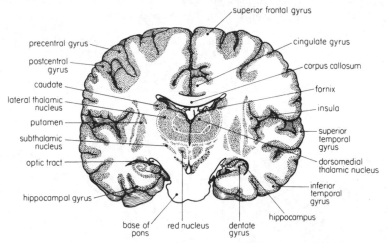

Figure 6.4. Coronal section through the adult human brain (Reprinted with permission of Macmillan Publishing Co., Inc. from *Correlative Anatomy of the Nervous System* by Crosby, Humphrey and Lauer[48]. Copyright © 1962 by Macmillan Publishing Co., Inc.)

marked off into *lobes* (Figure 6.5). These are not functional units, nor are they separate masses. They are mainly marked off by imaginary lines, except, for example the posterior border of the frontal lobe and the upper border of the temporal lobe which are formed by two deep crevices, the central and lateral *fissures* respectively.

The primary receiving areas for specific visual impulses lie at the tip or *pole* of the *occipital lobe* (area 17). This is surrounded by visual *association areas*, areas which are largely devoted to functions of analysis and integration of visual information.

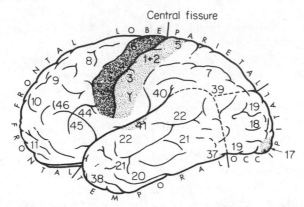

Figure 6.5. Lateral surface of the human cortex showing approximate location of some of the cytoarchitectural fields distinguished and numbered by Brodman. The numbering is mainly based on the order in which the fields were studied and bears no relation to their functional significance (Adapted from Penfield and Roberts, *Speech and Brain-Mechanisms*[194]. Copyright © 1959 by Princeton University Press. Reprinted by permission of Princeton University Press)

The primary receiving areas for somatic information (areas, 1, 2, 3) lie at the anterior end of the *parietal lobe*, bordering on the central fissure. These are surrounded posteriorly by the somatic association areas.

On the rostral side of the central fissure (and extending into it) lies the precentral *motor cortex*, (area 4) the primary cortical motor area. Although this region is by no means the only source of motor efferents from the cortex, it is most closely involved in voluntary movements and has a topographical organization on which it is possible to map local fields from which regionally organized movements may be elicited by electrical stimulation. The somatic sensory cortices, too, have areas with a topographical organization on which the various peripheral receptor regions may be mapped.

Continuing in the same direction along the frontal lobes we pass the *supplementary motor areas* which are mainly concerned in the automatic associated movements that assist in the implementation of voluntary motor activities. Finally we reach the association areas of the frontal lobe, the *frontal pole* and the *orbital* cortex, whose somewhat abstract functions are more difficult to epitomize. Very broadly one can say that in these areas sensory information from the posterior association areas and temporal lobes undergoes further processes of integration and also comes to be evaluated in the light of the motivational state of the organism.

The ventrolateral part of the brain is formed by the *temporal lobes*. These contain the primary auditory areas (41), the auditory association areas and also additional visual and somatic association areas. Some convergence of these separate modalities occurs at the anterior end of the temporal lobe, the *temporal pole*.

Hidden beneath the frontal and temporal lobes lies the *limbic 'lobe'* (cingulate gyrus, isthmus, uncus, hippocampal gyrus; Figure 6.4) which is entirely confined to the medial surface and runs around the root of the hemisphere in an almost closed curve. The *limbic system* also comprises the phylogenetically older parts of the cortex, the *allocortex* (hippocampus and other structures) which has a more primitive structure than the remainder of the cortex, or *neocortex*. This system includes some structures that are predominantly concerned with olfactory functions (the 'rhinencephalon'), but also important non-olfactory structures which are closely concerned in the elaboration of emotional behaviour and the motivational evaluation of sensory information of mainly cortical origin.

Also beneath the temporal lobes lies the *insula* (Figure 6.4), a circular area of cortex whose functions are closely integrated with those of the fronto-temporal complex.

Figure 6.6 illustrates some of the motor efferent pathways from the cortex and subcortical structures to the pool of motor neurons in the spinal cord.

The highest subcortical centres for somatic efferent signals are the *basal ganglia* (caudate nucleus, putamen, globus pallidus). This system of nuclei lies at the base of the hemispheres and together with various *brainstem nuclei* (red nucleus, substantia nigra and others; see also Figure 6.3) forms part of the *extra-pyramidal* motor system. This is paralleled by the *pyramidal* motor system, a tract of efferent fibres which runs from the cortex through the pons to spinal motor centres. About one third of its fibres originate in the primary motor cortex. Although the action of neither of these two motor systems can be considered in isolation, the extra-pyramidal system is mainly concerned with laying down the gross features of a behaviour pattern and with such automatic, associated movements as those involved in maintaining balance, whereas the pyramidal system deals with the less stereotyped and more finely adapted movement components.

Two notable pairs of structures on the dorsal midbrain are formed by the *superior* and *inferior colliculi*. These are correlation centres for visual and auditory information respectively. The superior colliculus, for example, is partly concerned with the detection of local changes in the visual field, e.g.

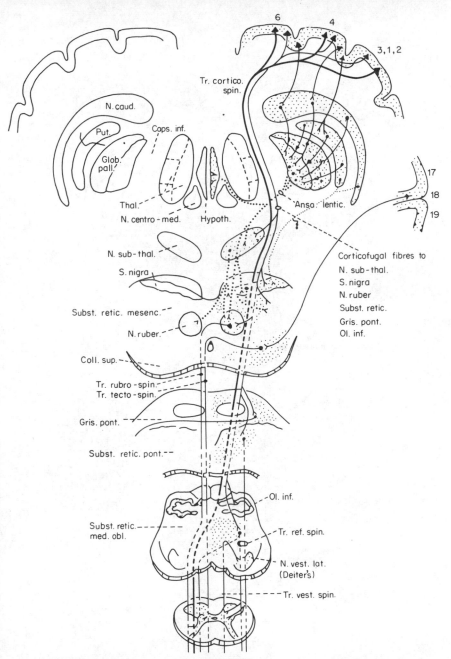

Figure 6.6. Some of the descending motor pathways passing from the cerebral cortex directly to the spinal cord or via various subcortical nuclei, including the reticular formation (From Brodal, *Descending Motor Pathways*[30]. Reproduced by permission of Acta Neurologica Scandinavica) Key: Ansa lentic., Ansa lenticularis; Caps. inf., internal capsule; Coll. sup., superior colliculus; Glob. pall., globus pallidus; Gris. pont., pontine grey matter; Hypoth., hypothalamus; N. caud., caudate nucleus; N. centro-med., centro-medial nucleus; N. ruber, red nucleus; N. sub-thal., subthalamic nucleus; Ol. inf., inferior olive; Put., putamen; S. nigra, substantia nigra; Subst. retic. mesenc., midbrain reticular substance; Subst. retic. pont., pontine reticular substance; Thal., thalamus; Tr. cortico-spin., corticospinal tract; Tr. ret. spin., reticulospinal tract; Tr. rubrospin., rubrospinal tract; Tr. tecto-spin., tectospinal tract; N. vest. lat. (Deiter's), lateral vestibular nucleus; Tr. vest. spin., vestibulospinal tract

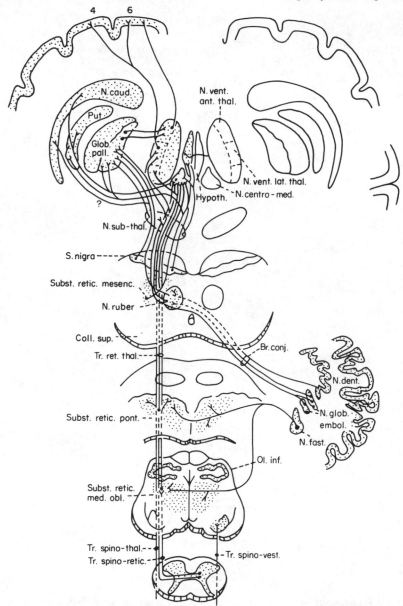

Figure 6.7. Some of the ascending pathways to nuclei that give off descending fibres (From Brodal, *Descending Motor Pathways*[30]. Reproduced by permission of Acta Neurologica Scandinavica) Key: Br. conj., Brachium conjunctivum; Coll. sup., superior colliculus; Glob. pall., globus pallidus; Hypoth., hypothalamus; N. caud., caudate nucleus; N. centro-med., centro-medial nucleus; N. dent., dentate nucleus; N. fast., fastigial nucleus; N. glob.-embol., globose-embolliform nuclei; N. ruber, red nucleus; N. sub thal., subthalamic nucleus; N. vent. ant. thal., ventro-anterior nucleus of thalamus; N. vent. lat. thal., ventro-lateral nucleus of thalamus; Ol. inf., inferior olive; Put., putamen; S. nigra, substantia nigra; Subst. retic. med. obl., reticular substance of medulla oblongata; Subst. retic. mesenc., midbrain reticular substance; Subst. retic. pont., pontine reticular substance; Tr. ret. thal., reticulothalamic tract; Tr. spino-retic., spinoreticular tract. Tr. spino-thal., spinothalamic tract; Tr. spino-vest., spinovestibular tract

detection of the direction and speed of perceived objects (largely regardless of the nature of the object). It receives afferents from the optic tract and the visual areas of the cortex and its efferents include projections to the oculomotor nuclei.

All the centres which participate in shaping the final pattern of excitations that reaches the motor neurons which energize the muscles, are supplied with afferent information from lower regions which monitors the general state of affairs and (by implication) the consequences of their activities. In essence, therefore, these afferents have a feedback character. Figure 6.7 shows some of the ascending connections to nuclei which give off descending fibres.

Some of the main sensory pathways originating in the spinal cord are illustrated in Figure 6.8. The free nerve endings (Fr. E) relate to temperature, pain and gross tactile sensibilities. They are supplemented by the special tactile corpuscles and by fine nerve endings serving general tactile sensibilities. A proprioceptive receptor and a vestibular receptor (VR) are also shown. We need not pursue these pathways in detail here. All are multisynaptic except the pathways that traverse the nucleus gracilis or nucleus cuneatus, which have only two relay stations on the way to the cortex. These are the fastest and most specific pathways to the cortex. By contrast the slowest and least specific pathway is formed by the collateral branches that enter the multisynaptic ascending system of the reticular formation (see below). The lateral spinothalamic tract is mainly concerned in projecting impulses relating to deep and superficial pain and temperature. The ventral spinothalamic tract projects impulses of tactile sensibility which relay in the grey. The interneurons of this relay area provide the anatomical background for the extensive central overlap of these sensory impulses.

Figure 6.8 also indicates some of the points at which the higher centres of the brain can exert a certain amount of more or less selective gating control over the ascending flow of sensory information.

The highest sensory relay stations on the way to the cortex are found in the *thalamus* (Figures 6.3, 6.4 and 6.7). However, the large neuronal mass of the thalamus is more than just a set of relay stations for afferent information. Within its domain the different sensory fibre tracks are regrouped and there are many opportunities for the interaction of different modalities. The regions receiving specific afferents are surrounded by nuclei actuated by diffuse multisynaptic and non-specific ascending pathways. Adjacent to both these regions there is a third region which has no direct source of extrinsic excitation but derives its inputs from inside the thalamus. These nuclei project to the association areas of the cortex. They are not the only nuclei participating in an intra-thalamic cross-flow. All internuclear boundaries (if one can speak of boundaries at all) are crossed by fibres, and often in both directions. A reflux system of corticofugal fibres enables each cortical area in turn to affect events in the associated thalamic nucleus.

At the head of the visceral system stands the *hypothalamus* (Figure 6.3), a small region of nuclei just ventral to the thalamus. It forms the main gateway through which visceral deprivations such as hunger and thirst initiate a rising

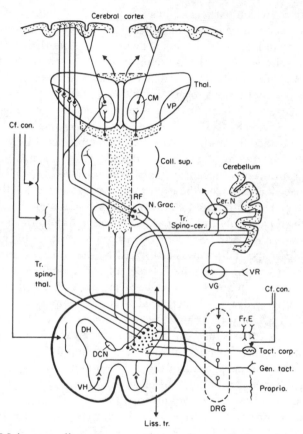

Figure 6.8. Main ascending sensory pathways from spinal cord to the cerebral and cerebellar cortices. Impulses in the peripheral nerves pass the dorsal root ganglion (DRG), which contains the cell bodies of the receptors, and enter the dorsal horn (DH) of the spinal cord. The fast, specific pathway for fine tactile and fine proprioceptive information ascends to the nucleus gracilis (N. grac.) or the parallel nucleus cuneatus (not shown) and finally relays in the ventro-posterior nuclei (VP) of the contralateral thalamus (Thal.). Centrifugal control or 'gating' over ascending pathways may be effected by a variety of descending fibre systems (Cf. con.). Some of these act on the reticular formation (RF, shown stippled) which provides the most highly convergent and polysynaptic ascending pathway. The most primitive tactile pathway and probably the one associated with generation of the pain sense ascends from free nerve endings (Fr. E.) via Lissauer's tract (Liss. tr.) and (lateral) spinothalamic tract (Tr. Spino. thal.); VR, vestibular receptors; VG, vestibular ganglion; Cer. N., cerebellar nuclei; DCN, dorsal column nuclei

activation which extends mainly to the thalamus and the limbic and frontal cortices and, through these and other pathways, comes to supply the motivational components of the ensuing behaviour patterns. Descending influences from the hypothalamus can act both on the motor system and the autonomous system. But interaction between the somatic and visceral systems may also occur at other levels, e.g. at the level of the basal ganglia and in the reticular formation of the brain stem. The hypothalamus also plays an important role in the elaboration of emotional behaviour. Stimulation at some hypothalamic foci elicits behavioural patterns of fear. Stimulation at other sites elicits aggressive reactions and symptoms of anger, including the concomitant autonomic adjustments (heart rate, blood pressure etc.)

The *reticular formation* (Figures 6.3 and 6.6 to 6.8) is a mesh of neurons with interspersed nuclei which stretches from the grey matter of the spinal cord up to the thalamic region. It receives convergent fibres from all sensory modalities and occupies a commanding position in the evaluation of non-specific sensory information, e.g. information relating to the intensity, duration, novelty and what may be called the 'general feeling' or 'tone' of a stimulus. It has both ascending and descending systems and plays an important part in various regulatory activities, such as the control of body temperature, neurosecretion, muscle tone and the state of arousal of the higher centres. In other respects, too, it is profoundly involved in the general programming of the nervous system.

The efferent stream of somatic signals may be modulated by the afferent stream at all the various levels of the brain I have mentioned and at each in its own particular way so that the final response pattern is the outcome of a great deal of parallel processing.

The *cerebellum* (Figures 6.3, 6.7 and 6.8) makes its own particular contributions to movement control. It is divided into the archicerebellum, the palaeocerebellum and the neocerebellum. Although these are phylogenetic distinctions they have broad functional counterparts. The archicerebellum is closely linked with the labyrinthine system and mainly concerned with the maintenance of balance. The palaeocerebellum deals mainly with the mechanism involved in preserving the normal position of the body at rest and in motion, and in maintaining the tonicity of the muscles necessary for normal body postures. The neocerebellum forms the largest part of the cerebellum and plays a crucial role in the coordination of movements and in the perfection of behavioural skills. Lesions in the neocerebellum interfere with the automatic flow of fast coordinated movements, thus forcing the patient to fall back on much slower and more deliberate cortical control. A patient with cerebellar lesions walks with his hemispheres, so to speak. Some of the cortico-cerebellar pathways relay in the *pons* (Figure 6.3), a mass of fibres and nuclei which forms the noticeable ventral bulge of the hindbrain.

Most movements of our limbs must be seen in their elementary form as modifications of postural responses which from spinal to cortical levels can be traced in various grades of refinement and adaptation to the requirements of, ultimately, the whole organism in relation to the whole environment. Whereas the spinal reflexes can mediate such reactions as limb withdrawal to noxious stimuli and elementary stepping reactions, only at the level of the brainstem and the pons do reactions become related to the rest of the body. The structures of the midbrain add the adjustment of posture to environment and the adaptive use of proprioceptive information, i.e. information derived from receptors in the muscles, tendons and joints.

At the level of the hypothalamus behaviour begins to show its characteristic motivational elements but even then it is still essentially blind behaviour. A cat with all structures above this level removed can show integrated rage reactions and it can walk, but it will blindly walk into any obstruction. The full use of the senses requires the cortex and so does the fully selective use of the muscles. Without the cortex an individual flexing of fingers is impossible. Discrimination and refinement, both in the evaluation of sensory inputs and the organization of motor outputs, are among the characteristic contributions made by the cortex. Thus the delicately balanced movements of the exploratory palpation by which the fingers may feel and explore the shape and texture of an object is in essence a refinement in which the cortex plays on the balance between a gross subcortical avoidance reaction and an equally primitive subcortical grasp reflex. The refinement is one learnt at the cortical level, but both subcortical reactions can be conditioned as is known from experiments with decorticate animals. Although in the latter case the acquired response disappears within a day, it yet shows that the plasticity implied in learning and conditioning cannot be expected to be a single localized affair, nor to be confined exclusively to the cerebral cortex.

Although the cortex plays an essential part in comparing particulars of a stimulus situation with those of situations previously encountered and is indispensable for evaluating the success or failure of an action, the shaping of the final responses relies on a substrate of subcortical contributions and the subcortical structures participate in the learning process. Investigations with microelectrodes show that throughout the learning process activity irradiates widely, involving for instance the reticular formation and even the autonomic system[126], and as new skills come to be acquired irrelevant movements drop out at all levels.

Decorticate animals can perform many routine reactions. Decorticate cats, for example, can walk and right themselves. They will accept milk while rejecting acid. They will adjust posture to gravity, pull the paw away from a pricking thorn and they can groom or nibble. But conditioning of decorticate animals can be achieved only with intense stimuli and after long periods, and is by simple association (i.e. contiguity of stimuli) only. Experiments with 'split-brain' animals in which the interconnections between the hemispheres are severed, show that instrumental conditioning proceeds independently in each hemisphere and must, therefore, be essentially a cortical function[234, 235].

Two important facts emerge even from this cursory account of the organization of the mammalian CNS. The first is that no motor activity is the product of any single action centre in the brain. Each and every movement is an integrated end product to which structures at various levels of the brain have made their own particular contribution. The stream of motor-efferent excitations receives tributaries from many levels.

The second fact is that the full realization of the learning capabilities of the CNS lies in the activities of the cerebral cortex. With the possible exception of the cerebellar cortex, the adaptive plasticity of the subcortical centres is small in comparison.

These two facts are rendered compatible by the nature of the control which the higher centres exercise over the lower ones. This is not one that could be likened to the formulation and imposition of commands spelling out the details of the actions required of the lower centres. Rather, it takes the form of a suppression of the gross motor reactions of the lower centres coupled with a selective release of particular components when the circumstances warrant it, plus a measure of modulating or sculpturing these reactions in order to achieve the precise matching of action to environment. This sculpturing may be effected either by selective excitations or selective inhibitions. In this manner the higher centres achieve the required level of discrimination in the evaluation of the stimulus situation and of articulation in the execution of the motor responses.

The suppression of the lower centres by the higher ones need not take the form of a direct inhibition. It may also be effected (and often is) indirectly by the release of an equilibrating excitation. The required effector activity is often achieved by a balanced system of contrary excitations. Both checks and balances between competing functions appear to be a fundamental feature of the CNS. Removal by surgical sections of one of the competing functions in the control of movement at any level results in the overaction of the other. The balance between the grasp reflex and avoidance reaction mentioned above is a typical example.

.6.4   PROPERTIES OF THE AFFERENT PATHWAYS

Throughout this volume we are mainly concerned with the logical relations between certain theoretical network configurations, the place they may occupy in the overall organization of the nervous system and their significance in relation to certain fundamental capabilities of the brain.

There are one or two general properties of the afferent pathways of the brain which are particularly significant in this respect. Foremost is the fact that owing to the structure of these pathways not even a simple stimulus applied to a single peripheral receptor causes a point-representation in the higher centres. So even in the case of simple environmental variables of which we have as it were a raw sensation, there is no isomorphic representation in the cortex. No region of the cortex acts like a television screen on which a true picture of the outer world unfolds.

In general there are at least two distinct ascending pathways to the higher centres of the brain. One is a modality specific, topographically organized, fast pathway involving only two or three relay stations; the other a slow multi-synaptic and modality convergent pathway involving the ascending system of the reticular formation. But despite its specificity and topographical organization even the fast pathways cannot be thought of as straightforward sets of telegraph lines resulting in a point for point cortical representation of the events occurring at the periphery. A considerable amount of transformation occurs on the way. Even when not stimulated some receptors have an idling rhythm of discharges and from the first relay station on neurons begin to fire repetitively even to a single presynaptic shock. Further transformations result from three common properties in afferent sensory pathways: *complementary innervation, afferent convergence* and *afferent divergence*.

By 'complementary afferent innervation' we mean that along the specific afferent pathways and in the receptor areas of the cortex we commonly find in the neighbourhood of any neuron that is excited by a peripheral stimulus another neuron which is inhibited by the same stimulus[174]. Now it is generally true that the axon-collaterals of a neuron will either only excite or only inhibit the neurons on which they impinge. If, therefore, an active afferent fibre is to excite one neuron and at the same time inhibit another (which is what we find) there must exist an (inhibitory) interneuron in addition to a source of spontaneous excitation. Thus in Figure 6.9 neuron *A* is excited and *B* inhibited by the stimulus *i*, *S* being a source of spontaneous excitation.

By *spontaneous activity* we mean no more than activity which arises independently of afferent stimulation. It is found in many structures of the brain,

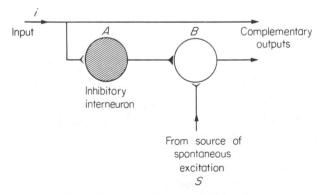

Figure 6.9. Complementary innervation

including the cerebral and cerebellar cortices. Penetrating into the cortical layers brings up units some of which are spontaneously active over the whole period of recording whereas others are silent and fire only to peripheral stimuli. It is a background activity which is often of the same order of magnitude as the signals the structures concerned have to handle. The sources of this spontaneous activity are unknown but they are probably of subcortical origin as there is no spontaneous activity in isolated slabs of cortex[36].

Even the fast, specific sensory pathways show *convergence* in the sense that each single cell within the receptive region of a higher centre is generally found to be responsive to point stimulations over a finite region of the periphery. Microelectrode studies in the receptive areas of the thalamus and cortex, for example, show that a cell activated by stimulation of the skin is responsive to stimulation within a certain limited area of the skin but with diminishing effects nearer the margins. Stimulation elsewhere does not excite the neuron.

The receptive peripheral regions of individual neurons in the higher centres overlap. In consequence we also find the converse relationship of *afferent divergence*: point stimulation at the periphery generally causes excitation over a finite region of the cortex or the intervening subcortical stations of the specific afferent pathways. This excitation generally has a maximum at the centre of the region and trails off towards the fringe.

The general biological significance of afferent convergence coupled with the overlap of receptive fields (and hence with afferent divergence) is obvious in one respect: it causes an established response to stimulation at one point of the periphery in some measure to transfer to stimulation at neighbouring points. This is obviously of biological advantage in all cases in which the exact location of the stimulus is of small significance. In the rarer cases in which the exact location of the stimulus is critical, the brain still has the necessary information available in the identity of the overlapping receptive fields which share the same stimulus.

The functional significance of reciprocal innervation is also obvious in one respect: in the control functions the brain has to perform the absence of a particular stimulus may be just as important in some cases as is the presence of the stimulus in others, and either must be able to elicit excitatory reactions if the need arises.

Afferent convergence may combine with inhibition in such a manner that the peripheral area from which a neuron belonging to an afferent pathway can be excited is surrounded by an area which, when stimulated, inhibits the neuron. Thus as a stimulus moves out of the centre of the receptive field of a cortical cell the excitation first declines, but then passes into an inhibition (suppression of spontaneous activity) as the stimulus crosses over into the inhibitory surround.

This pattern of central excitation and surround inhibition of the receptive fields appears to be a basic one for many afferent systems, including the special senses, e.g. the visual and auditory pathways.

Convergence, of course, does not only occur within a given sensory pathway. It occurs in all associative structures of the nervous system. An example may be taken from the scheme of convergence of visual, vestibular and reticulo-thalamic systems in the cat's visual cortex, as suggested by Jung *et al.*[130] (Figure 6.10). This diagram also illustrates some of the main features of the visual pathways which pass from the retina via the optic chiasma to the lateral geniculate nucleus of the thalamus to the primary visual cortex. At the optic chiasma in Man, the fibres that are connected with the nasal halves of the retina cross over to the opposite thalamus, whereas fibres connected with the temporal regions of the retina remain on the same side.

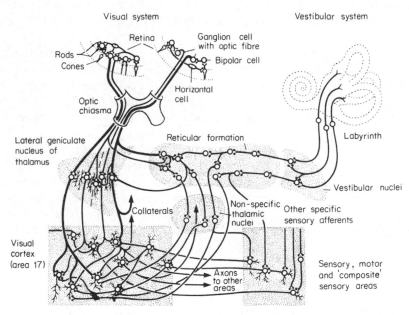

Figure 6.10. Scheme of the convergence of visual, vestibular and reticulothalamic systems in the cat's visual cortex as suggested by Jung (From Jung and Kornhuber, *Neurophysiologie und Psychophysik des Visuallen Systems.* Reproduced by permission of Springer-Verlag)

The outputs from the rods and cones which act as the receptive elements of the retina converge onto the bipolar cells which in turn synapse within the retina with the ganglion cells. Impulses from the latter pass in the optic nerve to the lateral geniculate body and thence to area 17 of the visual cortex. A considerable degree of lateral interaction already occurs at the retinal level. This is partly mediated by two layers of special cells, the horizontal cells and amacrine cells.

One of the net effects of these processes is that a diffuse illumination of the retina, even though it may affect every receptor in the retina, does not affect a retinal ganglion cell so strongly as a small circular spot of light of exactly the right size and covering exactly the receptive field centre. The main concern of these cells seems to be the contrast in illumination between one retinal region and its surrounding region.

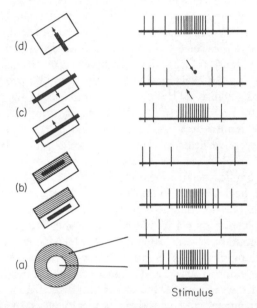

Stimulus

Figure 6.11. Schematic examples of specific cell responses in the visual system of the cat (Adapted from Hubel and Wiesel[118]) (a) Responses of retinal ganglion cell having small circular receptive field with inhibitory surround. Receptive field shown on the left; cell discharges following light stimuli applied to either part of the field are shown on the right. (b) Responses of 'simple cell' in primary visual cortex which has maximal sensitivity to black bar with specific orientation. Its narrow receptive field is flanked by an inhibitory area. (c) 'Complex cell' which is driven by movement in one direction of specifically oriented bar, but inhibited by opposite movement. (d) 'Hypercomplex cell' which responds maximally to a moving bar stopped at one end. A dark tongue 0·5° wide when introduced from below and advanced at 0·5° per second was here found to be equally effective anywhere within an activity region of 4° by 1·5° inclined at 15° to the horizontal

Each retinal ganglion cell thus comes to be driven from a circumscribed retinal region and has either an 'on' centre or an 'off' centre with an opposing periphery. Once again we meet an antagonistic centre–surround organization (Figure 6.11(a)). The same applies to the geniculate cells, but there is now an enhanced capacity of the periphery of the receptive field to cancel the effects of the centre. This means in effect that the lateral geniculate body increases the disparity between responses to a small, centred spot of light and to diffuse light.

In the visual cortex additional processes of convergence and inhibition achieve a variety of specialized effects. The chief of these result in cells, first discovered by Hubel and Wiesel in the cat, which respond maximally only to bars, slits or edges of light which have a specific orientation and location on the retina[118]. These cells are supplemented by cells in which only the orientation but not the location of the stimulus is critical. Thus Hubel and Wiesel distinguish between 'simple' cells, whose response depends both on the orientation and the exact position of the line-stimulus in the receptive field of the cell (Figure 6.11(b)), and 'complex' cells, which are much less discriminating as to the exact position of the stimulus provided that it is properly oriented (Figure 6.11(c)). Unlike simple cells they respond with sustained firing to moving lines. The firing may continue as the stimulus is moved over an extended area, the receptive field of the cell. Unlike simple cells, too, the receptive fields of the complex cells cannot be mapped into antagonistic 'on' and 'off' regions. These findings are consistent with the supposition that a 'complex' cell receives its inputs from a large number of 'simple' cells of the same field orientation and the same general type.

Although area 17 also contains complex cells the majority of these cells are found in the surrounding area 18 and area 19 beyond (Figure 6.5). These two areas also contain several categories of what Hubel and Wiesel have called the 'hypercomplex' cells. Some of these respond maximally to line-stimuli which are 'stopped' at one end (Figure 6.11(d)). If the stimulus extends beyond this limit the response of the cell is diminished. Evidently excitation and inhibition from complex cells here come together in one cell. Other 'hypercomplex' cells respond best if the line-stimulus is bounded at both ends, and others again if it contains a right angle or corner. Similar effects have been observed in the monkey[119].

Cells of all types responding to the same orientation of the line-stimuli in their receptive fields are generally found together within the confines of the same vertical segment or 'column' of the cortex. These columns are irregular in cross section and shape and they are not anatomically distinguishable. On the average they measure about 0·5 mm across. Disregarding the preferred orientation of the stimulus, which is common to all, the cells in a particular column tend to differ: some are simple, others complex; some respond to slits, others prefer bars or edges.

The main significance of these discoveries is that the visual cortex is now seen to be a highly specialized structure designed to factor out and emphasize the main features of optical inputs that are relevant in the perception of shapes and figures, viz. contours and their elements (lines, angles etc.). But, as Hubel and Wiesel themselves have stressed, these elementary feature detectors go only a little way towards explaining the complex processes of perception.

6.5   ATTENTION AND AROUSAL

The processes of attention are nature's way of overcoming the limitations of the information handling capacity of the nervous system. The solution of this problem meant developing mechanisms in the brain that could learn to distinguish between *relevant* and *irrelevant* classes of stimuli or internal representations in a given motivational and environmental situation. The relevant classes of stimuli or representations then have to be potentiated relative to the irrelevant ones. In theory this can be achieved either by facilitating the relevant stimuli or inhibiting the irrelevant.

Relevance as such is a very abstract property and the learning mechanisms which these processes of abstraction require presuppose a considerable degree of sophistication. It is not surprising, therefore, that the learning mechanisms concerned appear to draw upon some of the highest abstractive functions of which the brain is capable. In the primates, in particular, this means involvement of the frontal or frontotemporal cortices (Chapter 9). Moreover, to learn the relevance of a novel stimulus in a variety of situations is bound to be a complex process in which the brain passes through a number of intermediate stages.

To understand the workings of the brain it is again essential to realize that the nervous system functions simultaneously at a number of different levels. In all the internal or external reactions that a given stimulus situation elicits there are invariably some components which are appropriate in a great variety of situations and others which are appropriate only in the special circumstances concerned. Typically, these different categories of components are contributed by different parts of the brain.

This applies to most aspects of behaviour. In particular it applies to the reaction elicited by

  (i) novel stimuli,
 (ii) the need detectors of the brain,
(iii) the satiety detectors of the brain.

Thus the brain's reactions to novel stimuli contain some components which are appropriate in respect of all novel stimuli regardless of their modality, composition or context. A typical example is the change in alertness and arousal which novel stimuli tend to elicit.

Next there are reaction components which are appropriate only in relation to a single modality, such as pricking up the ears when the stimulus is an auditory one. Others are appropriate only in relation to the orientation of the stimulus object, such as turning the head or eyes. Finally, at the highest level of specificity, we have the potentiating reactions of focused attention in which both the exact location and the quality of the stimulus are relevant.

Similar distinctions can be made in respect of the reactions elicited by specific drive stimuli or the activities of specific satiety centres.

The most general components in all these reactions appear to be contributed by the mesencephalic reticular formation, whereas the more specific reaction elements are determined by the higher centres of the brain. These gross reactions of the mesencephalic brain are mainly innate, but during ontogeny they become conditioned via the higher centres to particular aspects of the stimulus situations. Thus, although the gross reactions to certain very general classes of stimuli are typically a function of the more primitive centres of the brain, the ultimate decision whether a specific stimulus should or should not be included in the respective class becomes the province of the higher centres and this decision will be profoundly influenced by experience and learning. In consequence the general reaction components contributed by the reticular formation become the focal point of intricate *reaction systems*, i.e. complex systems of partly innate, partly acquired connections through which stimulation comes to either excite or inhibit the reticular reactions as the case may be. Thus we arrive at a generalized orienting system, a generalized drive system and a generalized satiety system. A system of this kind may contain rather more specialized subsidiary systems which still have a high level of generality. For example we can think of the generalized aversive system as a subsystem of the generalized drive system.

As regards reactions to novel stimuli we can distinguish three main categories of reaction components. The first category comprises the typically reticular reactions which are independent of the nature and modality of the novel stimuli. These are exemplified in changes in arousal, general alertness and vigilance. The second category comprises that group of general but already somewhat modality-bound and place-specific reactions which Pavlov originally described as the orienting reflexes: pricking up the ears, turning head and eyes towards the stimulus source etc. We may distinguish these two categories as *general* and *special orienting reactions* respectively.

The third category is that of *focused attention*. These particular reactions go beyond the ones already listed in that they potentiate or disinhibit the specific stimuli concerned as potential cues for behaviour relative to other stimuli. In other words, they limit the set of cues which are taken into account, not necessarily in directing behaviour because no overt behaviour may ensue, but in the internal processes on which subsequent behaviour may be based. Whether in physiological terms this potentiation takes the form of an active facilitation of the significant set of afferents (or internal representations) or of an active inhibition of the remainder, is irrelevant in this context. The main point is that there is a redistribution of the relative weights of the stimuli.

With repetition of the initially novel stimuli these different components tend to drop out again (habituate) to an extent which depends on the significance the stimuli turn out to have in practice. If experience proves a particular stimulus to be significant in a given context of drive and environment, i.e. to have ecological consequences or accompaniments, the focused attention tends to remain. By that time it will have sharpened up into a highly selective function which is specific to the quality and location of the stimulus object. The habituation of the orienting reactions is therefore essentially a learning process, although the physiological mechanisms involved are bound to contain a number of stereotyped reaction complexes.

The term 'vigilance' was originally used by Head[103] to denote a state of readiness of mind and body. To differentiate this concept from the concept of 'arousal' we may go along with Berlyne[18] and equate vigilance with the total information flux which is absorbed from the environment and used in the overall control of behaviour. 'Arousal' may then be reserved for a particularly important complex of psychophysiological variables which are often found to be closely correlated. These variables relate to a variety of autonomic, somatic, electrocortical and behavioural indices. Typical autonomic variables are the galvanic skin response (the level of skin conductance), the heart rate, the respiration rate, pupillary dilation and vascular reactions. A prominent somatic variable is the muscle tone as measured by the muscle potentials of inactive muscles.

The relation of electrocortical potentials to other indices of arousal is a close one but not a simple one. The rhythms shown in EEG (electroencephalograph) recordings largely depend on the degree of synchronization of the individual neural events which run their course in the population of cortical cells below the recording scalp-electrode. The rhythms of the electrical background activities in these cells enable us to distinguish four main levels in the arousal continuum (Figure 6.12).

1. *Fully alert.* Continuous desynchronized fast-frequency, low-amplitude waves; stimuli produce no change.
2. *Alert but relaxed.* Synchronization produces the characteristic 'alpha rhythm' of 8–13 cycles per second. This is replaced by desynchronization when novel stimuli are given.
3. *Drowsy.* The desynchronized rhythm reappears with occasional 'spindle bursts' and slow high-amplitude waves. A burst of alpha rhythm may occur in response to a repetitive stimulus.
4. *Sleep.* Large irregular slow waves, interspersed with characteristic complexes produced by stimuli that are not strong enough to produce complete arousal ('K-complexes').

It can be seen from this that the significant EEG variables relate both to background rhythms and to the effect of stimulation.

The electrocortical, autonomic and somatic indices of arousal are not separate manifestations of identical central events. They represent separate complexes which may become dissociated in special circumstances. Thus atropine produces EEG rhythms characteristic of sleep, but the animal remains alert and responsive. Conversely, animals with nearly complete bilateral lesions of the hypothalamus cannot be behaviourally aroused, but cortical desynchronization may still be produced by stimulation of the midbrain reticular formation.

The general orienting reactions which are characteristically elicited by novel stimuli include most (but not necessarily all) the recognized indices of heightened arousal. Typically they also include some arrest of on-going activities and a state of instability in the mechanisms for controlling selective attention which manifests itself in scanning and searching. In extreme cases they take on a defensive character, as in the '*startle reactions*' that result when a subject is exposed to sudden and unexpectedly intense stimuli.

The qualities of the stimuli that are related to the orienting reactions have been described by Sokolov[229]. To evoke an orienting reaction stimuli need

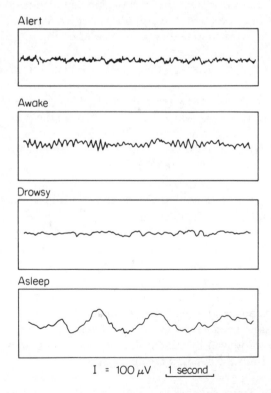

Figure 6.12. Changes in the normal electroencephalogram during alertness, relaxation, drowsiness and the early stages of deep sleep (From M. A. B. Brazier, *Electrical Activity of the Nervous System*[26]. Reproduced by permission of the author)

not be individually new but merely new in the context in which they occur. Changes in temporal patterns of stimuli may be effective as well as changes in intensity, quality or duration. The omission of an expected stimulus may be equally effective in eliciting orienting reactions. Another operative factor is the general character of the problem situation. When a discrimination is required between two stimuli the orienting reactions are stronger than when no discrimination is required, and the reactions increase as the discrimination becomes more difficult. Berlyne[18] and Nicky have shown that, in general, complexity, uncertainty and conflict attached to a stimulus increase the orienting reaction. Stimulus patterns making greater demands on the information-processing capacity of the nervous system produce more marked orienting reactions and heightened arousal. The work of Berlyne and Nicky also suggests that stimuli reducing these quantities are effective as positive reinforcers of behaviour.

Freedman, Hafer and Daniel[72] compared the EEG changes during learning with those found in a control group exposed to the same stimuli and response mode but without possibility of learning. Their results suggest that arousal was reduced as learning progressed whereas in the control group arousal increased due to frustration. These and other results underscore the close relationships between the orienting reaction and the normal processes of learning.

The biological function of the orientation reaction is probably best understood if it is seen as part of an integral process concerned in mobilizing the mechanisms of selective attention on which the control of behaviour largely depends. If attention is to be truly selective (and adaptably so) there must be a prior responsiveness to the domain from which selection is made, as well as an extension of that domain through scanning or searching. This calls for heightened alertness and arousal. The subsequent extinction of these general components as the appropriate responses to the (initially) novel situation develop, must be seen as an integral part of the development and finalization of the selective components. Selection means either inhibition of what is not wanted or facilitation of what is wanted in a particular situation. Both of these are internal reactions which we must expect to undergo adaptive modifications as an integral part of the normal process of learning appropriate behaviour.

The decline of the orienting reaction which follows upon the repetition of stimulus is a particular important example of the phenomenon of habituation. In one form or another habituation is found at all levels of the nervous system and, although we may think of it as a uniform phenomenon, it would be rash indeed to expect it to be produced by uniform physiological processes. In the form in which we are meeting it here habituation is a learned, stimulus-produced inhibition which has a specific (selective) and a general (intensive) component. The general component relates to the inhibition of the arousal reaction. The specific component relates to the inhibition of blockade of the classes of stimuli that come to be rejected as the mechanisms controlling selective attention stabilize their decisions.

As has been mentioned, habituation, at this level, is not a loss of sensitivity. It is a dynamic inhibition upon performance and mainly upon the degree of arousal released by and attention given to sensory stimuli.

Habituation is specific to the quality, modality or pattern of a given stimulus [158, 229]. When, for example, a response to an auditory stimulus of a given frequency and duration is habituated, the response may be restored by changing either the frequency or duration of the stimulus. The response may also return if the animal is distracted while the stimulus is presented—an observation which illustrates the involvement of the mechanisms of attention.

Normal cats can habituate a series of tones played in ascending order and then give orienting reactions if the same notes are played in descending order. This selective habituation to serial order is abolished by ablation of the auditory cortex (though some habituation to single notes still remains possible).

Situations in which a sequence of different stimuli occurs in a regular and predictable order are very common in our own lives. In these situations we habituate a serial order, and orienting reactions result if a stimulus at an unexpected point of the sequence occurs. In a method devised by Unger [258] subjects were presented with numbers in sequence (1, 2, 3, 4, . . .) at intervals of 5–25 seconds. Orienting reactions were recorded by finger vasoconstriction. Most subjects reacted to this situation and then habituated. But the orienting reaction returned if a number was presented out of sequence.

Sokolov has argued convincingly that these and similar phenomena are only explainable on the assumption that the cortex forms flexible and readily adaptable models of repeatedly occurring events or sequences. It must form complex neuronal configurations against which subsequent inputs are compared. Orienting reactions are elicited by stimulus patterns which fail to match these models. To habituate to a complex situation is to *register* the situation. The phenomena certainly show that habituation cannot be a simple one-stage process and, as Pavlov thought, a simple matter of higher thresholds of neurons resulting from a fatigue-like inhibitory process. There must be at least two stages: an initial stage of stimulus analysis followed by a second stage activating or blocking the orienting reactions.

Sokolov does not specify the neural structure of the cortical models beyond saying that they consist of chains of neurons which preserve information about the intensity, quality, duration and the order of presentation of the stimuli. On our analysis the activation of such models in consequence of a given stimulus situation is equivalent to the activation of a particular set of expectations. Orienting reactions are inhibited to the extent to which the stream of stimuli match the aroused expectations.

We saw in Chapter 2 that the concept of 'models' when used in the present sense relates to the expectations the brain forms of how certain things depend on each other in time. We also arrived at a broad idea of the general form such internal representations may take in terms of neural processes. This idea will be given greater precision in Chapters 7 and 9. I shall not linger with it here, except to point out that the habituation of the orienting reactions shows that these models are used by the brain to mediate appropriate inhibitions as well as appropriate activations in any given situation and, indeed, that we must expect them to be formed in order to serve the one purpose as much as the other.

Of the many investigations which have demonstrated the dependence of habituation on expectation, some simple tests devised by Fox are worth mentioning at this point. Fox[70] exposed monkeys to groups of regularly repeated flashes after 30 minutes in darkness. When the flashes were produced by the experimenter the evoked potentials in the visual cortex were found to habituate to criterion after about 8 flashes. When the flashes were produced by the monkeys themselves habituation occurred after only about 4 flashes. Virtually no habituation occurred when the flashes were given in random sequence.

As we have seen, complex learning mechanisms such as those concerned in the habituation of the orienting reactions must be expected to function at several levels of the brain. As regards the general arousal elicited by novel stimuli it has come to be generally accepted that the reticular formation mediates the global activating functions which this arousal implies. However, analysis of EEG records enables us to distinguish between two types of arousal:

1. A general (tonic) cortical arousal which is characterized by the desynchronization of EEG rhythms over the whole of the cerebral cortex. This is long-lasting but habituates quickly (typically after 10–15 trials).
2. A localized (phasic) cortical arousal in which the desynchronization is confined to the cortical area of the particular stimulus modality concerned. This reaction often remains after the general arousal has habituated. It is short-lasting and habituates rather more slowly (about 30 trials).

Sharpless and Jasper[219], as well as Gastaut[74], have suggested that these two types of arousal are mediated by the brainstem and thalamic reticular formation respectively.

Moruzzi[173] found that transection of the cat's brain at the upper pontine level abolished the generalized orienting reaction but the localized EEG desynchronization was retained. Similarly, Jus and Jus[131] found that when the brainstem in human adults is depressed by chlorpromazine injections the generalized desynchronization was abolished but the localized reactions remained.

The importance of the cortex in the control of habituation is now generally accepted, even though habituation is not exclusively controlled by the cortex. Some habituation of auditory stimuli has been obtained in decorticate dogs, for example. But habituation of the orienting reactions was greatly reduced.

Jouvet[129] has shown not only that lesions in the neocortex impair habituation but also that the smaller the amount of cortex left intact the greater the impairment. With total removal of the neocortex as many as 800 trials failed to habituate the orienting reaction. Jouvet sees the effect of cortical control as an inhibition exerted by the cortical mechanisms on the reticular formation.

Sharpless and Jasper have also shown that habituated stimuli may continue to elicit evoked potentials in the cerebral cortex. This indicates that the cortex itself is not inhibited during habituation. This observation also supports Sokolov's theory, since it shows that even habituated stimuli may reach the cortex for analysis.

Sokolov[229] believes that the orienting reaction depends on a twofold activation, viz. that the reticular formation is activated both by non-specific stimuli via collateral afferents and, in the case of novel stimuli, also by the cortex. With familiarization the cortex comes to withhold its excitation of the reticular formation and at the same time blocks the excitatory non-specific excitations from the afferent collaterals.

Moruzzi[173], whose hypotheses in many other respects resemble those of Sokolov, has adduced a considerable amount of evidence suggesting that the reduction of reticular arousal in habituation is mediated by inhibitory mechanisms within the reticular formation at the midpontine level. On this hypothesis, therefore, the cortex effects the habituation of the orienting reactions by activating the midpontine inhibitory system. However, Moruzzi does not commit himself as to the sites at which this inhibitory system asserts its influence over the ascending activations of the reticular formation.

A number of experiments conducted by Grastyan[90] and others have drawn attention to the possible role of mechanisms functioning at intermediate levels, viz. the limbic system and, in particular, the hippocampus.

Other structures of the limbic system also appear to be implicated. Orienting reactions are strongly affected by a variety of limbic lesions. The limbic system here appears to act in close association with the orbito-frontal insulo-temporal cortices (Chapter 10). Experimental stimulation of these areas can cause 'arrest', 'attention', 'search' and similar reactions.

6.6   LEARNING (1): CRITERIA OF SUCCESS AND FAILURE

In a very general sense 'learning' may be defined as the adaptive changes which the information-handling mechanisms of the brain may undergo as the result of experience. The precise and objective meaning which can be given to 'adaptive' in this context was discussed in Chapter 4. In the main we can consider the goal of these adaptive changes to be the enhancement of the organism's capacity for performing appropriate responses in different kinds of circumstances. Responses are 'appropriate' if they match the circumstances in which they occur in respect of the goals the organism pursues at the time.

Regardless of whether one subscribes to the old S–R theories or realizes the importance of 'expectations' and 'cognitive maps' in the organization of behaviour, one has to deal with the fact that if learning means lasting changes in the brain as the result of experience, some of these changes must be governed by the quality of the outcomes of behaviour, i.e. by the success or failure of the organism's responses. From the physiological point of view this raises a number of general questions. What indicators does the brain use for the appropriateness of a response or internal reaction? If, as we believe, the learning changes are synaptic changes, does the outcome of a response assert its effect through the direction in which these changes occur or through the identity of the changing synapses? How is the gap bridged between the time of the response and the time when its result will be known? Is the extinction of a failed response or false expectation a process symmetrically opposite to the reinforcement of a successful response or confirmed expectation? In the remainder of this chapter we shall deal with a number of issues that reflect on these questions. We start with the first question: the criteria the brain has available for monitoring the appropriateness of its responses.

Common sense suggests that the brain has certain obvious criteria available for detecting *a posteriori* whether a particular action sequence was or was not appropriate in the circumstances. When activities are prompted by hunger, thirst or other internal needs, for example, the brain has clear indications of success in the consummatory activities that result when food or water has been found and in the activity of the 'satiety' centres that indicate progress towards need reduction. Again, if a behaviour sequence results in pain or discomfort the experience of such noxious stimuli and stress conditions provides a clear indication that the antecedent behaviour was inappropriate. All these are definitive events which can serve physiological indicators of the appropriateness or inappropriateness of the actions that went before. But this is only part of the story, because in addition to such definitive events and terminal outcomes the brain needs a running check to monitor the appropriateness or otherwise of the individual steps in a behaviour sequence as each stage of the action follows upon the next. The assumption that reinforcement can directly strengthen responses which precede it by a time interval of more than a few seconds is contrary to the evidence and is not in fact made by any learning theory that has gained currency.

Grice[95] has shown that a delay of reinforcement of more than one second seriously impairs instrumental conditioning. Hence we cannot assume that when a rat learns to run a maze the consummatory events of finding food can directly reinforce more than the decisions made in the last second or so of the run. For simplicity let us say that they reinforce the choice made at the last choice point of the maze. What then reinforces the choices made at the penultimate choice point and at the earlier points?

At this point the psychological theories of the 1930s and 1940s brought in *secondary reinforcement*. Hull[121], for example, assumed that primary reinforcement could effectively act only on links in a chain of responses which preceded the final reward by not more than 5 seconds. Earlier links had to be strengthened by secondary reinforcement. This means reinforcement resulting from the fact that the reinforcing mechanisms (whatever their nature) may become conditioned to (previously neutral) stimuli whose traces are still extant during the final (consummatory) events. These stimuli themselves thus come to acquire reinforcing properties and, if they occur already during the earlier links in a chain of responses, they can come to effect reinforcement at those junctures. Some of the ambient constants of an experimental situation, for example, might come to act in this way. Hull also believed that fractional responses connected with the consummatory acts may advance along the antecedent response sequence (cf. Section 6.10). The stimulations associated with these 'fractional antedating goal-reactions' might also then come to function as secondary reinforcers.

The concept of secondary reinforcement still has currency today. But in the course of time learning theory has advanced beyond the hypothetical 'intermediate variables' constructed by Hull and his generation of investigators. The tendency today is to look at known physiological variables instead of trying to devise self-contained logical systems constructed in terms of measurable behavioural variables or stimuli plus hypothetical 'intermediate variables' which were restricted to whatever could be defined as symbolic constructs on these external variables only. At any rate, there is a tendency to be dissatisfied with such intermediate variables unless one can see their relation to known physiological variables.

We are also more conscious today of the limitations of the Principle of Effects in its original form (Section 5.4). There are forms of learning which it cannot explain, such as latent learning and learning by imitation. There is also the phenomenon of 'one-trial' learning. A familiar example is the phenomenon of 'imprinting'. Very young animals, usually only hours old, may form a highly specialized habit as a consequence of a single experience. Birds exhibit this phenomenon more strongly than most other animals. When young geese, for example, are reared from the egg in isolation, they react to their human keeper (or any other large moving object that they see) by following them as they would their parents. For the rest of their life they may retain a tendency to take to human beings as both parent companion and fellow members of the species to which sexual behaviour becomes attached later.

Expectancy theory was brought in to explain latent learning. According to this theory the animal learns as the result of experience that certain actions in certain situations will have certain consequences. However, a mere process of blindly recording all that has been experienced in the past would hardly meet the case. There must be some selection both in what is recorded and in the manner in which the records are put to use. These are functions that must be learnt. Expectancy theory, therefore, does not escape the problem of how appropriate reactions come to be strengthened and inappropriate ones diminished. But the theory does help to draw our attention to certain physiological variables which lend themselves as criteria for monitoring the appropriateness of current responses and thus for the running control of reinforcement. One of these variables is the difference in physiological arousal produced in a motivated animal by problem situations to which a ready answer has been acquired during previous learning compared with situations which have not yet been mastered to the same degree.

When the decisions made at the last choice point in a maze have been consistently successful and reinforced, the rat's experience at this choice point changes in character: the situation it meets at this point is no longer an unexpected and unfamiliar one. It no longer contains those elements of novelty and uncertainty which the motivated animal experiences when it runs in a problem situation to which it has not yet acquired a ready answer. At the physiological level those elements are represented by the reactions to novel stimuli we discussed in the last section. At the most general level these reactions include a transient rise in arousal coupled with a temporary arrest of activity and the substitution of scanning or searching behaviour. They habituate as the situation gains in familiarity. As we have seen, this habituation is of the nature of active inhibition of the orienting complex.

It follows from the definition of a 'novel' stimulus that no previously reinforced specific responses to it can exist in the repertoire of the organism. To the extent, therefore, to which novel situations are situations to which the organism has no ready answer immediately available, they contain elements which in a motivated animal amount to a state of *frustration*. This concept is frequently used in a restricted sense in which it denotes the omission of expected rewards. But there is also a wider sense in which it covers not only the unexpected absence of what in effect amounts to cues for consummatory action but also the unexpected absence of positive cues for further action irrespective of the nature of that action. In particular the concept may relate to situations in which the scanning or search elicited as part of the orienting reactions fails to produce such cues. Apart from pain and acute discomfort, this state of affairs is probably the most common indication of failure. At the physiological level it is detectable by the persistence of the orienting reactions. An *impasse* has been reached at this point: from one situation eliciting orienting reactions the organism merely passes to another. Mistakes made at the first move cannot be corrected at the next move. This contrasts with the case when a movement is inappropriate only in the sense that it misses its target with the first motor impulse but then homes on it with the second.

The hypothesis lies close at hand that once the rat has mastered the last choice point in the maze and the quality of its internal reactions at this point changes in the manner indicated above the rat's brain accepts this new quality as a positive reinforcer for the movements that took the animal to this choice point, i.e. for the decision made at the previous choice point. Similarly when the previous choice point comes to be mastered in consequence of these positive reinforcements, the new quality of the rat's internal reactions at this point may subsequently serve as positive reinforcers for the choices made at the preceding choice point—and so on, for each choice point in turn, from the goal backwards. On this hypothesis, therefore, reinforcement occurs in the absence of the type of arousal that attends the orienting reactions.

It is not unreasonable to expect that in monitoring current performance the brain should exploit such readily available indicators for determining whether recent responses have been problem-creating or problem-reducing.

The observation that rats tend to learn the blinds of a maze from the goal backwards could support this hypothesis as much as the hypothesis of secondary reinforcement. Possibly both influences function side by side. The two hypotheses are not mutually exclusive. The reduction of arousal may become conditioned. I have mentioned already that stimuli reducing orienting and arousal are known to be effective reinforcers.

6.7   LEARNING (2): CONDITIONAL VERSUS UNCONDITIONAL SYNAPTIC CHANGES

Assuming that the brain has adequate indicators available for signalling whether a given response has turned out to be appropriate or inappropriate, the question arises of how these signals of success or failure come to be effective in modifying the animal's subsequent behaviour. So far no plausible alternative has emerged in the neurosciences to the postulate that the learning changes in the brain take the form of processes which exert their effect through changes in synaptic conductivity. Granted that this is the case, an obvious hypothesis would be to assume that during learning the synapses that participated in producing a given response come to be upgraded if the response proves to be successful and/or downgraded if it does not. This hypothesis has to meet one particular difficulty. Invariably there is a time gap between the execution of a response and the first indications of its outcome. Thus by the time the indications of success or failure become available the response is a thing of the past; and yet the mechanisms that produced it must be modified.

One way in which this gap could be bridged would be to assume that the synapses which participate in producing the response remain earmarked for a few seconds in one way or another. They could then be singled out for the appropriate upgrading or downgrading when the indications of outcomes arrive. It is obviously important that the brain's reactivities should be modified at the appropriate sites only.

This 'earmarking' could take several different forms. One might suppose, for example, that the synapses which participated in the response (i.e. excited synapses in heavily discharging neurons) undergo some preliminary changes which result in lasting changes of conductivity if they are subsequently paired by signals related to outcomes. Or one might envisage more sophisticated mechanisms, mechanisms capable, for example, of sustaining a temporary record of on-going activities by some process of reverberation. The respective synapses would then be earmarked by virtue of their participation in this reverberatory process.

However, it is important to realize that to account for directive learning changes we may not necessarily have to assume that synaptic changes must be contingent on indications of outcomes. The necessity does not arise, for example, if one postulates that all learning is by contiguous association. The psychological learning theory first advanced by Guthrie[98] in 1935 is an outstanding example of a theory based on this principle.

Guthrie argued that all learning can be adequately explained on the parsimonious hypothesis that responses are reinforced simply because they occur. He postulated that a combination of stimuli which has accompanied a movement will on its recurrence tend to be followed by that movement. All learning, therefore, is by contiguous association and, according to Guthrie, each stimulus pattern gains its full associative strength on the occasion of its first pairing with a response. Increased habit strength with repetition results from an increase in the variety of stimulus situations and situation-details with which a given response becomes associated. ('Stimulus situation' here includes internal as well as external stimuli.) Rewards act by changing the stimulus situation, thus preventing 'retroactive inhibition': the reward prevents competing responses from becoming attached to the original stimulus situation simply by removing the stimulus situation. New stimuli with higher cue value have appeared on the scene. The whole situation and action of the animal is so changed by the reward that the pre-reward situation is shielded from new associations.

For the extinction of failed responses Guthrie relied mainly on interference. Thus an electric shock compellingly elicits withdrawal responses which are incompatible with approach. 'Sitting on tacks', Guthrie says, 'does not discourage learning. It encourages one in learning to do something else than sit. It is not the feeling caused by punishment but the specific action caused by punishment that determines what will be learned.' Thus punishments are effective by compelling a new action, an escape response let us say, which interferes with on-going activities. Through contiguous association with cues which are present at the time of the punishment the escape response can advance along the behaviour sequence and in due course become an avoidance response (cf. Section 6.8). Similarly, if in a succession of trials the animal is consistently punished for approaching a given object, the reactions elicited by the punishment become attached to the sight of the object and inhibit the approach response. Responses may also weaken through fatigue, for example, and then become permanently replaced by whatever other responses took their place.

According to Guthrie's theory, therefore, the brain's learning mechanisms require no neural traces of the kind we had to postulate above. It is an attractively parsimonious theory, but unfortunately Guthrie never developed paradigms of his learning mechanisms in sufficient detail to enable all their implications and presuppositions to be fully examined and put to the test. Guthrie's main ideas have since formed the basis of a number of more elaborate and more highly formalized theories. Both the postulational system of Voeks[263] and the stochastic models of Estes[60] have extended the range of predictions which could be derived from Guthrie's basic principles. However, in common with all other monolithic learning theories, these theories eventually had to rest their case without silencing the controversies that surrounded the subject.

On the theory of learning by contiguous association synaptic changes proceed unconditionally. But the brain nevertheless needs running indications of the appropriateness or otherwise of its activities. Since any intervening event can threaten a response, the degree to which positive indications of success can protect antecedent responses must depend on the temporal proximity of the responses concerned. This running information must be disseminated through those parts of the brain in which learning takes place. But at its various destinations it does not act by controlling synaptic changes. According to Guthrie it acts by changing the internal stimuli that form part of the overall stimulus input to which the responses become attached by contiguity in the respective structures of the brain. In physiological terms this means that neural pathways are strengthened whenever they are activated. Rewards act by changing the pathways (through changes in the stimulus situation) in a manner that prevents subsequently strengthened pathways from being of a kind that would inhibit or interfere with the action or effects of the old pathways. Failure, on the other hand, results in the subsequent strengthening of pathways that do inhibit or interfere in this manner.

Although Guthrie was an S–R theorist, his main ideas could equally be applied to responses formed as reactions to 'expectations' and 'internal models' activated by the sensory inputs. However, the main point is that Guthrie's theory does not affect the question whether there exist fibre tracts in the brain whose function is to disseminate information about success or failure (Section 6.9).

We have seen that in learning models which rely on conditional synaptic changes there is a short interval between responses and indications of outcomes during which the fate of the synaptic changes hangs in the balance. Guthrie in effect replaces this interim period by one of a different kind. The synaptic changes occur unconditionally and their fate, therefore, never hangs in the balance. Instead, their ultimate effect on behaviour hangs in the balance during the critical interval. Because, until the indication of positive outcomes remove the animal from the problem situation, other positive synaptic changes may occur which may radically change the responses elicited by the original internal stimulus situation in the given external circumstances.

6.8   LEARNING (3): REINFORCEMENT AND EXTINCTION

In one respect Guthrie's views are shared by a large number of other writers. This concerns his reliance on processes of interference to account for the extinction of responses with negative outcomes.

In theory, response decrements may result in two ways:

(i) through enduring negative changes in the potency of synapses participating in the production of the response, and/or
(ii) through interference by some other response which the learning situation promotes.

There is a considerable volume of evidence to show that the acquisition of a response and its extinction are not symmetrically opposite processes. It is well known that if a response has become maximally associated with a certain combination of exteroceptive stimuli (as when a rat has learnt to press a bar to release a food pellet) and then ceases to be rewarded, it gradually extinguishes. But it is also known that when it does so the original structure of the associations formed generally remains intact, only the response strength diminishes. The response is not forgotten. This is shown, for example, by the phenomenon of 'spontaneous recovery': a short period of rest usually suffices to resurrect an extinguished response complete with its original association structure. Again, an extinguished response may be resurrected by just one or two rewarded trials. The extinction of a response, therefore, does not generally signify its destruction.

There is also an *a priori* argument against the notion that response increments and decrements during learning are symmetrically opposite processes resulting from lasting increases and decreases in synaptic transmission respectively. The argument runs roughly as follows. If a response is successful nature's purpose would be adequately served if subsequently all synapses were facilitated which took part in the production of the response. On the other hand, if a response fails, nature's purposes would not be at all well served if all those synapses were diminished. Because in a failed response there are generally many parts that were right. There may be nothing wrong with the skill with which a rat runs towards the wrong foodbox. It would be fatal, therefore, if all parts of a failed response were to be diminished equally. Ideally when a wrong foodbox is chosen only the mechanisms for target selection should subsequently undergo revision, not the mechanisms for locomotion or for maintaining balance. On the other hand when the animal suffers a leg injury only the mechanisms for balance and locomotion should undergo revision and not those for target selection.

The problem does not arise if failed responses diminish through interference, partly because in this process responses diminish without being destroyed and learnt skills are not unlearned and partly for reasons we shall meet presently.

Facilitation of one response may cause extinction of another simply by virtue of the fact that in the last resort the overt responses of an organism depend on the balance of excitation in rival action systems and the facilitation of one response may tip the balance against another. This is true right down to the final rivalry between agonists and antagonists.

The origin of the interfering reactions which are elicited by failed responses and which eventually come to replace these responses, is often plain enough. Pain, for example, may radically change the drive state of the organism. Excitation of the aversive pathways in the brain may result in actions which interfere powerfully with on-going activities. With repetition such interfering responses tend to advance in the behaviour sequences which attracted punishment, thus progressively modifying antecedent behaviour as well.

In a classical experiment by Mowrer and Miller a rat is placed in a box with a grilled floor. Five seconds after a buzzer has sounded the grille is electrified. The rat can terminate the shock by turning a ratchet wheel. Having stumbled on this means to end the discomfort, the rat is seen to avail itself of the device with increasing alacrity as the trials are repeated. Then with further trials it gradually begins to anticipate the shock, and eventually it comes to turn the ratchet as soon as the buzzer is sounded. Generally speaking, in a succession of trials involving behaviour sequences with terminal punishment, the resulting alarm reactions and escape responses are seen to advance along the behaviour sequence, thus taking the form of fear reactions and avoidance responses respectively. As they advance along the behaviour sequence these reactions increasingly come to interfere with antecedent behaviour, thus modifying it and extinguishing the inappropriate approach response. I shall return to this question in Section 6.10.

Another possible source of interference is frustration. The frustration that results when the organism reaches an *impasse* or when expected rewards are withheld has general reaction components of an activating nature which may elicit responses that interfere with previously acquired behaviour patterns.

In terms of Tolman's expectancy hypothesis the main source of interfering reactions lies in the development of counterexpectancies. In this formulation conditioning consists of the establishment of an expectancy that the US will be followed by the CS. All that is necessary for extinction to occur is then to prove to the animal that this correlation no longer exists, in other words, to create interfering counterexpectancies. As with other aspects of expectancy theory the development of such counterexpectancies is a cognitive matter which does not require the performance of overt responses.

This theory also allows for the possibility of latent extinction: it should be possible to reduce response strength merely by exposing the animal to the goal situation in the absence of rewards. This effect has been demonstrated in the rat for maze running, pressing the bar in a Skinner box and for brightness discrimination.

Yet another way in which one activity may result in the extinction of another, involves the mechanisms of selective attention. Many forms of behaviour depend on selective attention being given to particular sets of stimuli. The eyes must focus on a target if it is to be pursued effectively. When an action sequence results in an unfamiliar situation to which no ready answer has been acquired during previous learning, orienting reactions result. As we have seen, these reactions are commonly coupled with uncertainty or instability of the mechanisms for selective attention. This is manifested in the scanning or searching activities which we observe as part of the orienting reactions. It follows from our assumptions that if any of the excursions of selective attention in this state of uncertainty result in actions which take the animal out of the problem situation concerned, these changes in selective attention will be reinforced. The mechanisms of selective attention can undergo learning changes as much as any other behavioural mechanism. But selection implies rejection. As one object is selected for attention another is rejected—and with it vanish the responses it used to evoke when attended to.

In this connection it is worth noting that the novelty of a situation is generally confined to particular subsystems of the brain. Thus an unfamiliar maze confronts the mechanism for target selection with novel stimulus configurations, but not the mechanisms for locomotion towards selected targets, nor the mechanisms for maintaining balance. On the other hand a sudden leg injury confronts the motor mechanisms with novel stimulus configurations but not the mechanisms for target selection. Any subsystem experiencing novel stimulus configurations is bound to be uncertain and fluctuating in its responses. Hence these subsystems will tend to be the main source of the random variations which trial-and-error learning requires. It follows that a brain which relies on general synaptic facilitation for the reinforcement of successful responses, but on interference for the extinction of unsuccessful ones, will minimize the amount of inappropriate unlearning following failed responses.

The upshot of this analysis is that one of the main modifiers of behaviour, one of the main factors which move the organism onto different tacks of behaviour, must be expected to reside in the interfering reactions which are triggered when the inappropriateness of a response results in noxious stimuli eliciting aversive reactions or in unfamiliar situations eliciting orienting reactions, or in the kind of *impasse* we identified with 'frustration' in Section 6.6. Some of these interfering reactions are specific, e.g. withdrawal responses; others are non-specific, such as those due to the general arousal elicited by the onset of pain.

The hypothesis that extinction is generally due to interference is also supported by the observation that conditions which increase inhibition generally tend to accelerate the process of extinction. However, I have mentioned that in theory there is also another way in which aversive reactions may assert their effect on learning. It is conceivable that some generalized internal reaction to the onset of pain may somehow prevent facilitatory synaptic changes in the neurons responsible for the antecedent responses—or prevent their physiological consolidation. (Possibly they may even effect a reversal of the synaptic changes.) It is conceivable that, if a tentative response executed in a trial-and-error situation is followed by pain, some global (perhaps humoral) effects of the pain reactions prevent the lasting facilitatory changes for which the synapses involved in the execution of the response had been earmarked.

I know of no conclusive evidence to either confirm or refute this hypothesis. However, the general impression still stands that the main mechanisms of extinction probably operate through the interference caused by the stabilization (and possible advance along the behaviour sequence) of incompatible responses or internal reactions elicited by pain, fear or frustration.

As regards the reinforcement of successful responses we are left with a number of elementary options:

1. All responses are synaptically facilitated simply because they occur. Responses are extinguished through the stabilization of incompatible, competing responses or through other interfering reactions of the types mentioned above. This in essence is Guthrie's position, but formulated at the physiological rather than psychological level.
2. All responses are synaptically facilitated only when there are indications of positive outcomes such as those listed earlier. They are extinguished as before.
3. All responses are synaptically facilitated except when there are indications of negative outcomes. They are extinguished as before.

On the first and third hypotheses rewards act only indirectly, viz. by preventing the interference that threatens all responses from a variety of sources. They prevent unlearning. All three hypotheses require detectors for monitoring the appropriateness (or otherwise) of on-going activities and also fairly global systems for distributing this information throughout the brain (cf. Section 6.6). On the second and third hypotheses this messenger system could be humoral, but it will be evident from the discussion of Guthrie's theory in Section 6.7 that this can hardly be assumed under the first hypothesis.

It might be thought that it should be easy to devise experiments for deciding between the alternatives I have listed above. In practice, however, these issues have proved to be extremely recalcitrant. One reason is that until one comes to grips with the neurophysiology of the processes involved and the details of the particular networks concerned, it is virtually impossible to distinguish between an excitation of a neural process and an inhibition of an inhibition upon the process. Thus global signalling of 'success' could effectively be mediated by an inhibition upon global 'failure' signals and vice versa.

It must also be remembered that these three hypotheses are not necessarily mutually exclusive. At the physiological level it is quite conceivable, for example, that the phylogenetically older and the phylogenetically newer structures of the brain rely on different mechanisms.

Explorations with microelectrodes have brought up cases in which the stimulation of an identifiable pathway (e.g. the perforant pathway to the hippocampus) was followed by lasting increments in conductivity[151]. But until the exact functional role of the pathway is known, this does not settle the question whether the observed synaptic facilitations occurred conditionally or unconditionally in the sense discussed above.

In the sequel I shall adopt the obvious course in connection with the structure in which the question arises. This is to adopt the simplest hypothesis, i.e. the first hypothesis, unless profounder considerations dictate otherwise. We shall see in Chapter 7 that the first hypothesis need *not* be tantamount to the assumption that synaptic potencies can only increase during learning, never decrease.

6.9   REWARD AND PUNISHMENT SYSTEMS

I have mentioned before that the processes involved in the realization of particular brain functions frequently contain general components which are common to an entire class of functions. Thus orienting, aversion, attack, attention etc. all have internal reaction components which are common to the various behaviours that fall into each of these categories. These general components must be contributed by structures which are activated by appropriately convergent inputs and whose outputs have appropriately global effects. The indications are that the reticular formation and the hypothalamus play a leading part in this.

Important discoveries made in the 1950s suggest that the organism's internal indicators for positive or negative outcomes similarly act through central and generalized reaction systems and that these generalized reaction systems are closely interrelated with the generalized approach and aversion systems.

The existence of these systems came to light in 1954 when reciprocal regions were identified in the brain stem and limbic areas of the rat at which direct experimental stimulation produced all the features of reward and punishment respectively. These results have since been confirmed for other species, including the primates. In Man stimulation of the reward centres produces feelings of ease, relaxation and great satisfaction. Stimulation of other centres may cause feelings of anxiety, restlessness or fright.

Prima facie we would expect that the system activated by rewards acts through a 'general satiety' centre and the system activated by punishment through an 'aversion' centre. However, the experimental data in the rat and other species suggest that the truth is not as simple as this. The punishment system indeed appears to act through an aversive system. But the reward system appears to act primarily through centres which occupy a systemic position more akin to an 'approach' centre. This is perhaps not surprising if we remember from the discussions in Section 6.6 how closely the internal indicators of success are linked with internal reactions of the 'go ahead' type.

Working with rats, Olds and Milner[185] discovered that there are regions in the brain where the application of a small electrical stimulus through implanted electrodes acts as a reinforcer to any activity to which this stimulus is added. If the stimulation was administered whenever the rat happened to go to a particular corner of its box the animal seemed to experience an enjoyable sensation from the injection of the current and soon developed a consistent behaviour pattern of coming back to the corner for more. If the rat is given the chance of self-stimulation through pressing a lever, the animal would take to pressing the lever several thousand times an hour without any sign of satiation. With electrodes suitably placed in the brain the animals would press the lever until physically exhausted. Even a starved rat would prefer this self-stimulation to the food that has been made available. A surprising result of these and subsequent experiments was the extent of the brain areas in which suitable foci could be found. These include the basal tegmentum of the midbrain, the hypothalamus, the amygdala, the septum and other limbic areas. The lateral hypothalamus was the most sensitive area. The reward system thus appears to be a very diffuse system, or, rather, a central system whose effective action comes to be subject to a wide range of less central influences.

That the reward system forms an integral system is shown by the observation that once a reward zone has been found and the animal has been trained for self-stimulation, other reward zones require no further training.

In the same year Delgado, Roberts and Miller[49] discovered the punishment system. Electrical stimulation in these particular zones produces aversive reactions and manifestations of fright, frustration or pain. The stimulation can provoke reactions of extreme intensity. If electrical stimuli are administered to an aversion zone which the animal can only terminate by pressing a lever, it will work for hours to minimize the amount of unpleasantness it experiences, often with after-effects characteristic of severe illness. At any stage during this process the pattern may be rapidly reversed by applying stimuli to a reward zone instead.

Further investigations have led Olds and others to the view that there is a primary reward system which is localized around the drive centres of the lateral hypothalamus. The association of neural reward in its strongest form with brain points where basic drives are also induced has been confirmed by a number of experiments related to hunger, thirst and sexual responses. This primary reward system can be inhibited by the activities of a central aversion system which is mainly based on the midbrain tegmentum. This inhibition is not reciprocal. However, according to Olds, there is also a secondary reward system which is based on the limbic brain and one of whose effects is to inhibit the aversion system, thus achieving rewarding effects by disinhibiting the primary reward system. These interactions, Olds believes, occur in the hypothalamic region, whence their net effects are distributed to the palaeocortex, neocortex, thalamus and midbrain. These systems also have generalized reaction components in the reticular formation.

Thus the anatomical study of brain rewards shows a relatively unified system to be involved, consisting of the limbic system and the hypothalamus. The upper part of this system had already previously been connected with 'emotional experience', whereas the lower part, the hypothalamus, was known to be connected with the basic drives related to food, water, sex, temperature and so forth.

Stimulation has the strongest and most stable rewarding effects when applied to the lateral hypothalamus bundle, the main pathway connecting this unified system together. This tract is well placed to be affected by receptors of physiological need in the central core of the hypothalamus. The reinforcing effects of stimulating the limbic zones, i.e. the secondary reward system, are weaker than those caused by stimulating the primary reward system and they wear off more quickly after repetition. Stimulation of this system also diminishes arousal and the effects of conditioned fear. Pain becomes more bearable in humans. By contrast, stimulation of the primary reward system may increase arousal, as does stimulation of the aversive system. Food rewards and the alleviation of fear through reassuring stimuli appear to act through the secondary reward system. Fear itself acts through the aversion system.

It may seem paradoxical that stimulation of some hypothalamic drive centres, for example some which elicit eating or drinking, should sometimes have rewarding effects and, similarly, that stimulation of the satiety centres which cause cessation of eating or drinking may have aversive effects. On the face of it one would expect drive inducing stimuli to have aversive effects and drive reducing stimuli to be rewarding. (In fact Olds has also discovered centres in the dorsal part of the medial hypothalamus where stimulation causes eating and aversion.)

These apparently paradoxical results show that it is important to be clear about the meaning of 'drive centres' and 'satiety centres'. The paradox arises only if these terms are understood in so liberal a sense that they include not only the primary detectors of a physiological need or of satiety, but also the derivative centres involved in mediating or organizing the appropriate action programmes (or the cessation of these programmes). The activity mediated or organized by a 'drive centre' of the derivative kind can be expected to have a generalized component of a 'go ahead' type, with positively reinforcing qualities. Conversely, the activity mediated or organized by a 'satiety' centre of the derivative type can be expected to produce an aversive disposition (towards food or water, for example, thus bringing eating or drinking to a halt) which has a generalized aversive component with negatively reinforcing qualities. From this point of view, therefore, the terms 'Go' and 'No go' system, used by some writers, appear to be the better choice[165].

6.10 SHORT-CIRCUITING

The gradual perfection through practice of any skilled activity commonly results in an increase in the speed with which the movements are performed. Frequently there is also a concomitant increase in the economy of the movements executed. Part of the increased speed can be explained in terms of the reduced latencies which result as the routine becomes familiar and the remaining orienting reactions are progressively eliminated. Another part is due to a process which is commonly known as *short-circuiting*. By this we mean the case when a reaction originally elicited at one point in a behaviour sequence appears gradually to move forward in that sequence and occur in an anticipatory fashion. We met examples of this in Section 6.8.

This tendency of responses to advance is to be expected in any learning situation in which there are cues that overlap with the beginning of the action or in which there are antecedent internal reactions that leave traces overlapping with the action.

If stimuli leave short-term traces within the neural networks in which the stimulus–response associations are formed, then it is to be expected that as a response becomes conditioned to a particular set of stimuli it also becomes conditioned to the traces of the stimuli that preceded this set. Eventually, therefore, the response may come to be triggered already by the earlier stimuli. And so it advances within the behaviour pattern. The earlier stimuli have taken over as adequate releasers for the response. This *principle of adequate stimulus substitution* may also result in one modality gradually taking over control from another.

When we learn a new motor skill our initial movements are apt to be slow, deliberate and disjointed, and they appear to rely mainly on visual clues. A child learning to tie his shoelaces is a typical example. After each initial move-ment the child may pause, examine the situation and then try the next move. But as the skill improves with practice the importance of visual clues recedes. More and more proprioceptive clues take their place. Whenever any part of the body is moved receptors in the muscles, tendons and joints are activated and deliver their characteristic signals to the higher centres. In the shoelace-tying situation there are also additional clues such as changes in the location and intensity of the cutaneous sensations. As the skill develops these clues progressively take over control of the child's movements. In other words, the clues produced by preceding movements become adequate clues for the release of succeeding movements. They have become adequate stimulus sub-stitutes for the visual clues used previously. Concomitantly there is a reduction in delay and a speeding-up of the whole sequence. The whole action becomes more and more automatic as the principle of adequate stimulus substitution takes effect and permits the highest centres to be relieved by lower ones. It is probable that the cerebellum plays a large part in some of these processes and in effecting some of the necessary stimulus substitutions. Lesions in the cere-bellum may cause the execution of skilled movements to revert to something very much resembling the early fumbling stages of a new skill.

An important consequence of short-circuiting is the straightening out of approach-paths to a goal (hence, in fact, the name) and a greater economy of movement as skills come to be perfected. In the early stages of training, skilled movements will be punctuated by errors: the target may be missed by over-shoot, undershoot or lateral errors. After each error some correcting action will be required. During learning this action will advance, and as it advances it will tend to diminish the original error and be diminished itself. If in learning to ride a bicycle I begin by oversteering, each initial steering movement will be followed by an opposite, corrective movement. As this corrective movement advances along the behaviour line it will begin to cancel part of the oversteer by interference and it will itself subsequently come to be partially cancelled by the same process. The result is a straighter course.

Of course, reactions may advance along a behaviour sequence in circum-stances in which this prejudices the outcome of the activity. When a rat is rewarded for pressing a bar the response of ducking down to the food dish elicited by the food is incompatible with that of standing up to press the bar. Miller[165] has reported that anticipatory ducking responses indeed sometimes intrude and interfere with pressing the bar. However, when anticipation reaches this point the resulting failure or frustration evidently prevents its reinforcement, possibly by eliciting interfering reactions which inhibit the action should it tend to occur too early in the sequence.

6.11   CONCLUDING REMARKS

In our earlier chapters we established the key concepts of directive correlation and internal representations of the outer world. The concept of directive correlation formalized the directiveness of appropriate behaviours. Internal representations were interpreted as aggregates of expectations, mainly of how sensory inputs transform as the result of movement, and in Section 2.2 we were able to form a general idea of how such expectations may be registered in neural terms.

The development during learning of the appropriate directive correlations and of the internal representations which mediate appropriate behaviours calls for lasting changes in the nervous system as the result of experience which may be active or passive. *Hence the question of reinforcement and extinction is not one that concerns S–R theory only. It equally concerns the development of expectations and the manner in which the organism reacts to them.*

In Section 6.6 we considered the physiological criteria the brain may use for monitoring whether a response was or was not appropriate in the circumstances in which it occurred. We noted the importance of the novelty of an experience in this context and we also noted that in certain circumstances novelty can serve as a criterion for the inappropriateness of a response or expectation. The question of the time-gap between a response and first indications of its appropriateness was also considered. In Section 6.7 we noted how some theories, such as Guthrie's, get around this problem and proceed on the assumption that synaptic changes happen unconditionally. Next we compared the general nature of reinforcement with that of extinction and noted that in physiological terms they do not appear to consist of symmetrically opposite processes (Section 6.8). However, the mechanisms mediating both effects appear to have general reaction components which can be activated by experimental stimulation of narrowly localized foci. These reaction components appear to be closely interrelated with the general reaction components of approach behaviour and aversion respectively (Section 6.9). A short digression on short-circuiting drew our attention to the importance of 'adequate stimulus substitution' in the further development and perfection of learnt behaviours (Section 6.10).

CHAPTER 7

Significant Operations and Network Configurations

7.1 INTRODUCTION

By contrast with the last chapter the present chapter deals with fiction rather than fact. It is an exercise of the imagination. The question is simply this: how can we imagine the main system-properties of the brain that have aroused our interest in Part I of this volume to be generated by the known properties of neurons and by the types of connectivities that are known to exist between neurons? This is clearly a very open-ended question with scope for a multitude of answers. We can narrow this scope considerably by searching initially only for the simplest possible ways in which the known properties of neurons may generate the kind of advanced operations we are interested in.

This type of speculative modelling is not in our time a fashionable pursuit among neurophysiologists or anatomists. The extreme caution the working neurologist has to observe in the interpretation of his results discourages flights of fancy. While this is right in certain contexts, those whose interests focus on the functions of the brain as a whole and those who like to keep an eye on the whole when searching for new hypotheses to explain the operations of the parts, see the matter in a different light and often feel that any model that is consistent with the bulk of the evidence can act as a valuable stimulus to further research.

For the greater part of this section we shall be looking at ideal learning systems which combine maximum plasticity with maximum simplicity and output contrast. We shall see that, if such systems are composed of units which have the basic properties of neurons, they must have certain structural features, such as input sharing and some form of lateral inhibition. A theoretical system of neurons satisfying these conditions and capable of undergoing plastic changes will be called a 'lambda system' and the input sharing neurons of the system will be known as 'lambda neurons'.

From the point of view of the higher brain functions the most important system-properties of the brain are

(i) the development of goal-directed behaviour, i.e. of executive directive correlations, and

(ii) the development in the brain of neural representations or 'models' of external objects, events, properties or relations.

As we have seen, observable behaviour in the higher orders of the animal kingdom can often be explained only on the assumption that the brain constructs some kind of internal model of the outside world. And, of course, we know from introspection that the human brain, at any rate, has advanced capabilities of this kind.

The neurology of these processes is still unknown territory. My aim in this chapter, therefore, is to look at the most elementary forms of information processing through which the brain may in theory achieve such capabilities and, with the aid of simple models, to illustrate some of the elementary ways in which systems composed of neurons may accomplish the required operations. In these models I shall confine myself to the lowest level of organization at which the required system-properties can be seen to emerge, if only in rudimentary form.

I aim no higher than to make the reader aware of the elementary capacity of certain neural properties and connectivities to perform required types of operation. This is primarily an analytical aim. The simple models I shall introduce, therefore, can do no more than give us a glimpse of possible ways in which things may hang together in the complex operations of the living brain. But in our present state of ignorance about the mechanisms of the higher brain functions even this must be counted as a gain, quite apart from the value of having that kind of knowledge available at the back of the mind in the search for new hypotheses or new experimental approaches. To the extent to which this type of analytical exercise succeeds in uncovering the potential contribution known properties of parts of the brain can make to the known capabilities of the whole, it helps to guide our thoughts in the quest for further information or in the design of new experiments.

The theoretical models we meet in this chapter are not therefore to be regarded as concrete hypotheses. They are merely heuristic devices designed to illustrate certain elementary logical implications of particular neural properties or interneural relationships. Moreover, they are based on an abstract view of the nervous system in which the digital aspect of neural mechanisms is lifted out of its context and treated in separation from the analog aspect (see below).

It is clear from the start that the naive notion of the neuron as a single-input, single-output switching device is quite inadequate for the kind of operations we have to consider. Even if the neuron is conceived as a multiple-input device which is capable of showing selective preferences for particular input patterns and of modifying these preferences as the result of experience, this is too narrow a concept. The responses of central neurons are frequently modified by lateral interactions with neighbouring neurons which share some or all of the afferent information, so that the responses of a single neuron cannot fruitfully be thought of as single-valued functions of such information. Hence if we are to have any hope at all of eventually arriving at an interpretative model of the brain, or parts of the brain, in terms of functional units whose outputs can be explained as functions of their inputs it would not be plausible to expect such elementary organizational entities to be anything less than a multiple-input, multiple-output network of neurons.

If the information handled by such networks relies on line-labelling, the learning function of the network becomes that of learning to produce the appropriate spatial pattern or distribution of excited output fibres in response to any given spatial distribution of excited input fibres.*

We shall see in due course to what extent line-labelling is an acceptable assumption for the main functions with which we shall be concerned. We know that even if at the peripheral receptors input intensities are critical (as in the difference between light pressure and painful pressure) these soon become line-labelled higher up the afferent pathways as specific neurons are mobilized when critical intensities are reached. But along the efferent pathways the converse happens and relative intensities once again assume critical significance (Section 6.1).

In computer terms the operations of the central networks of the brain appear to be partly analog and partly digital. They are analog in so far as they depend critically on the degree of excitation in the nerve fibres, i.e. on the impulse frequencies of the volleys propagated in the nerve fibres. They are digital in so far as they depend critically on line-labelling, i.e. on the identity of the activated fibres rather than the impulse frequency. When the digital aspect prevails we need to think of fibres only as either active or quiescent and it would suffice to represent the current state of activity of a set of fibres simply by a set of binary digits, e.g. 01101 for a set of five fibres, where '0' and '1' would denote 'quiescent' and 'active' respectively.

In the decision making processes of the higher brain centres the digital element appears to prevail but in the dynamic implementation of the decisions the analog element reasserts itself. A couple of examples may serve to illustrate this.

Examining the responses of individual neurons in the motor cortex of the cat to flashes of light, O'Brien and Fox[183] found that in 79% of the cells the response was reversed when the light flashes were paired with somatic shock. Previously facilitated cells now showed inhibition and previously inhibited cells now showed activation. This is a typically digital picture. It suggests an information flow in which (say) output 10011 changed to output 01101 when the second stimulus was added to the first.

---

* This concentration on the input–output relations of certain hypothetical networks should not, of course, be interpreted as a tacit return to the S–R concept for the organism as a whole.

The analog element is illustrated by the following example. If a dog is conditioned to lift the left forepaw when given a particular signal and strychnine is then applied to the exposed cortical area that controls the right hind limb, the dog will lift the right hind limb instead of the left forepaw when given the usual signal.[73] This behavioural change results from the facilitatory effect of strychnine on the dendritic synapses of the cortical neurons. It shows the degree to which relative levels of excitation in mutually antagonistic movement organizations can be decisive in determining final behaviour. Other examples will be found in Chapter 10.

In this chapter I shall concentrate exclusively on the digital aspect of brain functions and temporarily assume, therefore, that in the brain functions we are about to study all essential information is coded in terms of the identity of the excited fibres. In other words, we shall move to a level of abstraction at which the digital aspect is lifted out and the analog aspect temporarily disregarded. In these abstract models, therefore, any input fibre is assumed to be either silent or to be excited at a frequency of (say) 100 impulses per second. These simplifying assumptions are harmless provided we do not lose sight of the fact that we have made them and that certain aspects of the matter thus come to be temporarily ignored. These aspects include 'noise' and certain forms of redundancy. Since in the digital models one fibre may be active while its neighbour is silent, for example, we are temporarily disregarding the redundancy that is implied in the lateral diffusion of afferent excitation, i.e. in afferent convergence.

We shall see presently that the main network capabilities we are interested in require a number of special processes or operations, such as contrast enhancement, adaptive changes in the patterns of outputs elicited by a given input pattern, the progressive acquisition of a new set of stimuli as adequate releasers of an output pattern previously triggered only by another set of stimuli ('adequate stimulus substitution'), and the telescoping of temporal (i.e. serial) patterns of neural events into spatial patterns of neural events. (Contrast enhancement may seem the odd man out on this list since one tends to think of it primarily in connection with analog operations. But, as we shall see, if contrast enhancement is driven to the point at which it results in all output channels being either fully active or entirely quiescent, it becomes an essential instrument for maintaining the digital character of a network.)

To illustrate these operations at the lowest levels of organization our models require neurons whose synaptic potencies can undergo plastic changes which increase the sensitivity of these neurons to particular input configurations. In addition they require neurons which can function in the manner of (inclusive) logical OR gates, that is to say neurons subject to such threshold parameters that significant discharge rates can result already if no more than one of several possible input channels is fully activated. Finally we require neurons which function in the manner of logical AND gates, i.e. neurons in which significant discharge rates result only if two or more input channels are fully activated.

The main difficulty encountered in groping for a functional interpretation of the actual connectivities known to exist in the brain is that one has to advance on two fronts simultaneously. We cannot in our thinking segregate particular neural networks as distinct functional units without making some reference to the contribution each is assumed to make to the overall organization of the brain. On the other hand we cannot think of the overall functional organization of the brain except in terms of the functional units over which it disposes. The growth of fruitful hypotheses, therefore, depends on the mind constantly switching between two points of view: looking at the supposed functional units from the point of view of the whole and looking at the whole from the point of view of the supposed functional units. This is pertinent, for example, when we ask ourselves how much adaptive plasticity we must expect to find in particular local networks in the brain.

In this chapter we shall think mainly in terms of coherent localized networks which we treat as distinct functional entities and which we shall examine from the standpoint of particular functional properties such as adaptive plasticity, the ability to convert temporal patterns of excitation into spatial patterns etc. We approach these questions in each case by developing hypothetical networks, ideal models, in which a realization of the property we are interested in is illustrated at an elementary level of organization.

At a later stage these ideal models may then be compared with actual structures in the brain in the hope that they may advance our understanding of these structures, or, at any rate, suggest new questions to ask in the experimental investigation of the structures concerned. But at that stage we shall have to look again at the functional organization of the brain as a whole. It would be premature to conclude out of context that because particular structures in the brain have certain features in common with one of our models, these structures must necessarily be realizations of the models.

7.2 THE POWER OF RECURRENT INHIBITION AND COMPLEMENTARY CODING

Our first investigations concern the general conditions in which a multiple-input, multiple-output network of neurons could achieve optimal plasticity and resolution. By this we mean that in theory the network could learn to produce any stipulated output pattern in response to any given input pattern or set of input patterns. Since we are temporarily thinking in digital terms only, 'input pattern' here means any given combination of fully active and entirely quiescent input fibres.

Continuing with the digital concept, it is clear that the internal connections of such a network must be such that (a) any output fibre is potentially excitable by activity in any input fibre and (b) any output fibre is potentially inhibitable by activity in any input fibre. Of these two requirements the second is the more exacting.

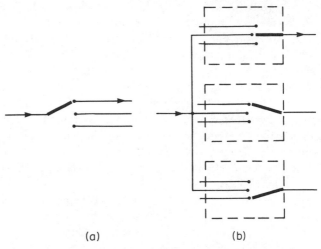

(a)   (b)

Figure 7.1. Channel switching by (a) selective projection and (b) selective acceptance

In consequence of the fact that neurons have multiple input channels but each only a single output channel, the information flow in neural networks differs in one crucial respect from that in a telephone exchange, for example. In the telephone exchange the problem of directing the flow of information to alternative destinations is solved by the telephone selector. Figure 7.1(a) symbolizes a selector for one input channel in relation to three alternative output channels. The method may be described as one of 'selective projection'. By way of contrast neural networks can achieve similar functions only by a method of 'selective acceptance', symbolized in Figure 7.1(b). A minimum of three neurons would be required to provide for the same alternatives as those envisaged in the previous diagram. In other words, learning changes in a neural network can only result in a redirection of information flow to different output channels if the neurons change their selective preferences for particular input configurations. Figure 7.1(b) demonstrates a significant consequence of this: there must be *input sharing* between sets of neurons in the learning network. That is to say neural learning systems in digital functions must *begin with a divergent (i.e. distributive) afferent inflow.*

In consequence of this input sharing one of the main problems an optimal learning system composed of neurons must solve is how to keep quiescent those output fibres which the desired output pattern requires to be quiescent. Each output fibre must be the axon of a neuron and each of these neurons must be potentially excitable by each of the many input fibres of the system if any possible input–output combination is to be obtainable in practice. Since during learning (or at any other time) no excitatory synapse can change into an inhibitory one, any system of this kind would have to rely on internal inhibitory circuits to keep some output fibres inactive while others are activated by the given input pattern. In essence, therefore, the required inhibition has to function as a type of *contrast enhancement* which causes output fibres to be either fully active or entirely quiescent. These inhibitory circuits might be either of a feedback or feedforward type. As we shall see, feedback inhibition or 'recurrent inhibition' is the more powerful of the two. The abundance of recurrent inhibition in the cortex and many subcortical structures thus assumes particular significance from this point of view. Well-documented examples of forward inhibition are found in the cerebellum (Chapter 8).

The contrast enhancing effect of recurrent inhibition may be illustrated by the observations made by Brooks, Kameda and Nagel[32] in the motor cortex of the cat. If the recurrent inhibitory system of the pyramidal tract neurons in this area is given an extra impetus by antidromic stimulation via the pyramidal tract, it is seen to subtract a roughly constant number of impulses from the responses of single tested pyramidal tract neurons to peripheral test stimuli of various strengths. It follows that the percentage depression is greater for weak test responses than for strong ones and contrast is enhanced.

Figure 7.2 illustrates two simple, theoretical input-sharing networks subject to (a) recurrent inhibition and (b) forward inhibition respectively. The mode of operation of either system of lateral inhibition offers a considerable number of theoretical possibilities, depending on the special assumptions one would care to make about the various network parameters. There is considerable scope for mathematical speculation here, but for our purposes it suffices to outline just three possible modes of action which illustrate both the inherent capabilities of lateral inhibition and the diversity of the theoretical possibilities. In each of these modes of action the function of the lateral inhibition is to favour the discharges of those neurons whose synaptic potencies are most receptive to a given pattern of inputs, as against the neurons which are less excited by the input pattern. The difference between them lies in the exact nature of these contrast enhancing effects.

First a few definitions. In the future I shall designate as a *lambda system* any network of neurons in which

   (i) a number of input channels are shared by all excitatory neurons of the network;
   (ii) the excitatory neurons are subject to some form of recurrent or forward inhibition with lateral spread which favours those that are most receptive to the given pattern of inputs;
   (iii) some or all of the synapses of the shared input channels can undergo lasting changes as the result of experience.

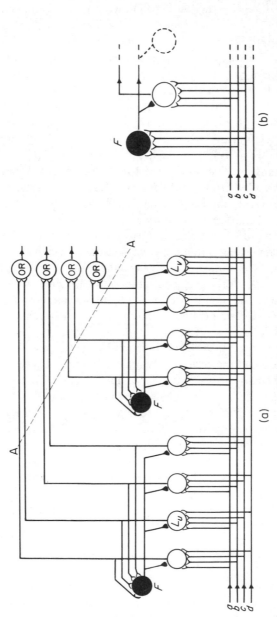

Figure 7.2. 'Lambda systems' are defined as systems of input-sharing neurons which are subject to some form of contrast enhancing lateral inhibition. (a) Simple lambda system using recurrent inhibition. Two 'modules' are shown, each consisting of four 'lambda neurons' governed by a single inhibitory neuron (*F*). The OR gates shown to the right of the line A–A are not included in the definition of the system since their function may be performed implicitly by follow-up systems. (b) Inhibitory segment of lambda system using forward inhibition. For explanation see text

The input-sharing excitatory neurons in the lambda system will be known as *lambda* neurons. If the lambda neurons can be partitioned according to the inhibitory neurons controlling them (as instanced in Figure 7.2), these groups will be called *lambda modules*.

To understand the particular operation of recurrent inhibition which I intend to illustrate it must be assumed that the distribution of synaptic potencies on the lambda neurons differs from neuron to neuron, so that each neuron has selective preferences for particular input patterns, and also that this synaptic potency distribution can change as the result of learning. Given these assumptions the general effect of the inhibitory neuron *F* is readily visualized. The EPSP generated in each lambda neuron by any particular input pattern differs from neuron to neuron. Via the recurrent collaterals that impinge on it neuron *F* is excited by the aggregate discharges of the lambda neurons. Its inhibitory synapses on these neurons generate IPSPs which are tantamount to a rise in threshold of all the lambda neurons of the module. Given appropriate system parameters the thresholds can rise to a point at which the net excitation in a number of lambda neurons remains subliminal and their output fibres are held silent. Obviously the thresholds cannot rise to a point at which *all* net excitations become subliminal, for the discharges of *F* would then cease and the inhibition vanish altogether. The question is at what point equilibrium occurs. This decides the number and identity of the discharging lambda neurons and of the activated output fibres.

Clearly there are a number of theoretical possibilities here which could be explored in depth. But since there is a large choice of parameters and we lack a great deal of relevant information it is best not to tie ourselves down and to keep as many options open as possible. The purposes of this chapter are therefore best served if I merely give a couple of examples to illustrate the kind of effects recurrent inhibition can achieve in theory. These will then be followed by a single example to illustrate a possible mode of operation of forward inhibition. For ease of reference these three theoretical examples will be called Models I, II and III respectively. Thus Models I and II employ recurrent inhibition whereas Model III relies on feedforward inhibition. Models II and III are stochastic models and probably the most realistic. Model I has been chosen because it illustrates the extreme power inherent in recurrent inhibition and because it lends itself particularly well to simple simulations of learning processes of a deterministic kind.

Model I

As our first model we take the extreme case in which the recurrent inhibition illustrated in Figure 7.2(a) functions as a maximum intensity filter, in the sense that all net excitations of the lambda neurons remain subliminal except that of the *one* neuron in each module which receives the strongest excitation from the given input pattern—the net excitations of the other neurons being held subliminal by the IPSPs generated by the inhibitory neuron F.

The mathematical conditions for recurrent inhibition to function in this manner are given in Appendix B. They are not particularly stringent conditions. When the parameters of the system satisfy these conditions all lambda neurons in a given module remain quiescent except the one that receives maximum excitation from the current input pattern. This then fires at a frequency high enough to produce what we understand by a 'fully activated' output fibre or a digital '1'. In future we shall simply say that the respective lambda neuron 'responds', 'discharges' or 'fires'.

A system functioning under these extreme assumptions constitutes the highest grade filter which the lambda configuration can provide. In lower grade systems more than one lambda neuron would respond in each module, given suitable input conditions. We shall meet such systems when we come to consider lambda systems function according to Model II and Model III later in this section.

The neurons to the right of the broken line (A–A) in Figure 7.2(a) are taken to function in the manner of logical OR gates. This means that these neurons discharge at a rate identifiable as a digital '1' whenever one or more of their input channels is active at a frequency qualifying as a digital '1'. These OR gates are added to our theoretical model to satisfy the postulate that, if required, the system must be able to produce the same final output pattern in response to two or more dissimilar input patterns. In particular cases, of course, the required OR functions may be performed implicitly by the follow-up systems into which the outputs of a given lambda system feed.

To account for learning changes in the lambda systems we assume that if the outcome of a response is favourable the required positive reinforcement consists of an increase in synaptic potency of the excited synapses in the neurons responsible for the response (the discharging neuron in each module) *relative* to the potency of the unexcited synapses in the same neuron (which are assumed to decrease in proportion). When the outcome is unfavourable (punishment and frustration) these changes are suppressed or possibly even negatived.

The reason for this assumption is a purely heuristic one. Although, as we have seen in Section 6.7, it is possible that complex learning systems may conceivably achieve adaptive changes if stimulus–response associations are reinforced irrespective of outcomes (Section 6.7), in a simple isolated learning system whose functions one may wish to visualize or to simulate electronically, some direct feedback effect of outcomes must be assumed. The reason why we postulate relative rather than absolute synaptic changes will be explained in Section 7.3. Relative changes would result, for example, if the potency of the excited synapses is increased while that of the non-excited synapses is decreased.

The inputs to a lambda configuration may consist of what in Section 5.6 we have distinguished as 'contingent' and 'demand' inputs respectively. Provided the lambda system comprises a sufficient number of modules and each module a sufficient number of lambda neurons, its final response patterns will then tend to become directively correlated to the ambient circumstances reflected in the contingent inputs in respect of the goals reflected in the demand inputs. It is also clear that the system can learn and store directive correlations in respect of as many alternative goals as there are alternative demand input patterns between which it can learn to discriminate.

The power of discrimination possessed by lambda configurations functioning according to our Model I depends on the largest permissible difference between the excitation of the most powerfully excited neuron and that of the next most powerfully excited neuron.

Another limitation is common to all systems whose power of effective discrimination depends on the selective preferences of constituent neurons for particular input patterns. This limitation can only be removed by the use of complementary coding (Section 6.2). Suppose that lambda neuron A is the most receptive neuron for a stimulus combination $S_1S_2S_3$. This neuron will then also be the most receptive neuron for the combination S_1S_2—unless the input channels use complementary coding. The mere omission of activation in one or more fibres cannot cause a different neuron, B, suddenly to become the maximally excited one. Hence the responses of the system cannot effectively discriminate between $S_1S_2S_3$ and S_1S_2. But if reciprocal coding is used the absence of S_3 entails not only the absence of excitation in fibres which were previously active but also the emergence of excitation in fibres which were previously quiescent. Now it is possible for a neuron to be more powerfully excited by S_1S_2 than by $S_1S_2S_3$. Thus complementary coding of inputs enables lambda-type systems to discriminate between the absence and the presence of a single stimulus among several others.

The simplest conception of a digital input system using complementary coding is one in which the input channels are thought of as paired in such a way that always either the one or the other member of each pair is active. If one channel in each pair is labelled '1' and the other '0', the total input pattern at any time may then be visualized as a set of binary digits, e.g. 11010, but each digit now specifies the current state of a *pair* of channels.

The OR gates in Figure 7.2(a) were arranged to preserve this reciprocal coding. Since there are two OR gates per lambda module, always one output fibre will be active while the other is quiescent.

Model II

We may now turn to a theoretical example which shows recurrent inhibition functioning in a different way. In this model each set of lambda neurons under control of a single inhibitory neuron (each lambda module) is conceived as a statistical population of input-sharing neurons in which any given input pattern sets up a variety of different EPSPs depending on the potencies of the individual synapses concerned in the individual neurons. For any given input pattern, therefore, we can then imagine a histogram which gives the frequency distribution of different levels of EPSPs generated in the neurons of the module (Figure 7.3).

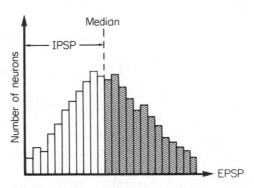

Figure 7.3. Imaginary histogram showing the number of neurons of the lambda population in which a given stimulus elicits the respective level of EPSP. If for simplicity we ignore the inherent threshold of the cells, the number of discharging neurons (shaded area) will be the number of cells whose individual EPSP exceeds the common IPSP. In Model II it is assumed that the inhibitory neurons generate IPSPs which are equal to the median value of the elicited EPSPs. Thus approximately half the population of neurons would actively respond to any given stimulus

We now demand that the inhibitory system functions in such a manner that in response to any given input pattern approximately half the neurons respond (viz. those which receive the highest EPSPs) while the others remain silent. In other words, the IPSPs generated by the inhibitory neuron must be so controlled that for any given input pattern in half the population the *net* excitation (EPSP − IPSP) remains subliminal.

The advantage of this arrangement would be that the outputs of the system would then have a far greater information content than in Model I, while the overall plasticity of the system would remain virtually unimpaired. Functioning according to Model I a lambda module containing N lambda neurons has N possible and (if its history is unknown) equally probable output patterns. Thus the information content per output pattern is

$$\log_2 N \text{ bits}$$

In Model II the number of possible (and, by the same token, equally probable) output patterns equals the number of ways in which $N/2$ digital '1's can be distributed over N places. This equals the binomial coefficient

$$\binom{N}{\frac{N}{2}}$$

and the information content (in bits) of the output pattern would be the logarithm (to base 2) of this number.

A glance at Figure 7.3 shows that the stipulated conditions will be met if the inhibitory neuron generates IPSPs which are equal to the *median* value of the EPSPs in this frequency distribution. Only the neurons which fall into the shaded area of the histogram would then discharge, and by definition this is half the total population of the module. (For simplicity I am ignoring the intrinsic threshold of the cell, in the absence of externally generated IPSPs.) Bar a scaling factor, this condition will be met if the output frequency of the inhibitory neuron is proportional to the *number* of discharging lambda neurons, i.e. to the *number* of *activated* axon collaterals impinging on it, regardless of the intensity of that activation. In theory the inhibitory neuron could function in this manner if the packets of disposable transmitter agent in each presynaptic terminal were few in number, quick to exhaust and slow to regenerate.

The difference between Model I and Model II is highlighted if we examine the type of correlation that would be found in sampling the activities of adjacent or closely spaced neurons in input-sharing systems in which there exists (a) no lateral inhibition, (b) recurrent inhibition functioning according to Model I, and (c) recurrent inhibition functioning according to Model II. In case (a) the correlation would tend to be positive by virtue of the simple fact of shared inputs. In other words outputs would be more or less *synchronized*. In case (b) the correlation would be negative because the recurrent inhibition here functions in a manner which precludes simultaneous discharges in two closely spaced neurons (strictly: in any two neurons belonging to the same module). In case (c), on the other hand, there would tend to be a complete decorrelation. The activity of say one lambda neuron in Model II can tell us nothing about the discharge probabilities of any other. In other words, outputs would be *desynchronized*. These observations are pertinent in view of the correlation studies regarding the activity of closely spaced neurons which have been carried out by Noda and others in the hippocampus and neocortex. We shall return to these in Chapter 8. The question of the synchronization of neural discharges also occupies a central position in the interpretation of EEG records.

Model III

Finally we come to our third illustration of the possible modes of action of lateral inhibition in input-sharing systems. In this particular mode of operation forward inhibition is used (Figure 7.2(b)) instead of the recurrent inhibition we have considered so far.

According to the assumptions we have made about learning changes in lambda systems, only those neurons undergo changes whose discharges result in successful responses. It is assumed that in these neurons the potencies of the excited synapses increase while the potencies of the non-excited synapses decrease in proportion. In this manner particular lambda neurons thus come to develop appropriate preferences for particular input patterns. Meanwhile let us also assume for the sake of argument that before learning began all synaptic potencies throughout the lambda population were equal.

Suppose now that the inhibitory neurons in the system of Figure 7.2(b) discharge at a rate which is proportional to the total activity occurring in the input channels (as may plausibly be assumed since they receive collaterals from all input fibres). The IPSPs generated at the lambda neurons would also then be proportional to the total input activity. It follows that with a suitable choice of parameters the system could function in such a manner that only those lambda neurons reach a firing level which during learning have developed some degree of selective preference for the given input pattern. In these conditions we would then have a system in which only learnt input patterns would be effective, while unlearnt patterns (and 'noise') would be ignored. Since before learning began all patterns would be unlearnt, the system could not begin to function unless it were to operate in conjunction with a supplementary system of 'forcing' or 'facilitating' inputs which could force or facilitate cell discharges even in the absence of adequate excitation from the shared inputs (Section 7.4). As this is precisely the case in the only well-documented example of an input-sharing system with forward inhibition (the Purkinje cells in the cerebellum) this theoretical model is not as far-fetched as it might appear at a first reading. A system functioning according to this model would be effective in a case in which the desired effect of learning is that one source of inputs (the shared inputs) should gradually come to substitute for a second source (the supplementary inputs) as adequate, appropriate and possibly anticipatory releasers of the responses originally triggered by the second source.

Enough has been said to give a broad idea of the kind of effects lateral inhibition can achieve in input-sharing systems—even though we have only looked at a few of the many theoretical possibilities. All the theoretical network configurations we shall look at in this chapter are basically of the 'lambda' type. All therefore presuppose input sharing and some form of lateral inhibition which favours the neurons whose synaptic potency distribution best matches the given input patterns. We shall not pursue the details of this contrast enhancement any further. The particular effects required of it will be evident in the particular applications we shall consider. They will remain well within the capabilities of the inhibitory systems I have illustrated above.

To simplify the graphical representation of lambda systems it is expedient to use special ideograms. When the input connections to all lambda neurons of a given lambda configuration are taken to be the same, it is superfluous to draw the complete configuration. Instead it suffices to show merely one or two lambda neurons whose connections may then be taken as representative for the whole system. Nor will the inhibitory system be shown explicitly. The existence of some form of appropriate lateral inhibition, i.e. contrast enhancement, will be taken for granted.

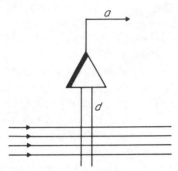

Figure 7.4. Symbolic representation of lambda neuron. It is assumed that input fibres (*i*) synapse with dendrites (*d*) and these synapses can undergo lasting changes; *a*, axon. Black bar symbolizes the lateral inhibition which is one of the defining characteristics of lambda systems

Figure 7.4 shows the ideogram to be used for single lambda neurons—generally in order to typify the connections to or from the lambda system. The triangle represents the soma of the neuron and the heavy bar on the left symbolizes the inhibitory component of the configuration. Frequently, too, we shall omit the subdivision of a lambda configuration into modules, since the required partitioning can usually be inferred from the context. The vertical lines *d* symbolize the dendrites of the lambda neurons which make synaptic contacts with the shared input fibres *i*.

7.3 THE LAMBDA CONFIGURATION AS A POSSIBLE LEARNING SYSTEM

It will not be suggested that all learning systems in the brain are necessarily based on lambda configurations or that those which are based on such configurations necessarily exploit their capabilities to the limit. But lambda systems of the type illustrated in Figure 7.2(a) can serve as a basis of simple models whose action is comparatively easy to visualize and which can help to clarify a number of theoretical issues. The models can also demonstrate a

number of features which are common to all learning systems depending on
competitive principles. In our 'Model I', for example, the competitive principle
lies in the assumption that within each module the lambda neuron receiving
the greatest synaptic drive from the input pattern presented to the system fires
to the exclusion of the remaining neurons in the module. As the inputs to the
system are assumed to be equally distributed to all lambda neurons, the neuron
which defeats its competitors must be the one whose synaptic potency distribution provides the best match to the particular input pattern in question.
As the system could not function selectively over any considerable length of
time if the synaptic potencies of all its excitatory synapses could drift towards
a common maximum, the most realistic assumption is that during learning
synaptic potencies can decrease as well as increase—perhaps maintaining
some constant average over each individual neuron. (Hence the term 'synaptic
potency distribution' used above.)

Any assumption that during learning synapses can only *increase* in potency
would be unrealistic in the sense that it is difficult to see how these changes
could be large enough to have perceptible overt effects and at the same time
small enough to avoid the neuron reaching saturation in a very short period
of time. This is particularly true if we think of the many readjustments to
changing environmental parameters we have to learn over a period of time
in the many routine skills we have to exercise in our daily transactions with
the environment. Since both positive and negative changes in synaptic potency
have been observed in various parts of the nervous system our hypothesis is
not unreasonable. There is also the question of stability to be considered.
Milner[169] has pointed out that a nervous system containing only synapses whose
potency was increased by usage would be highly unstable. But, as already
mentioned, the nervous system is very stable and maintains a surprisingly
constant overall level of excitation.

Unfortunately we still lack empirical evidence of any systematic way in
which synaptic changes occur as the result of learnIng. Some indirect evidence
comes from studies of the cortical anatomy of rats kept in a lively, free-
ranging environment compared with rats kept in an impoverished environment in which each rat lives alone in a cage.[210] Most of the synaptic contacts
between nerve cells in the cortex are made on the branchlike dendrites of the
receiving cells or on small projections from the dendrites, the spines (Section
6.2). Albert Globus found that the pyramidal cells of the rats reared in an
enriched environment formed more spines, particularly on the basal dendrites.
Several investigators have found that in the visual cortex there is an increase
in the size of the synapses in enriched-experience rats, but that this increase
in size is associated with a decreased number of synapses, whereas decreased
size of synapses is associated with an increased number. This suggests that
during learning synapses may undergo either positive or negative changes in
either size or number. It would appear then that memory changes may be

encoded in the brain either by selective addition of contact between nerve cells or by selective removal of contact and that both processes may go on at the same time.

To provide for appropriate learning changes in our theoretical lambda systems the most plausible postulate would seem to be that when the system has responded to a particular input pattern with a particular spatial pattern of outputs and the outcome is positive, synaptic potencies are subsequently changed only in the neurons which discharged at the time and so produced the respective output pattern. This postulate would minimize retroactive interference, i.e. interference with other input–output associations which may previously have become established via other lambda neurons in connection with different input patterns (see below).

Accordingly we may tentatively postulate that under conditions of *positive* reinforcement

(i)   only those lambda neurons undergo learning changes which participate in the production of the response (in Model I, for example, this is in each module the neuron whose synaptic potency distribution provides the best match for the given input pattern);

(ii)   the potency of the excited synapses increases while at the same time that of the non-excited synapses decreases.

The question of the effect of *negative* outcomes must be left open. The reader who recalls the upshot of our discussion of reinforcement in Chapter 6 will appreciate that whereas in models of localized networks one may hope to formulate realistic postulates about learning changes following positive outcomes, one cannot do the same in respect of negative outcomes. The reason is that the most significant changes following negative outcomes may not occur in the systems responsible for producing the original responses. As we saw at the time, the most telling changes of behaviour that follow failed trials may result from changes which are produced elsewhere in the nervous system and which extinguish the original responses simply by interfering with them somewhere along the line to the final effector organs. In consequence one cannot use models of localized systems (for example, the electronic models of lambda systems the writer has built from time to time) to simulate *realistic* trial-and-error learning without introducing purely ad hoc and often unrealistic rules for synaptic changes following failed trials.

On the above hypotheses a repeated presentation of the same input pattern, each followed by the same and (we assume) successful response, causes the synaptic potency distribution of the lambda neurons eliciting the response gradually to approach an optimum distribution for this input pattern. For these neurons the respective input pattern would thus become a specific *trigger feature*.

Thus if a particular input pattern consists of the activation of the input fibres *a*, *b* and *c* (Figure 7.2(a)) and at each occasion this causes lambda neuron L_u to fire in the first module of the system and L_v in the second module, then (assuming this output pattern to mediate a successful response at each presentation) our assumption is that the synapses of the *a*, *b* and *c* fibres at those particular neurons increase their potency while all other synapses at the same neurons diminish theirs. In future this process will be called the *alignment* of the respective lambda neurons on the given input pattern.

On our hypotheses for positive reinforcement alone the only way in which the alignment of a lambda neuron on any particular stimulus pattern can subsequently again be destroyed is by a series of positively reinforced trials in which a succession of small changes in the input pattern (none large enough to change the identity of the responding lambda neurons) causes a succession of correlated realignments in the same lambda neurons. Thus the system favours small and gradual modifications of responses but resists their sudden destruction. For particular modelling purposes it may be necessary to introduce stronger hypotheses, for instance that a failed response destroys or randomizes previous synaptic alignments.

If the system has to function in isolation and has to discover each required input–output association by pure trial and error, it would be a slow system indeed. But, as we shall see later, in the manner in which we envisage such systems to be integrated with other systems, the pure trial-and-error situation is the exception rather than the rule.

The assumption that the responses of a lambda system are determined by the lambda neurons whose synaptic potency distribution best matches the given input pattern, conforms to one very general characteristic of the brain as a behaving whole. This is that the responses the brain makes to any new, but not wholly unfamiliar, stimulus situation tend to be those it is accustomed to make in similar circumstances to whatever familiar and previously assimilated stimulus pattern most closely resembles the given one. This applies particularly to those internal 'responses' of the brain which we know as perception and recognition. It explains why the brain tends to spell out our visual perceptions in terms of the basic forms and figures on which the eye was trained or to which it innately tends to respond most readily.

Another general feature of the lambda system may be illustrated with reference to our Model I. Suppose that in consequence of a repeated presentation of a stimulus pattern S_1 in a series of positively reinforced trials a given lambda neuron L_x has become fully aligned on S_1, yielding the response R_x. L_x, we may say, has been *captured* by S_1. If then a different stimulus pattern (S_2) is presented to the system the resulting response depends on the similarity between S_1 and S_2. If the initial synaptic potency distribution in the system was random, then the chances are that if S_1 and S_2 are dissimilar the lambda neuron whose potency distribution best matches S_2 will not be the same as the one that was captured by S_1. A new response R_y results and if this is subsequently reinforced in a number of successive trials a new association S_2–R_y is added to the repertoire of the system without detriment to the existing S_1–R_x association.

But if S_2 closely resembles S_1 then L_x may be captured by S_2 and R_x generalizes to S_2. If in repeated trials L_x now realigns on S_2, the probability of R_x following S_1 is diminished. Thus the new learning has come about at the cost of some unlearning. But this type of *retroactive interference* is precisely what we must demand of a system which is expected in the course of its working life to make running adjustments to the gradual changes in the parameters that affect the implementation and effectiveness of its responses. Such gradual changes are bound to happen as the organism matures or its environment or circumstances change in character. As already mentioned, this unlearning by retroactive interference is the only type of direct unlearning through defacilitation which the lambda models offer on the simple assumptions we have made for them.

On the debit side this type of interference means that every act of learning in a lambda system also implies a certain element of unlearning. What matters in the long run, of course, is that the average amount of learning per rewarded trial should exceed the average amount of unlearning. This depends on the extent to which the number of uncommitted lambda neurons in the system exceeds the number of committed and aligned ones. This sets a ceiling to the learning capacity of the lambda system. When this point is passed new learning drives out old learning to an extent which results in no net overall gain.

Another important property of the lambda system is *stimulus generalization*. If the system has acquired a maximal association between a particular stimulus pattern and a particular output pattern, the probability of a different stimulus pattern eliciting the same response varies inversely with the difference between the respective stimulus patterns. The more they differ the fewer will be the number of lambda neurons which are aligned on the first and yet respond to the second.

7.4   RESPONSE MODULATION, ADEQUATE STIMULUS SUBSTITUTION AND FORCED ACQUISITION

A number of models have been introduced above to illustrate how certain capabilities may arise from comparatively simple properties of neurons and their connectivities. In these models all afferents to the lambda neurons enter on equal terms. But we know that this is not the rule in real neurons, certainly not in large and complex neurons such as the pyramidal neurons of the neocortex or hippocampus, or in the Purkinje cells of the cerebellum. It was pointed out in Section 6.2 that the efficacy of synapses must in some measure depend on their topographical location on the surface of the postsynaptic cell and that the influence of a presynaptic fibre depends also on the number of contacts it makes with the cell. Synapses on the soma, for example, may exert more effective control than synapses located at the terminal branches of the dendrites. The multiple synapses of climbing fibres and pericellular nests confer similar privileges. Nor need it necessarily be the case that all synapses on a neuron have the same degree of plasticity—if indeed they have any.

In this section I shall use the class I model to illustrate a select number of possibilities that arise when a lambda system acts under control of two different input systems with independent signal distributions and different controlling powers over the postsynaptic cells. Three particular cases will be considered.

Case 1

The first case is illustrated in Figure 7.5. The lambda system receives one set of inputs (b) which act on the lambda neurons in the same way as in our previous models. This input system uses complementary coding, and therefore the number of excited input fibres remains constant. A second set of inputs (a_1, a_2, a_3) consists of afferents each of which innervates one specific lambda module only and serves the sole function of controlling the level of excitability of the module in a facilitatory manner. All thresholds in the module are depressed by equal amounts if this fibre is active. Finally we assume that in the absence of this facilitation all net excitations induced in the lambda neurons by inputs to the b fibres remain subliminal.

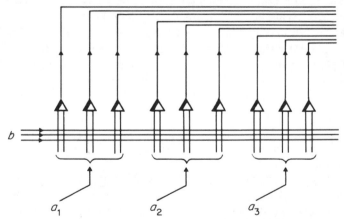

Figure 7.5. Lambda system illustrating response refinement. The response pattern in the a fibres is 'refined' or 'modulated' by the b inputs. For explanation see text

These assumptions give us a system in which the b inputs *modulate* or *refine* the responses arriving along the a fibres in the sense that the identity of the activated a fibres determines the *group* of output fibres in which excitation result, but the synaptic alignments of the lambda neurons within the respective module determines *which* fibre within the respective output group will be the excited one. This is a digital form of response modulation or refinement. It can be improved by learning if we assume that the *b* synapses can undergo learning changes in the manner discussed in Section 7.3.

It is important to realize, therefore, that even in the digital aspect of brain function (with which this chapter is mainly concerned) there is a sense in which we can talk about the 'modulation' or 'refinement' of particular reactions.

The physiological implications of the above assumptions would naturally depend on the exact type of lambda system concerned (cf. Models I, II and III, Section 7.2). In Chapter 8 we shall meet evidence which suggests that in the actual structures of the brain the type of group-facilitation we have envisaged above takes the form of processes which facilitate the information-transfer capacity of the group rather than its overall firing probabilities.

Case 2

The second case is based on a similar type of organization. The essentials of this imaginary configuration are shown in Figure 7.6. Two lambda systems are envisaged (*A* and *B*) in which the outputs of the first act on the lambda modules of the second in the same manner as in the previous case, except that we shall make one additional assumption: when the synaptic potency distribution of a *B* neuron is fully aligned on a given input pattern to the *b* fibres, this neuron will discharge even in the absence of facilitation by the *a* fibre innervating its module.

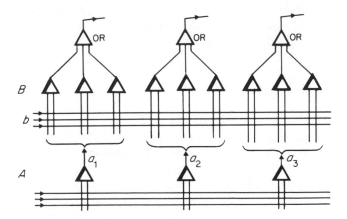

Figure 7.6. Lambda system illustrating the process of 'adequate stimulus substitution'

In consequence of the convergent OR gates shown the synaptic alignments of the B neurons have no effect on the nature of the final outputs of the combined systems. However, on the assumptions we have made, repeated trials under conditions of positive reinforcement enable stimuli applied to the B system to come to *substitute* for stimuli applied to the A system as adequate releasers of particular responses. Let S_A and S_B denote particular patterns of inputs applied to system A and B respectively. Assume that S_A elicits discharges in a particular set of a fibres. Each activated a fibre causes one or more B neurons to fire in the associated B module (depending on the exact type of lambda system envisaged) and thus elicits an output from the associated OR gate. If S_B is consistently paired with S_A the responding B neurons gradually align on S_B. On our assumptions the time must then come when S_B suffices to trigger the same B neurons even in the absence of facilitation from below, i.e. in the absence of S_A.

This hypothetical mechanism has an obvious resemblance to *conditioning*. But to avoid making rash generalizations I prefer to use the neutral phrase *adequate stimulus substitution* for the effects we have here imagined. Note that the a fibres are specifically related to individual groups of B neurons and that their effect in each associated group is that of a locally uniform excitability control. Such facilities for adequate stimulus substitution are particularly important when the b inputs are of a 'global' or 'contextual' type which reflects a wide range of possible input conditions or, for example, the general context in which a particular response occurs. As we shall see later, there are many aspects of learning in which it is important that a response which becomes established to a particular stimulus configuration in a particular set of circumstances should progressively be able to generalize to a wider range of input conditions or to alternative sets of circumstances. We shall see that to form internal representations of external objects or events the brain needs mechanisms through which 'the context in which an internal reaction is consistently triggered by specific stimuli can eventually come to substitute as adequate releaser of the reaction.

Case 3

The third hypothetical case is a special version of the last system. In this new system each a fibre acts only on a single neuron of the B system (Figure 7.7) and we assume that its connection with this neuron is such that activity in the a fibre invariably forces discharges in the respective B neuron. We can imagine these fibres forming pericellular nests around their B cells or engaging them in the manner of climbing fibres (Section 6.2). This forcing function is symbolized in the diagram by an arrow to the 'soma' of the B neuron. To distinguish this case from the previous one we shall say that the adequate stimulus substitution here results through *forced acquisition*.

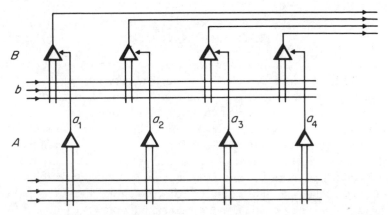

Figure 7.7. Adequate stimulus substitution through 'forced acquisition'

The lambda systems envisaged in the three hypothetical systems introduced in this section may function along the lines of any one of the three models discussed in Section 7.2. But, as was mentioned at the time, a Model III system cannot function unless supported by auxiliary inputs of the kind illustrated in the systems outlined above.

Looking back over these systems we note that

(i) the synapses of the b inputs were assumed to undergo learning changes; the adaptive scope of the B system therefore depends on the possible variety of the b inputs;

(ii) the synapses of the a inputs undergo no learning changes;

(iii) the effect of the a inputs was taken to be either a local facilitatory one or a direct forcing one which compelled responses in the postsynaptic cell concerned (cf. Figure 7.7).

These contrasting features assume particular significance in some of the systems we shall use as illustrative models later on. On the basis of these models we may distinguish three particular categories of inputs which will be called 'contextual', 'biasing' and 'forcing' inputs respectively.

By *contextual* inputs I mean inputs similar to those assumed for the b fibres in the above examples. They have a high variety and enter through synapses which can undergo enduring changes during learning. In some cases their main function is to await assimilation as adequate stimulus substitutes for excitations arriving through the biasing or forcing fibres (see below).

By *biasing inputs* I mean inputs which have a local facilitatory action and enter through synapses which undergo no learning changes (similar to the a fibres in Figures 7.5 and 7.6). *Forcing inputs* are similar to biasing inputs except that they can force discharges in the neurons on which they impinge (Figure 7.7).

7.5 THE RECOGNITION AND REPRODUCTION OF TEMPORAL SEQUENCES

In Section 7.2 we saw how powerful an instrument of dynamic control *negative* feedback loops can become when they take the form of recurrent inhibition in input sharing systems. The *positive* feedback loop, too, has contributions to make which exceed those that are immediately obvious. One obvious capacity of positive feedback loops is to re-excite the structures in which they originate, thus producing reverberation and a state of excitation which outlasts the stimulus that triggered it. This may be a condition of many brain functions. A short stimulus applied to the reticular formation and lasting no longer than one millisecond can cause potential changes in the cortex lasting as long as one second. The brainstem and limbic system appear to play a particularly important role in the mechanisms on which the brain must depend if the experience of a short stimulus is to trigger patterns of behaviour which extend over significant periods of time. If a transection is made at the intercollicular level, for example, the emotive reaction to a brief painful stimulus cannot outlast the duration of the stimulus. A strong case can also be made out for the view that reverberation of one kind or another bridges the gap between the occurrence of an event and its final registration in the memory systems of the brain.

These are questions of gross organization to which we must return later. Meanwhile there are possibilities to be considered which relate to the fine organization of brain structures and which are not always fully appreciated. The most important one of these concerns the power of positive feedback loops to yield networks which can distinguish between different *temporal* sequences of events, as distinct from the merely *spatial* patterns which we have considered so far.

Despite their extensive capabilities the lambda models we introduced above are still deficient in one essential respect. They can only learn to discriminate between different spatial patterns of inputs, whereas many of the most important capabilities of the nervous system depend on its power to distinguish between different temporal patterns as well. It is therefore important to realize that the addition of positive feedback loops allows the lambda configuration to be extended in a manner which removes this limitation.

The function of recognizing a particular temporal sequence of inputs must not be confused with the function of temporal summation. In temporal summation, X followed by Y elicits the same response as Y followed by X, whereas in the recognition of a temporal sequence the *order* in which the inputs occur is critical. However, to the extent to which temporal sequence recognition requires a neural mechanism which can convert a temporal pattern of inputs into a distinctive spatial pattern, temporal summation is likely to enter into the process at one stage or another.

As our main interest at present lies in the adaptive plasticity of the nervous system, the only forms of temporal sequence recognition relevant in the present context are those acquired by learning. We are not here interested in stereotyped networks in which (say) neuron *A* fires only if neuron *B* is excited before neuron *C* but not vice versa. And we must reject from the start any hypothesis that the recognition of the many types of temporal sequences on which certain powers of the brain critically depend can be accounted for in terms of such preformed networks. The assumption that for any combination and permutation in the sequences of inputs that may occur in any particular sequence of events there exists some innate neural chain in the brain which has a wired-in responsiveness to just that particular order of events must be ruled out on account of the obviously astronomical demands it would make on the number of such chains required to meet all possible contingencies. Far from being the simplest hypothesis it would in fact be the most complex and unattractive one to pursue. A more reasonable hypothesis is to assume that the brain is not prewired to detect every possible combination and permutation of inputs that *might* occur in temporal sequences of one kind or another, but that it learns to recognize the temporal sequences that *do* occur by forming patterns of connectivities characteristic of those sequences as and when they occur.

By introducing some form of *associative feedback* into the lambda systems in a way which I shall illustrate presently we can make these systems achieve just that. The process requires first a conversion of temporal patterns to spatial patterns and then a system for classifying and recognizing these spatial patterns.

A simple lambda configuration capable of converting temporal patterns of events into spatial patterns is shown in Figure 7.8. The contingent, e.g.

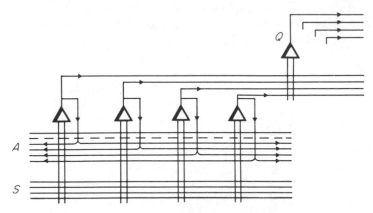

Figure 7.8. Segment of lambda system capable of translating distinctive *temporal* patterns of inputs into distinctive *spatial* patterns of outputs. For explanation see text

sensory, input channels (S) are here supplemented by 'associative feedback' channels (A) which consist of branches of recurrent collaterals of the axons of the lambda neurons.

In consequence of this arrangement the synaptic excitation received by each lambda neuron depends not only on the sensory input but also on which lambda neuron was the last to discharge—provided, of course, we assume that this discharge either left a trace at all the synapses of the recurrent collaterals of the discharging neuron or that the discharge itself was reverberatory in consequence of the positive feedback loops the system contains. If during learning any given lambda neuron aligns its synaptic potency distribution on a particular input configuration, e.g. on a sensory input S' and the traces left by the previous discharges of a lambda neuron X', it acquires maximum sensitivity for S' only in a sequence of events in which S' is preceded by the discharges of X', i.e. by the stimuli on which X' is aligned. In consequence the output patterns of the lambda system will tend to become distinctive not only of the sensory inputs occurring but also of the temporal order in which they occur. A temporal pattern has been converted into a spatial pattern. The outputs from this system might then be fed into a second lambda system Q (Figure 7.8) capable of forming synaptic traces lasting long enough to register the characteristic spatial distribution of a temporal sequence of lambda neurons firing in the primary system. As the lambda neurons of Q align on such specific input patterns (and traces) this system comes to yield output patterns which are specific to particular temporal sequences of inputs to the primary system. In other words, Q can learn to discriminate between specific temporal sequences of inputs to the primary system and it can learn to attach specific responses to them. The system requires that the temporary excitation of a synapse can leave enduring traces. But, since it is known that a transmitter substance like acetylchol may have decay times extending over seconds or even minutes, this is not an unrealistic assumption to make.

By virtue of its positive feedback loops a simple lambda system of this type could also function as a *reproductive memory system*. Suppose that in a series of positively reinforced trials the input patterns S_p, S_q, S_r, S_s (when occurring in that order), become established as triggers for the lambda neurons L_u, L_v, L_w, L_x. Then if we imagine the threshold of all lambda neurons to be lowered by some agency so that they could fire in response to the activation of the associative feedback channels only, the triggering of L_u by any event could release the whole sequence L_u to L_x as an independent chain reaction. We shall meet more powerful systems of this type presently.

A combination of associative feedback and forced acquisition (Section 7.4) can give a reproductive memory system which functions on two levels instead of one. The schematic is given in Figure 7.9. The responses of a normal lambda system A are taken out via forcing fibres (ff) which activate the associated neurons in lambda system B. This second system is a purely associative feedback system: in positively reinforced trials any activated neuron in the *B* system aligns its synaptic potency distribution on the concomitant dendritic inputs, and these are here determined by the *B* neurons that fired before.

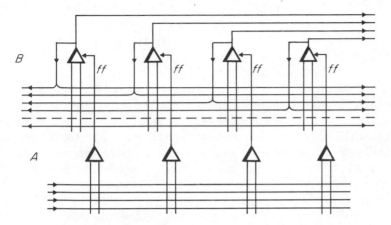

Figure 7.9. Two-tier reproductive memory system

In consequence of this arrangement, if the thresholds of the upper system are lowered by some extraneous factor, a learnt sequence of responses can come to run its course spontaneously and without the instrumentality of system *A*, provided the first responses of the sequence are somehow triggered to start with (by *A* or otherwise). A system of this kind was used by the writer in a small electronic model in which a mechanical 'rat' was first trained on a small maze under guidance of 'sensory' inputs identifying the choice points of the maze. The device could then learn to run the same maze 'blindfold', i.e. without any sensory identification of the choice points it had reached. The 'rat' could be trained either by trial and error learning or by being taken along the correct route and learning the correct responses in one single guided tour through the method of forced acquisition.

In this system it is easy to visualize a state of affairs in which a lowering of the thresholds of the upper level results in a triggered chain release (via the associative feedback channels) of any sequential pattern of responses which the lower level neurons may have come to attach to a given sequence of sensory inputs during previous learning. Since this triggered chain-release of the response sequence may run a faster course than the sequence of sensory inputs that would normally have released the responses, a system of this kind may also be visualized in an important *anticipatory function*: each response now anticipates the sensory input that would normally have released it.

If we imagine the outputs of the upper system to have no direct motor effects but merely to be of the nature of internal responses with no more than potential motor effects, we can picture temporal association networks of this kind in yet another role, viz. as networks suitable for anticipating the outcome of a behaviour sequence before the agent embarks on the sequence. In the temporal association system of Figure 7.9 a chain reaction of the upper system would be tantamount to an 'imaginary' run through a given behaviour sequence, and it is not impossible to picture an arrangement whereby the decision to embark on the sequence is influenced by the terminal events of such an imaginary run.

One essential point of detail remains to be mentioned. The simple schematics of Figures 7.8 and 7.9 are obviously too simple in one respect. If the associative feedback channels are to accomplish the task we have allotted to them, the recurrent collaterals concerned must have a very wide lateral spread. In turn, each lambda neuron must be reached by the recurrent collaterals of a large number of other lambda neurons belonging to the same system. And yet we are postulating that discharges in only a small fraction of these can be sufficient to cause the neuron to fire provided it has an appropriate synaptic potency distribution. It is difficult to see how this could become a realistic proposition except on the assumption that there exists an *intermediate coding network* between the recurrent collaterals of the (upper level) lambda neurons and the inputs to these neurons which distributes the excitation of each recurrent collateral over a characteristic set of numerous input channels. In the sequel I shall take some such coding system for granted in all associative feedback circuits.

With this section we conclude an important stage in our programme. We shall see presently that the lambda configurations introduced in Sections 7.2, 7.4 and in the present section suffice to model a wide range of network capabilities which are of particular interest in connection with the higher functions of the brain. Some of these capabilities will be discussed in the remainder of this chapter. Others will be added in Chapters 9 and 10. The following is a review of the basic lambda configurations we have envisaged.

We began with three models of learning systems which illustrated the latent capabilities of *recurrent inhibition* (Figure 7.2(a)) and *forward inhibition* (Figure 7.2(b)) in input-sharing systems (Models I, II and III, Section 7.2). We then added certain types of auxiliary input to these basic systems and arrived at elementary models for *response modulation* (Figure 7.5) and *adequate stimulus substitution* (Figures 7.6 and 7.7). Finally we added positive feedback and arrived at systems for *temporal sequence recognition* (Figure 7.8) and *reproductive memory* (Figure 7.9).

The reader should note that the elaborations and refinements we have here added to the basic lambda configuration do not depend on whether this configuration functions according to Model I, II or III.

7.6   REPRODUCTIVE MEMORY CIRCUITS AND 'IMAGINATION'

At no point in this volume will it be suggested that the brain is just a large assembly of either simple or compound lambda systems, but in exploring the possibilities inherent in comparatively simple networks of this kind it is none the less profitable to consider one or two particularly suggestive possibilities.

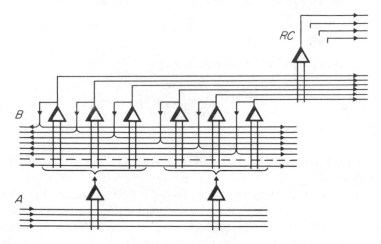

Figure 7.10. Alternative system for the registration and subsequent recognition of distinctive temporal sequences of inputs, i.e. of the serial order in which inputs occur

A simple hypothetical arrangement in which one lambda system (*B*) modulates the responses of another (*A*) was discussed in Section 7.4 (Figure 7.5). A particular application of this method yields an alternative system for the registration and subsequent recognition of temporal sequences (Figure 7.10). In this arrangement the *B* inputs consist of an associative feedback system from the *B* outputs. If the *B* inputs leave a trace of sufficient duration the system integrates the *A* outputs with signals reflecting the temporal sequence in which the *A* neurons are activated, since responses of the lower system will be treated differently in the upper system according to the temporal order in which they occur. For example if the *A* neurons fire in a regular sequence *X*, *Y*, *Z*, *W*, this will be registered in the *B* system by a different set of neurons than a sequence *Z*, *Y*, *X*, *W*, despite the identity of the *A* neurons concerned.

A special application of this principle is shown in Figure 7.11. In this system the neurons of row *A* receive both sensory (contingent) inputs and demand inputs. All *A* neurons shown belong to the same lambda module. The identity of the *A* neuron responding to any particular combination of these stimuli determines whether the final output of the system is O_1 or O_2. The outputs

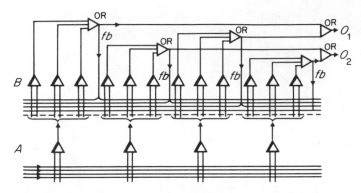

Figure 7.11. Reproductive memory system capable of registering specific stimulus–response routines

(many more in any real system, of course) determine the motor response of the organism. But the identity of the response-mediating neuron within the respective group of lambda neurons in row B is determined by the temporal order in which the stimulus–response combinations occur. For the dendritic inputs to the B system are derived from feedback fibres (fb) each of which is activated by a particular stimulus–response combination. Hence which B neuron responds in any group facilitated from below depends on the stimulus–response combination that went before. Any particular *temporal* sequence of particular stimulus–response combinations, therefore, comes to be registered in the B system as a distinct *spatial* pattern of responding neurons.

This spatial differentiation has important applications. It lends itself for the anticipatory release of responses in a learnt stimulus–response routine as a function of the *S–R combinations* that went before. Above all it lends itself as a reproductive memory circuit capable of recalling such routines.

This system has also been used in one of the mechanical 'rats' designed by the writer. Assume that the system has learnt a particular routine, a maze-routine for example, and that the lambda neurons concerned have aligned their synaptic potency distributions on the dendritic inputs consistently occurring in the routine. Then any threshold depression of the B system which enables these neurons to fire even in the absence of facilitation from below, will permit chain reactions in the B row which recreate the responses occurring in the routine in the correct order and in the absence of sensory inputs to the system. Moreover, the system can assimilate a number of different routines even if the same stimulus–response combination occurs in more than one routine—provided always that there is a sufficiency of B neurons to accommodate the different possibilities. Thus, when given a particular starting position and command input (relating to the goal to be reached in the maze) the mechanical 'rat' could run 'blindfold' through the sequence of responses appropriate to the maze routine concerned.

This is a reproductive memory system of a particularly important type. Since the identity of a responding B neuron is determined both by a particular stimulus–response combination and the temporal sequence in which this occurs, the spatial pattern of outputs from the B neurons in a triggered chain reaction *maps the entire drama* of the stimulus–response sequence, and not just the temporal sequence of either the stimuli or the responses.

An interesting alternative is one in which the demand signals are removed from the lower level and added to the upper level. This entails extending the B level groups facilitated by the A neurons, as the choice of responses must in part be determined by the demand signals. In this system a chain discharge triggered in the upper system can be changed in its course by a change in demand signals even while it is in progress. If the overt responses of the system are suppressed the resulting covert 'runs' through the maze can be called *imaginary* runs in a sense more closely related to the common meaning of the term. If the demand signals are freely changed during the triggered discharges the resulting events are not unlike what we mean when we say that someone is imagining walking through a familiar garden. Once again we have the rudiments of a system which can explore the consequences of its actions by means of hypothetical experiments before engaging on them. It is also conceivable that, if the thresholds of the upper system are lowered sufficiently, spontaneous train-discharges may occur which jump from the terminal point of one train to the initial point of any other. This would add an element resembling the free play of the human imagination.

All this, of course, is just playing games—whether, to stir the pot, we actually build such mechanical toys or merely think around them. There are too many options open and we lack the physiological information we would need to decide between them. Nevertheless they are important games to play because they explore possibilities inherent in the basic properties of neurons and so stimulate the formation of hypotheses and the search for the physiological or behavioural data that might decide between alternative possibilities.

The concept of memory is often vague and ambiguous. In a broad sense any lasting change in the nervous system resulting from experience and affecting subsequent behaviour may be called a memory change. Any redistribution of the synaptic potencies changes in the lambda neurons of the kind we have considered so far qualifies as a memory change in that sense. But in the manner in which temporal sequences of events may become registered in the upper network of the system shown in Figure 7.11 we have a new form of information storage, and one which conforms more closely to the narrower concept of memory in which the term implies capabilities of structured retrieval and playback of events experienced before. It is a reproductive and particulate memory as distinct from the merely cumulative changes involved in learning appropriate

214 Logic of the Living Brain

responses. We have the equivalent of playback, of course, in the triggered chain discharges of the upper system of Figure 7.11 which we mentioned at the time. It may be objected that this playback in the form of triggered chain discharges in the upper system would not amount to a structured recall of the original sensory inputs. But this objection overlooks the fact that no memory recall ever amounts to a recreation of the original sensory inputs. It never reactivates the respective peripheral receptors. What it does reactivate is the set of internal analysing and categorizing reactions which those sensory inputs elicited at the time of the original events.

An interesting problem arises in connection with the speed of alignment that should be postulated for the upper level units. How many times must the same temporal sequence of inputs be presented to the upper level network before full alignment of the respective lambda neurons is achieved? If a large number of repetitions are required the system loses its usefulness for the quick registration of brief events. But if we insist on only a few repetitions or even single trial learning, the storage capacity of the system will soon be exhausted. This illustrates a real dilemma.

On the evidence it seems that the nervous system resolves this dilemma by having both types of registration, fast and slow: one with high-speed alignments but short expectation of life for the registered patterns, the other depending on repetition but achieving greater permanency. In Man at any rate there exists a *short-term* memory side by side with a *long-term* memory. The former is of the order of minutes and is unstable in the sense, for instance, that traumatic events like concussion may irretrievably destroy it. This is not the case with long-term memory which may indeed become inaccessible for shorter or longer periods but is never totally destroyed.

In the lambda model both types of memory could be accommodated within the same system if we assume that the initial alignment of the neurons is unstable and decays with time unless it is consolidated by repetition. In reality this repetition could result simply because attention remains riveted on the same stimuli over an adequate period of time. Or it could occur in consequence of reverberation and playback.

The idea that the recollection of past events involves facilitated chain discharges finds support in Penfield's well known observations on patients with a past history of epilepsy. Penfield found that in these patients electrical stimulation of the temporal lobes sometimes forces into consciousness detailed recollections of past events, and these then roll off in strict temporal order. When the electrode is withdrawn they stop. Absent from the recollections are the sensations ignored at the occurrence of the original events. Presumably the stimulation did two things: it triggered the chain discharges and at the same time maintained thresholds at the low levels required for their continuation.

7.7   THE PRINCIPLE OF REAFFERENCE

The power of the brain to recognize not only spatial distributions of inputs but also the temporal sequence in which particular inputs may occur is undoubtedly one of its most fundamental qualities. This is evident from our own ability to recognize spoken words, melodies, gestures etc. But the matter goes very much further than this. The inputs that form the elements of a temporal sequence may be wholly exteroceptive in origin, as in the examples just quoted. However, they may also contain movement information and temporal sequences of this kind take us into a realm of cognitive processes of the utmost importance.

Of such things as colour, heat, pressure, smell etc. we may say that we have a raw sensation in the sense that we have peripheral receptors which are sensitive to these things. But we have no such raw sensations, for instance, of the shape of an object, of its position in space or of its hardness or elasticity. We discover properties of this kind by evaluating the transformations that our sensations undergo when we move, or when we act on the object or environment in certain ways. Thus we discover the elasticity of a rubber band by extending it and noting how the muscular effort varies with the extension achieved. We discover the hardness of an object by pressing on it, we detect its weight by lifting it. A blind person discovers the shape of an object by exploring its contours with the finger tips and, although a seeing person acquires a more direct awareness of shape, in the formative stages of vision contour-following has a distinctive part to play and in the later stages it probably remains the ultimate test for the correct assessment of a shape by other means (Chapter 9).

Similarly, we discover the spatial relations prevailing in our environment through the way in which our sensory inputs transform as we move our eyes, head or body. And even when we have some additional source of information, such as ocular accommodation and binocular parallax, we learn to interpret that information only with reference to what in effect we discover independently through the way our sensory inputs transform in response to our movements. This is not surprising, seeing that the final test for the efficacy of our mental processes must be whether they enable us to anticipate such transformations correctly. The now acknowledged role of expectation in the activities of the brain has highlighted the importance of these factors.

It may be urged that an object is the sum of its properties. So how does the system know that it is experiencing an object Q before it has any properties for it? If it does not, why does it attend to Q and channel the inputs into the correct place to build up the property? I do not see any difficulty here. It is the question whether the hen came before the egg. It is easy to imagine that in early infancy we initially attend only to raw sensations: mere sounds, patches of light and dark, tactile stimuli etc. As the result of exploration and experience expectations build up as to how stimuli change as the result of movement. Thus properties begin to build up. As properties link up objects build up. As the objects gain control over attention more properties can build up, and so on.

The principle of extracting information about the environment through self-induced movements is known (after von Holst and Mittelstaedt[114]) as the *principle of reafference*. The information is extracted from neural excitations following stimulation that is systematically dependent on movements initiated by the sensing organism. This is undoubtedly the most significant process of achieving object-reference in the higher organisms. However, the method is sometimes obscured by the fact that although our first discernment of a property may be based on active explorations and on the reafference principle, we may later on learn to infer the property from instantaneous cues. This appears to be the case, for example, in the mechanism for visual shape recognition.

The principle of reafference finds its most sophisticated realization in the operation methods of the experimental sciences. In scientific experiments we discover the properties of an object by systematically interfering with the object, subsequently integrating information relating to the nature of the interference with information relating to its observable effects. Activities like searching, exploring, probing, scrutinizing, scanning etc. are specifically designed to produce reafferent sequences of sensory inputs which contain the clues required by the nervous system to achieve the necessary object-reference in the behavioural responses it controls. We may distinguish two main types of exploratory activities which provide the nervous system with such clues.

In the first method the subject allows its exploratory movements to be guided by the object to be explored and registers the nature and temporal sequences of the resulting movements. The necessary clues about the object property are then contained primarily in the movements required to maintain some particular relation to the object. When, for example, we discover the shape of an object by tactile exploration the clues are contained in the sequences of movements which the object permits subject to the condition that light tactile contact is maintained with the surface of the object throughout the palpation. This information, of course, may be supplemented by registering the special landmarks (corners, protrusions etc.) we meet in the course of the exploration. The same applies to visual shape recognition by contour-following. Here the overriding condition is that the line of vision remains locked on the contour.

In the second method the exploratory movements actively interfere with the object or situation to be explored, or with its sensory projections, thus effecting a transformation of the sensory inputs derived from the object or situation. The brain then registers the nature of the transformation and evaluates this information in conjunction with information relating to the nature of the interfering movements. We meet examples of this in everyday life when we discover the elasticity of an object by bending or stretching it, its weight by lifting it, its inertia by moving it, its stability by disturbing it, its force by resisting it etc. This is a particularly important application of the reafference principle—and the one I shall follow up in the next section.

7.8   THE RECOGNITION OF PROPERTIES

In this section I want to construct a simple model which illustrates the application of the reafference principle according to the second method outlined above and which helps us to see how information about properties or relations in the physical world may be extracted from the sensory inflow and stored in the nervous system.

We have met the principle of reafference as the main instrument through which the organism can detect object properties which transcend the immediate evidence of the senses. We have also seen that the principle is needed to check the significance of the immediate evidence furnished by the senses.

In dealing with physical properties or relations we are dealing with ways of classifying objects. In the reafference case we are dealing with the classification of objects according to the manner in which they (or their sensory projections) transform in response to a particular class of actions. In general a class of exploratory movements which suffices to detect a particular property of this kind is specific to the nature of the property concerned (stretching or bending for elasticity, pressing for hardness, contour-following for shape etc.).

The neural mechanisms required to form an internal representation of a given property must begin by registering what members of the appropriate class of movements effect what kind of transformation of the object or of its sensory projections. A simple model, formulated in terms of discrete elements, will show what this implies and what type of network organization can store information of this nature.

Suppose that to represent the property P of an object Q the brain must register what transformation a variable E undergoes in response to a particular (discrete) set of exploratory actions $A_1, A_2, \ldots, A_n$. E need not be a simple variable. It could be a complex feature of Q or of the sensory projection of Q, or of particular experiences we incur in handling Q. But we shall assume that it is an instantly recognizable variable in the sense that the brain already has the power to form internal representations of its current values. Let e_1, $e_2, \ldots$ be the internal representations of the values $E_1, E_2, \ldots$. For simplicity we assume that the actions $A_1, A_2, \ldots, A_n$ form a discrete set and that each action is defined (and internally represented) not by the movements executed but by the commanded end-states of the exploring action-system. Let a_1, $a_2, \ldots, a_n$ be the internal representations of these commanded end-states. Finally we assume that the property P is adequately determined by the transformations the internal representations of E undergo in consequence of actions defined by the specified internal representations of A. In other words, we assume that the property P is adequately determined by the function

$$e = f(a)$$

As mentioned in Section 2.2, the internal representation of such a functional relationship (in the mathematical sense) must be envisaged as a set of simultaneous neural events which can be mapped on an adequate sample of the set of ordered pairs of elements which the function denotes. In the present case this calls for

  (i) the internal representation of an adequate sample of pertinent combinations of the variables e and a, as experienced during the investigation of the object Q;

 (ii) the formation of associative connections which eventually enable this set of individual representations (or any set of neural events which can be mapped on them) to be activated simultaneously.

A representative section of a type of network configuration which could achieve these results is shown in Figure 7.12. Row A consists of neurons which function in the manner of logical AND gates. Each of these receives one input which is specific to a particular value of the e variable and one which is specific to a particular value of the a variable. Each of these neurons, therefore, discharges upon the occurrence of a particular combination $a_x e_y$.

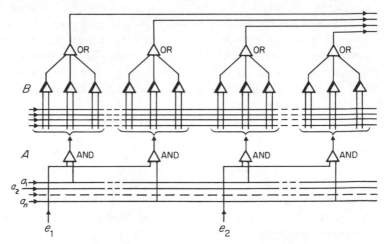

Figure 7.12. Segment of elementary network suitable for the recognition of properties on the reafference principle

Row B consists of a stimulus-substituting network of the type previously discussed in connection with Figure 7.6 (Section 7.4). The simple operational principles of this network were given at the time. The upshot of this mechanism is that although initially the outputs O are solely determined by the outputs of row A, in due course they become conditioned to any regularly coincident stimulus pattern in the horizontal inputs to row B. In other words, the horizontal inputs to B are grafted on the effector arcs of row A.

Finally we assume that the horizontal inputs to row B consist of stimulus patterns which are specific to the object the organism explores, in this case object Q. In due course, therefore, the perception of Q comes to act as an adequate trigger for any B neuron which during learning came to respond in consequence of the facilitation its module received from the associated A neuron, i.e. from an *experienced* combination of a and e. Thus when learning is complete the perception of Q releases simultaneously a set of outputs O which represents the experienced samples of the ordered pairs of elements denoted by the function $e = f(a)$.

This set of outputs is distinctive of the property P provided only that the registered sample of experienced combinations $a_x e_y$ is sufficiently representative of the function $e = f(a)$ as a whole to prevent confusion with similar functions. *Thus a neural representation of the property P can now be triggered without the subject having to perform any of the exploratory activities through which the property was detected in the first instance.*

On our assumptions it is possible also for other objects to come to elicit the same final output pattern if they have the same property. If each B module contains an adequate number of lambda neurons, there is scope for different neurons within each module to align their synaptic potencies on different stimulus configurations in the horizontal input fibres. How many such associations can be accommodated within each B module would depend both on the number of lambda neurons per B module and on the exact mode of operation of the lambda systems concerned. The most economical system would be one operating according to our lambda model type I (Section 7.2), since this permits only one lambda neuron per module to respond at any one time and thus can accommodate the greatest variety of appropriately assimilated patterns of B inputs.

Although the above neuronal model is only a simple paradigm it makes some important points and we can also use it to illustrate a number of important concepts.

In consequence of the fact that a variety of different objects (having the same property P) can elicit the same final output pattern, the outputs of the system amount to a classification of the perceived objects according to properties revealed by the exploratory actions $A_1, \ldots, A_n$.

The synaptic alignments which occur in the B system during the learning stage constitute what may be called a *latent representation* of the property P. By way of contrast the actual set of discharges which the perception of the object subsequently elicits in the output channels O, may be called the *active* representation of P. Thus the *active* representations which the perception of objects comes to elicit in this system are based on the *latent* representations which have formed as the result of prior experience. The latent representations are the *stored* form of the information extracted from the prior experiences. The *activation* of any latent representation by the subsequent perception of an object amounts to a *categorizing reaction* or *classificatory response* in respect of the object. This is the *read-out* of the memory system, if you like.

The activated representation of the property P in our system may also be said to amount to an *expectation* of the way the variable E transforms in consequence of the action $A_1, A_2, \ldots, A_n$. The use of 'expectation' here conforms to the objective sense in which this term may be understood (Chapter 5). 'Expectation' in this sense denotes a state of adaptedness which matches the fact that in the circumstances particular events are consistently followed by another particular set of events—in this case that particular actions performed in relation to Q consistently result in particular transformations of certain sensory inputs or internal representations. The pattern of discharging OR gates in system B is the neural correlate of the aggregate of expectations of how E transforms in consequence of actions $A_1, \ldots, A_n$. It is the neural correlate of a what-leads-to-what expectancy which has been formed as the result of past experience and against which current inputs may be matched when we experiment with similar objects.

In this example we have assumed for simplicity that each value of E and A is represented by activity in only one specific e and a fibre respectively. This is not a necessary condition. The network could function equally if each value of E and A were represented by a specific spatial distribution of excitations over the set of e fibres and a fibres respectively. This indeed would be the more economical method. In binary coding and using complementary innervation, 10 e (or a) fibres could signal 2^5 different values of E (or A) and the neurons of row B could assimilate up to 2^{20} different properties.

It should be noted that owing to the wired-in, cross-modal specificity of the AND gates assumed in our model the original a or e information can be recovered from the outputs of the system.

It is also worth noting that the functions of the AND gates shown in our model might conceivably be performed by the dendritic apparatus of the B neurons, so that no separate neurons, no A system, would be required to discharge these particular functions. However, since the primary purpose of these models is to help us visualize the logical significance of certain operations and to illustrate simple ways in which neurons may accomplish these operations, we shall continue to assume separate units for these functions.

Finally we must note that the system of Figure 7.12 could feed into a further learning system in which single cells become selectively responsive to particular patterns of outputs from the B system so that eventually the presence of the property P is indicated not by a specific pattern of outputs, but by exclusive activity in one or more final output fibres.

7.9   THE RECOGNITION OF RELATIONS

Many of the things that have been said above about the internal representation of those properties of objects of which we have no raw sensation apply also to the internal representation of *relations* between two or more objects. In a sense the internal representations that occupied us in the last section were in fact representations of relations—e.g. the relation $e=f(a)$. In essence, therefore, we have already covered the main principles governing the internal representation of external relations. In this section I want to illustrate the application of these principles with the aid of a few rather more specific examples, and also make a number of additional points.

To say that a particular 'relation' exists between two objects means formally that the objects belong to a particular class of ordered pairs of objects. Whereas, for example the *property* 'green' denotes a particular class of either single or plural objects, the *relation* 'to the left of' denotes a particular class of *pairs* of objects which are *ordered* in the sense that if the members of any pair are interchanged in any representation (symbolic, physiological or otherwise) of the relation, the pair will cease to belong to the respective class (unless the relation is symmetrical).

Any operation which consistently generates a particular class of ordered pairs generates a relation. Thus if the eye is successively trained on each of a given set of objects and at each stage can select another object by moving upwards, a set of ordered pairs of objects is generated which represents the relation *below* between the first and second member of each pair and the relation *above* between the second and first member of each pair. We could indeed say that the very first time this was done by any observer the relations 'above' and 'below' were *generated* by the upward movements of the eyes (and the converse relations by downward movements). If we now take this relation as given and if then a second observer learns from the first observer to classify objects in the same way we may then say that the second used the movement of the eyes to *detect* the given relation. Hence the question whether particular operations 'generate' or 'detect' relations is merely a question of context which we can safely ignore in the matter we have in hand. Nor need we become embroiled in philosophical arguments about the intrinsic nature of 'relations'. It suffices to accept that the world is such that the objects it contains can be paired off in a multitude of different ways.

Relations, of course, may exist between more than two objects. Thus the relation 'between' denotes a class of ordered triplets (of which two can be interchanged without prejudice to their class-membership).

Relations may associate types of elements belonging to very different categories. On the one hand, for example, the word 'relation' may be used to refer to physical associations such as between stimuli differing in size, intensity or position. On the other hand it may refer to conceptual associations such as associations between synonyms and antonyms. In this case the 'operations' which generate the ordered pairs are complex conceptual operations involving comparisons between the meaning of sentences when one word is substituted for another. However, in the present context, we can confine the discussion to physical relations. The most important of these are the spatial relations on which our internal representations of the outer world critically depend.

In the laboratory the power of a subject to discern particular relations is commonly studied in terms of *transposition phenomena*. By transposition we mean the transfer of a response from one set of stimuli to another which apparently results from learning to respond to particular relations or sets of relations pertaining to the stimuli. Shape transposition is a particularly important example. Many investigators work with unidimensional relations. The most common type of problem used is the 'two-stimulus' problem. In a typical experiment of this type the subject first learns to choose one stimulus of a pair and is then tested with a pair which differ in absolute qualities but in which the relation between the stimuli is the same as in the training stimuli. A typical pair, for instance, might consist of two shapes of which one is always larger than the other.

To learn to discern a particular relation is to learn to select and order pairs of objects in a consistent and appropriate manner—or, if the pairs of objects are selected by the experimenter, to learn to order the pairs consistently and in the appropriate manner. What this implies in precise neurophysiological terms, of course, must depend on the type of relation concerned.

In a number of simple spatial relations ('above', 'below', 'to the left of', 'to the right of', 'inside', 'outside' etc.) the appropriate ordering may require no more than that the subject should be able to alternate attention between the two objects and register the nature of the actions (e.g. eye movements) associated with this 'comparison behaviour'.

The basic logical operations the neural networks must perform in this case are again similar to those we discussed in Section 7.8. But the action variable now has fewer relevant values. In learning to discern the relations 'X above Y' or 'Y below X', for example, the only relevant values would be 'moving eyes upward', 'moving eyes downward'. The sensory input variable also has only two relevant values: 'perceiving object X as a centralized image' and 'perceiving object Y as a centralized image'. The brain then has to register first that fixation on Y after X is conditional on a downward movement of the eyes while fixation on X after Y is conditional on an upward movement. Foremost, therefore, the brain would need a set of four AND gates in each of which discharges are conditional on one of the four possible combinations of a relevant action value with a relevant sensation value respectively. Two of these would then be activated by experiencing this particular relation. Secondly, the brain would need a stimulus substitution network, similar to that of row *B* (Figure 7.12), in which the simultaneous perception of the two objects, regardless of the point of fixation of the eyes, can be assimilated as an adequate stimulus for triggering a set of neurons associated with the activated AND gates. Thus when learning is complete the excitation of a pattern of outputs representing the relation concerned ceases to be conditional on the prior execution of explicit comparison behaviour. The relation can now be detected instantaneously.

Although the number of relevant values of the action variable and sensation variable is small, it is evident that the complexity and domain of these input variables must be very large if the system is to be able to cope with an adequate variety of relations and possible stimulus objects. The same applies to the number of neurons and number of inputs required in row *B* of the model. In fact it would be misleading to think of the required neural networks simply in terms of enlarged copies of our simple model. Rather, the model of Figure 7.12 should be interpreted as no more than a convenient way of symbolizing in neural terms the logical operations which the internal representations of this type of physical relation require. The actual physiological processes yielding these logical operations may well be dispersed over, or embedded in, complex neural systems extending over extensive regions of the brain.

In many other types of relation it would not be sufficient if the brain merely registers the nature of the actions contained in the overt comparison behaviour. To effect the appropriate ordering of the pairs of objects concerned the brain in addition may have to register specific changes in the quality of the sensory inputs which accompany the alternation of attention between the two objects. It may also have to register changes in stimulus intensity, colour, size of retinal image, distance of object etc. In many of these 'transitional experiences' only the direction of the change has to be registered. Relations like 'larger than', 'brighter than' and 'further than' are typical examples.

A simple way in which this might be achieved would be an arrangement in which the brain forms two reciprocal reactions. One of these is facilitated by the record of the first attended stimulus object in proportion to the intensity (size, distance etc.) of the stimulus, and inhibited by the subsequent perception of the second stimulus object (again in proportion to intensity, size, distance etc.). In the other reaction facilitation and inhibition are reversed. In conjunction with a record of the attentional shift the net excitation resulting in this system would then suffice to order the objects in the appropriate manner along the particular stimulus dimension concerned. The outputs of this system would have to feed into the AND gates we envisaged in our model network.

It is evident from these considerations and simplified examples that the internal representation of diverse physical relations cannot depend on a class of compact and uniform physiological mechanisms. In general it must involve the integrated activity of a number of more or less complex representational

systems operating at different levels of abstraction. Our model merely illustrates the general nature of these interactions. In particular it suggests how
representations which initially depend on explicit acts of comparison between
the two objects by a vigilant and attentive subject may in due course come to
be elicited instantaneously and without prior comparison behaviour. Attention to the parts of the whole formed by the two objects becomes superfluous
in these later stages of training. Thus the trained subject may eventually come
to respond appropriately to the whole without explicit examination of its
parts.

We know, of course, from introspection that relational judgments can be
made without explicit comparison between the stimuli. In the literature this
has often been allowed to obscure the fact that during the initial training
explicit comparisons may be necessary. Indeed it could be argued that they
must occur if the resulting discriminations are to be truly relational and are to
transpose consistently and appropriately to new situations.

It follows that restricting the direct comparison of stimuli in the initial
stages should interfere with relation perception. Since in successive discrimination problems the opportunity to compare stimuli is restricted it follows that
there should be less transposition following successive discrimination training
than following simultaneous discrimination training. The results obtained by
most investigators bear this out. However there are also contradictory data.
In some of these cases the observed transpositions have been explained in
terms of stimulus generalization rather than relation perception.

One point which has clearly emerged in the last two sections is that what we
commonly regard as specific external properties or relations really stand for
unique families of sensory transformations. The nervous system learns to
represent such families by unique patterns of excitations. In particular this
applies to the shape of objects. As the Gibsons have pointed out, the face of a
solid object is usually given to us not as a unique form but as a unique
family of transformations to which the nervous system learns to establish a
unique internal reaction[80]. These transformations may be brought about
through movements executed by the observer, as when we move to inspect an
object from different angles or when the eyes move between two objects
offered for comparison. Or they may occur if the object moves while the observer remains stationary.

I remark on this to remind us that despite the importance of the reafference
principle, passive observation also has a part to play in the classification of
objects. However, in this case too, the nervous system has to register what
transforms into what and in what circumstances. But the circumstances are
not now defined by particular sets of self-induced movements or changes of
attention.

7.10   THE NEURAL REPRESENTATION OF PROPERTIES AND RELATIONS: SUMMARY

The above analysis has been conducted in terms of simple models and 'formal' neurons only. The networks shown were designed only to illustrate the kind of neural operations and connectivities that might yield the type of basic brain functions we are interested in. In fact, *the reader should regard these models as no more than a graphic way of setting out the logical operations required for particular functions in a manner which brings out the possible contributions particular neural properties or connectivities can make towards these functions.* The models have demonstrated how a number of obviously relevant functions can in theory be generated from only a very small set of basic neural properties.

A number of generally valid principles have emerged. The most important of these concern the nature of the internal representation of the properties of external objects and of the relations between such objects or their parts. The kind of physical properties we have in mind in the first instance are attributes of which we have no direct sensations, such as solidity, inertia, hardness, elasticity, shape etc. The most important relations, of course, are the spatial relations between objects or their parts. It does not particularly matter in this context whether we think of shape as a property in its own right or as a set of spatial relations between visually salient elements. What matters is that from either viewpoint shape is given to us as a family of transformations of sensory inputs which satisfy particular conditions.

We have seen that the internal representations of properties and relations may be interpreted as aggregates of expectations concerning the way objects or their sensory projections transform in particular circumstances, especially the way they transform in response to our own movements or comparison behaviours. On our analysis the neural correlate of these expectations in turn consists of neural representations of functional relationships of the type $s = f(m)$, where m here stands for the transformation-controlling circumstances (e.g. self-induced movements and comparison behaviours) and s for the resulting sensory transformations or object transformations.

The question arises what our notion of how the brain forms internal representations of external realities adds to our traditional ideas of the physiological mechanisms that mediate the connection between, on the one hand, the flow of afferent information generated by the stimulus situation and, on the other, the flow of efferent signals which determines our overt responses.

We know that the brain can produce responses which are conditional on the occurrence of particular stimulus configurations in one or more modalities. We also know that in suitable circumstances such responses can subsequently become conditioned to an almost unlimited variety of other stimulus patterns. The results of our analysis suggest that to be able to form internal representations of external properties or relations, the brain must use these powers in respect of particular organizational elements and in a particular manner:

1. It must be able to form internal reactions which are each conditional on the occurrence of a particular combination (m, s) of stimuli (m) representing movements or comparison behaviours and stimuli (s) representing the resulting sensory input transformations (cf. the AND gates in Figure 7.12).
2. These reaction systems must be able to cover an adequate domain of (m, s), i.e. provide for an adequate variety of possible combinations of m and s.
3. Appropriate aggregates of reactions of this kind (i.e. reactions representing samples of the experienced combinations of movements and sensory transformations) must jointly become conditioned to the diverse sensory projections of the objects, events or situations which have the respective property or stand in the respective relation (cf. the upper networks in Figure 7.12).

As our simple paradigm has illustrated, in this manner the sensory projections of an object (event or situation) can come to trigger a pattern of outputs which is a unique representation of the external property or relation. That is to say, we arrive at a pattern of outputs which can be mapped on a representative sample of the ordered pairs of elements denoted by the function $s=f(m)$ which we took to be characteristic of the property or relation concerned (cf. the patterns of outputs of the OR gates in Figure 7.12). This pattern then constitutes an active *neural representation* of the function and thus of the property or relation. The activation of this representation may also be viewed as the activation of the set of *expectations* regarding the way s transforms as a function of m. In this sense, therefore, the sight of an object or set of objects may come to trigger neural events representing expectations which have formed as the result of prior experiences of the object.

It is not difficult to imagine these paradigms to be extended to expectations covering the behaviour of s as a function also of time, e.g. $s=f(m, t)$. The A system of Figure 7.12 would then have to be replaced by networks capable of registering temporal sequences. The type was illustrated in Figure 7.11. We shall meet simple paradigms of this kind when we return to the subject in Chapter 9.

Although these abstract organizational conditions for the neural representation of properties or relations appear to be pretty uniform, they leave room for a great deal of diversity in the manner in which they come to be realized in the brain. A couple of additional examples will serve to illustrate this point.

One of the foremost functions of the visual system is to construct a stable image of the world from the stream of sensory projections that cross the retina as our eyes move in their sockets. The words on this page do not leap about when the reader flicks his eyes across the page. The stable image may be thought of as a stable set of expectations which are aroused by looking at one point of the page and relate to what the eye will see when it looks at any other point. In this case, therefore, our m variable denotes excitations relating to eye-movements and our s variable denotes complex sets of visual stimulations.

Compare this with the expectations which are aroused when I see a ball flying towards me and evaluated as I prepare to catch it. These are no longer expectations of how primary sensory inputs transform in response to primary movements. They are expectations of how a three-dimensional scene will transform in consequence of three-dimensional movements. Our m and s variables now relate to sophisticated internal representations of solid objects, distances, body postures etc.

In concrete terms, therefore, the broad organizational conditions formulated above cover a whole spectrum of cases in which the domain of m and s relates to primary movements and primary sensory inputs at the one extreme and to complex internal representations of body postures or movements and of complex external objects or situations at the other extreme.

In general, of course, the brain has to classify objects not on the strength of a single property but on an aggregate of several distinct properties or relations. This means that the outputs from the representational systems we have considered must feed into adaptive convergent systems where the appropriate final categorization can take place. Some of these properties will be more derivative than others. The concept of the elasticity of a rubber band, for example, presupposes the concept of length. We must assume, therefore, that some of these systems derive their inputs (directly or indirectly) from the outputs of other systems of the same formal type and, in turn, feed into further analysing and categorizing systems.

Since the operations of these convergent systems are categorizing operations they amount to a process of *abstraction*. The systems *abstract* particular properties of objects presented to the senses. If, as suggested above, the outputs of one such system may furnish the inputs to another, we arrive at processes of *progressive abstraction*. In particular, abstraction of visual form thus appears to be a staggered affair involving cascades of progressive specifications which may begin already in the primary visual cortex. Additional degrees of abstraction, of course, may be introduced if a convergent network intervenes between the outputs of one such system and the inputs to another. One fact emerges plainly from this discussion: the complete neural representation of even simple shapes or objects in our environment is likely to involve diffuse and widely dispersed processes in the brain.

Some of the evidence we shall meet in Chapter 10 suggests that in physical terms these processes of progressive abstraction run in the cortex in a rostral direction—starting with the lowest level of abstraction in the primary visual cortex and passing forward through the visual association areas and the inferior temporal lobes to reach the highest levels of abstraction in the association areas of the frontal cortex.

As we have seen, one of the main biological functions of the expectations which the brain forms as the result of experience, is to enable it to anticipate the consequences of an action before it is begun. In Man the anticipation of possible consequences of his actions reaches levels of abstraction in the frontal cortex which extend also over the social consequences of the actions. The observed effects of frontal lesions, at any rate, suggest that these regions are closely implicated in forms of awareness or anticipation which we may identify with the 'social conscience' or the Freudian 'superego'. (It may jar to see such psychological concepts mentioned in this particular context. But since the concept of directive correlation also enables us to express the abstract properties of social integration in objective terms, there is no real discordance here.)

Since the more abstract levels of anticipation must dominate the more concrete levels in the overall decision-making processes of the brain, we must expect the primary impact of the physiological drive-state of the organism to occur in the frontal rather than posterior association areas. The close association of the frontal areas with the limbic system and the hypothalamic drive-system is particularly significant in this respect. An interesting example of the anatomical separation of the various processes of abstraction is furnished by the fact that brain lesions have been reported in which the patient can only recognize animate objects but not inanimate ones.

7.11 SOME RELEVANT PHYSIOLOGICAL OBSERVATIONS

Although for a fuller discussion of the modelling activities of the brain the reader must be referred to Chapter 9, a few particulars may be considered already at this point.

The external properties and relations of which the brain can form internal representations have a diversity which is bound to be reflected in the character of the movement information on which these representations depend.

In some cases the movement information has to relate only to the movement of the eyes. Such information could be derived from 'corollary discharges' related to the internal generation of the eye-movements, i.e. from a central loop connecting oculomotor and visual centres, as was first suggested by Helmholtz[108] to account for visual stability during eye movements. Interaction between saccadic eye movements and visually evoked responses has been demonstrated by a number of investigators. Indeed, Noda, Freeman and Cruetzfeldt[181] have reported cells in the visual cortex which respond only during saccadic eye movements. Orban, Wissaert and Callens[186] have reported that in the cat stimulations applied at mesencephalic and anterior pontine levels at which they elicit eye movements also affect the response of visual cortex neurons, and they do so even when the respective movements are prevented by curare. They have argued that these effects can not be attributed merely to reticular activation.

In other representational functions the required movement or position information may have to be very much more complex or sophisticated. It may, for example, have to relate to the body schema as a whole (cf. Section 9.7), or it may have to relate to the goals and anticipated end-states of movements rather than to the details of their execution. My expectations of how the scene in this room will transform as I move about must be governed by *where* I move rather than *how* I move.

It is evident, therefore, that so far as concerns the question of the neural organization of internal models we cannot expect to find a single formula to cover all cases. However, the main principles summarized at the beginning of Section 7.10 seem clear enough. It is essential to grasp these principles if we are eventually to arrive at a clearer understanding of the functional organization of the nervous system.

We are still far removed from the stage at which one could marshal systematic evidence regarding the details of the connectivities through which these principles work out in practice. But already at this very general level of discussion the principles throw light on phenomena which have puzzled neurologists.

One of these phenomena is that visual information appears to be uninterpretable to an animal that lacks information about the posture and movements of its own body. Visual agnosias have been known to follow lemniscal lesions in which only afferent information relating tactile, proprioceptive and nociceptive stimuli is disrupted.

Thus Sprague, Chambers and Stellar [236] observed in the cat that unilateral lesions in the spinal lemniscus unexpectedly showed drastic visual defects even though visual pathways were not directly involved in the lesions. Transection of the lemniscal pathways in the midbrain, sparing much of the reticular core, produced a picture of sensory disregard and a loss of comprehension for things seen and felt. The lesion resulted in failure to respond to the large temporal visual field on the contralateral eye and to the nasal visual field in the ipsilateral eye. Moreover, the defect was not so much a simple sensory deficit but a failure to interpret sensory information, to attend to relevant stimuli and to localize them in space. The cat would pursue a mouse appearing on the ipsilateral side and would lose and forget it when it entered the contralateral field.

With bilateral lesions the same defect appeared on both sides. Behaviour now became generally docile and devoid of emotional responses. At the same time the animal fell into a state of hyperexploratory activity in which the head and eyes made constant and stereotyped searching movements.

Denny-Brown[52] has observed similar phenomena in the macaque monkey. Unilateral removal of that part of the superior colliculus which comprises lemniscal afferents for tactile, proprioceptive, nociceptive, gustatory and auditory modalities, gave complete restriction of vision to one lateral half of the binocular visual field (hemiopia). Bilateral removal similarly resulted in profound disturbances of visual and general behaviour. One animal remained wholly unreactive to visual stimuli. Another could reach out for a stationary object for the first time after five weeks. Postoperatively the animals collided with walls and other objects, fell off tables etc. They appeared to be totally unaware of events in their environment.

From the effect of similar, but rather more localized, lesions in the chimpanzee, Porter and McK. Rioch[198] concluded that loss of ascending influences on the cerebral cortex must be held to account for the observed defects rather than the loss of any integration of incoming signals at the site of the lesions.

It is significant to note in this connection that EEG records of the primary visual cortex show no abnormalities following lesions of this nature.

Exceptionally interesting results have recently been obtained by Gross, Rocha-Miranda and Bender[97] regarding the response to complex visual shapes of single neurons in the inferotemporal cortex of the monkey. I shall return to these studies in Section 9.6. At this point, however, it is worth noting that in the course of their investigations the authors have been impressed by the possibility that 'stimulus adequacy' for some inferotemporal neurons involved in visual shape recognition depends on more than retinal stimulation. It may depend, for example, on the orientation of the animal relative to the stimulus. In this connection the authors draw attention to the fact that besides input from the visual cortex and surrounding areas the inferotemporal cortex receives projections from the pulvinar (a thalamic nuclear complex) which in turn receives projections from the superior colliculus. It is conceivable, therefore, that information about the relation of visual stimuli to the position or movement of the eyes and head may be projected to the representational cortex from the pulvinar and that these cortical areas integrate analysing functions of the primary visual areas with orientation functions of the tectofugal system. The additional suggestion that these integrating functions are learning functions is supported by the observation that visual discrimination deficits resulting from inferotemporal lesions are known to depend on several non-sensory factors, such as the animal's prior experience, the training procedures used and the type of reinforcement.

7.12 CONCLUDING REMARKS

In this chapter we have given free rein to the imagination, as the reader will be well aware. We have tried to imagine the simplest networks that could give us the main system properties we are interested in, viz. the development during learning of particular directive correlations and the formation as the result of experience of sets of linkages in the brain which amount to internal representations of features of the real world. Since we regard these representations as aggregates of expectations of how sensory inputs transform as the result of movements of the eyes, head or body, the key problem was how networks could register in a permanent way the manner in which one variable depends on another. This was illustrated in the paradigm of Section 7.8.

The reader will also recall that we have introduced these paradigms only as a symbolization of the logical steps (AND operations, OR operations, adequate stimulus substitution etc.) which can lead from the known properties of neurons to the desired system-properties. They do not claim to be concrete hypotheses. Their object was merely to point to certain logical connections which it may be useful to have at the back of the mind in the search for specific hypotheses.

In the orderly progress of research one begins with the formulation of hypotheses and computes a set of predictions that would follow from them. Next one would compile a list of the ways in which these predictions appear to agree with the already known facts of neurophysiology and behaviour studies, i.e. the fact the model was designed to explain. Most important of all one would search for predictions of new experimental results for which the usefulness of the model could be tested. Finally one would examine whether this is the only model that would do the job.

To arrive at concrete hypotheses that could be applied to actual networks in the brain and tested in this way, one would have to add a number of special assumptions to the very general assumptions on which the lambda paradigms were based. This belongs to the province of the specialist. Marr's theory of cerebellar function is a good example of a theory in which the formal order of the steps I have listed is clearly exposed. However, I do not propose to advance to that stage and tie myself down to that extent. The very introduction of the special assumptions required would take us beyond the realm of the generally valid logical relations which I aim to expose in this volume. The lambda paradigms served to illustrate some of these. Above all they have drawn our attention to the possible significance of certain logical operations (AND functions, OR functions) and certain network features such as input sharing and lateral inhibition. It is not asserted that these operations must necessarily be performed in the brain by neatly separated units that can be identified with the formal neurons used in our paradigms. In the next chapter we shall indeed examine whether there are networks in the brain resembling our lambda systems. This is naturally of interest in the context and, to the extent to which such networks are found, helps to focus our thoughts in the search for fruitful hypotheses. I shall even hint at some possible hypotheses. But to go further would be to usurp the functions of the specialist.

One final point must be dealt with. The fact that in the discussion of the lambda paradigms we examined outputs as functions of inputs does not, of course, mean a tacit return to the old S–R concept for the organisms as a whole. Our lambda systems were paradigms of local networks whose fictional inputs may or may not have been taken to relate to sensory inputs and whose outputs may or may not have been taken to relate to motor functions, but which were never conceived as the sole link between peripheral inputs and motor efferent outputs. They dealt with special functions somewhere along the line of complex processes that intervene between peripheral inputs and motor outputs. Briefly, our picture of these processes is the following. The animal learns what to expect in a variety of situations in which its own role may be passive but most importantly is active. Aggregates of such expectations are stored in the brain and jointly constitute the brain's neural models of the real world. Sensory stimuli activate the respective models and the animal reacts to these activations with particular motor functions, depending on its current drive state. Learning changes occur all along the line, and our paradigms have tried to illustrate the logic of some of the mechanisms that may here be involved.

The totality of these learning changes progressively extends the combinations of sensory inputs capable of creating goals that are related to the animal's current drives. How, as the result of learning changes, sensory inputs come to create goals was illustrated at a very simple level by the elementary machine model introduced in Section 5.6. When the machine has learnt to respond to the inputs listed in the second table with the outputs listed in that table, the combination of 'drive' input D_2 and 'sensory' input L' results in outputs which are directly correlated to the environmental variables H, I, J, K in respect of the goal SG. In the living organism the equivalent of D_2 would be a set of inputs reflecting the physiological state of the organism, L' would relate to internal representations of particular features of the environment which are changed by the action, and H', I', J', K' to representations of a host of contingent variables which affect the outcomes of the action.

CHAPTER 8

Selected Structures

The last chapter has shown how networks of neurons which share the same presynaptic inputs and which are subject to certain forms of lateral inhibition may yield network properties which, if conceived on a more elaborate scale, could meet some of the more important requirements of the higher brain functions. In particular we have seen how in theory even comparatively simple networks can register relationships between stimulus variables and movement variables in a way which amounts to registering expectations of how stimuli will vary as the result of movement. This is the essence of the way in which the brain builds up internal representations of the properties and relations that characterize the physical world.

All this becomes more than an academic exercise only because, so far as we can tell, all the essential neural elements, connectivities, feedback loops etc. are abundantly present in the higher centres of the brain. Although the available evidence does not suggest that the real processes in the brain are accurate copies of our lambda models, the models serve to focus attention on anatomical and physiological features which may eventually prove to hold the key to a solution of the problem and they highlight the functional potential of these features.

The application of theoretical models to any actual structure of the brain can only be done profitably if the structure is discussed in relation to the overall organization of the brain. For the benefit of the general reader, therefore, I shall attempt to give a brief outline of these organizational relationships at the appropriate points of the chapter. At the same time I shall try to fill in some of the background of fact and theory that is relevant to topics we shall reach later.

8.1 THE CEREBELLUM

In searching for evidence of lambda-type systems in the brain the cerebellar cortex is one of the first structures to draw our attention. This is partly because it is known to participate in learning behaviour and partly because there is no other structure of comparable complexity in the brain of which we have such detailed anatomical knowledge.

The three main divisions of the cerebellum were mentioned in Section 6.3. In the following pages I shall confine myself to the neocerebellum, but much of what I have to say applies equally to the palaeocerebellum. We know that both these divisions are capable of some degree of adaptive plasticity. This is evident not only from the manner in which the nervous system can adapt to changes in some of the basic parameters on which the successful activity of the cerebellum depends, but also because it can be shown that the cerebellum itself is involved in the compensatory changes that occur if any part of it suffers extensive lesions or other deficiencies.

To the neuroanatomist the cerebellar cortex has traditionally been a more rewarding subject for study than the cerebral cortex. It has a simpler structure with more clearly demarcated cell types and an exceptionally uniform architecture throughout [59, 71].

Externally the cerebellar cortex consists of many long narrow folia, all essentially alike in structure (Figure 8.1). The main afferent inputs to the cere-

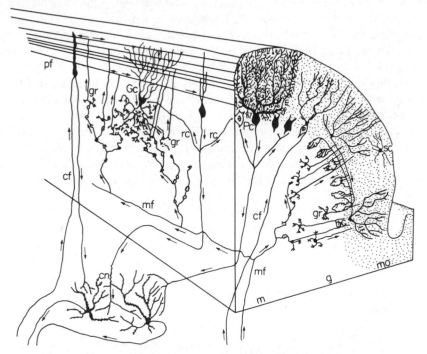

Figure 8.1. Schematic view of a folium showing the interneuronal connections of the cerebellar cortex (Reprinted with permission of Macmillan Publishing Co., Inc. from *Correlative Anatomy of the Nervous System* by Crosby, Humphrey and Lauer [48]. Copyright © 1962 by Macmillan Publishing Co., Inc.) Key: bc, basket cells; cf, climbing fibres; cn, deep cerebellar nuclei; g, granular layer; Gc, Golgi cell; gr, granule cell; m, medullary layer; mf, mossy fibre; mo, molecular layer; Pc, Purkinje cell; pf, parallel fibre; rc, recurrent collateral; sc, stellate cell

bellar cortex are provided by the *mossy fibres* (mf) and the *climbing fibres* (cf). Both sets of fibres can carry information about the sensory periphery as well as about what goes on inside the nervous system. But their mode of action within the cerebellar cortex is very different.

Some mossy fibres have small and modality specific peripheral fields, relating specifically to stimulation of skin, muscle or joints, for example. Others have fields that comprise several modalities and vary widely in size and pattern. Additional mossy fibre inputs derive from the cerebral cortex and certain subcortical structures. The cerebral signals relay in the pons.

The mossy fibres have moss-like terminals that are clasped by claw-like dendrites of the *granule cells* (gr) in bushy structures known as the cerebellar *glomeruli*. Each granule cell may send dendrites to 3–6 glomeruli and each glomerulus may receive dendrites from about 20 granule cells. Each granule cell sends a bifurcating axon for some distance parallel to the long axis of the folium. These axons form the *parallel fibres* (pf) which supply inputs to the dendritic trees of the *Purkinje cells* (Pc). These are the efferent cells of the cerebellar circuit. Each parallel fibre may contact up to 500 Purkinje cells and the intensely ramified dendrites of these cells enable each to contact a number of parallel fibres that runs into many thousands.

Two other important cell types draw inputs from the parallel fibres: the *Golgi cells* (*Gc*) and the *basket cells* (*bc*). These also receive recurrent collaterals from the Purkinje cells. A few of these collaterals also go to other Purkinje cells where they exercise an inhibitory function. The function of both the Golgi cells and basket cells is also inhibitory. The axons of the Golgi cells exercise a negative feedback on the granule cells, those of the basket cells an inhibitory feedforward on the Purkinje cells. Each basket cell exercises its inhibitory function over a horizontal region of something like 10×20 Purkinje cells. Beyond the basket lies a region of *stellate cells* (sc) which are also inhibitory. But whereas the basket cells act on the soma of the Purkinje cell, the stellate cells act on the dendrites. The main relations between the cell types mentioned are shown diagrammatically in Figure 8.2.

The Purkinje cells are also acted upon by the afferent climbing fibres (cf). By contrast, these fibres stand in a close one-to-one relationship with the Purkinje cells, each climbing fibre acting on one cell only through a set of intimate climbing contacts. The overriding control function a presynaptic fibre may derive from such climbing contacts was mentioned in Section 6.2. The climbing fibres originate in the olivary nucleus, a brainstem nucleus which receives fibres from the cord, the reticular formation and from certain nuclear masses of the midbrain associated with the extra-pyramidal motor system (Section 6.3).

The neocerebellum is heavily involved in the coordination of movements and the development of practical skills. Lesions in this area have striking effects on voluntary activity. They may produce severe errors in the rate, range,

force or direction of movements (apraxia). Sometimes the resulting movements have an uncertain and stepwise character suggestive of hesitant trials
followed by cerebrally computed corrections (intention tremor).

The precise function and exact mode of action of the cerebellum are still
unknown. The sole outputs from the cerebellar cortex come from the Purkinje cells. These outputs then loop back and distribute to the motor apparatus via the cerebellar nuclei and the red nucleus on the one hand, and via the

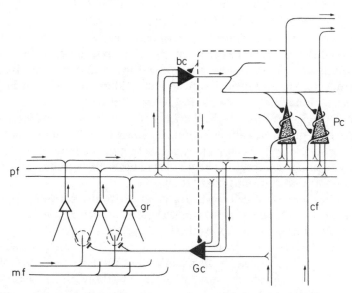

Figure 8.2. Schematic presentation of the main relations between some of the cell
types mentioned in Figure 8.1

cerebellar nuclei, the ventrolateral nucleus of the thalamus and the motor
cortex on the other (Figure 8.3). There are also projections to the sensory
cortex. Stimulation of the cerebellar nuclei causes evoked potentials in the
sensorimotor and association areas of the cortex.

The effect of the Purkinje cell axons on the cerebellar nuclei is purely
inhibitory. These nuclei receive a coarse-grained excitatory input from diffuse
fibre systems of pontine, spinal and olivary origin, and this excitation is modulated or 'sculptured' by the fine-grained, selective inhibition exercised by the
Purkinje outputs. The main excitatory input to the cerebellar nuclei is of
mossy fibre origin, bypassing the cerebellum. The impulse frequency of this
excitatory input is large compared with the inhibitory impulses arriving from
the Purkinje cells.

Very precise and somatotopical patterns project from the primary motor
cortex and the somatosensory areas of the centre to the pontine nuclei, which
in turn project to the cerebellum via the pontocerebellar tract. Extensive

connections from the sensorimotor cortex also project to the olivary nucleus, which is the source of the climbing fibres to the Purkinje cells. The olivary nucleus also receives movement information from the basal ganglia, various nuclei of the midbrain, the reticular formation and the spinal cord. In a sense the cerebellar circuits therefore form part of a giant closed loop from the cortex and extra-pyramidal motor system through the pontine nuclei and olivary nucleus to the cerebellum and back to the extra-pyramidal motor system and cortex (Figure 8.3). They also form part of an open loop which depends on feedback from the motor outputs via the peripheral receptors. Opinions differ as to the relative importance of these two loops.

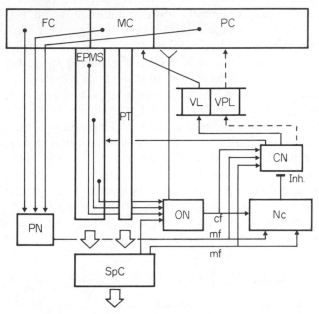

Figure 8.3. The cerebellar loops. Key: CN, cerebellar nuclei; EPMS, extra-pyramidal motor system; FC, frontal cortex; MC, motor cortex; Nc, neocerebellum; ON, olivary nuclei; PC, posterior and temporal cortex; PN, pontine nuclei; PT, pyramidal tract; SpC, spinal centres; VL, nucleus ventralis lateralis of thalamus; VPL, nucleus ventralis posteromedialis of thalamus

Opinions also differ about the intrinsic difference between the mf inputs and cf inputs. Both systems convey information about approximately the same peripheral receptors and in both systems the information may be either phasic or tonic. Eccles[59] therefore feels that there is no essential difference between the two input systems. Oscarsson[187], on the other hand, believes that each climbing fibre path carries information about nervous activity related to particular motor mechanisms, different for different zones, whereas each mossy fibre path carries more general information, either about the evolving movements as signalled by the proprioceptors and exteroceptors or about the sum total of the motor effects. Braitenberg[24] has suggested a more sophisticated difference: owing to their length and small diameter the parallel fibres may introduce different delays into the propagation of signals to the Purkinje cells. This may enable the cerebellum to perform special chronometric functions; for example, to interpose delays between the various components of rapid voluntary movements. Many activities, such as the rapid movements in handwriting, sports, music, etc., require extremely critical timing. According to Braitenberg's model the cerebellum could provide such temporal definitions with an accuracy better than milliseconds.

Kornhuber[141] has also recently drawn attention to the importance of pre-programming the fast muscle movements required in the exercise of practical skills. Rapid movements like saccadic and ballistic movements cannot be regulated continuously but must be preprogrammed in systems in which inherent time delays may be critical. In the case of complete recruitment of motoneurons the energies needed for different movements must be translated into different burst durations for these neurons. In Kornhuber's view the function of the cerebellar cortex is to calculate and preprogramme these burst durations. This is a distortive function which requires the integration of a great deal of phasic information. The required 'distortions' would be accomplished by the modulation the Purkinje outputs effect in the cerebellar nuclei. Eccles, on the other hand, tends to think in more general terms and believes that modulation of the outputs of the cerebellar nuclei by phasic integrations performed in the cerebellar cortex forms a basis for the dynamic improvement of ongoing or evolving motor activities.

8.2   LAMBDA CONFIGURATIONS IN THE CEREBELLUM

Looking at the schematics of Figure 8.2 in the light of the forcing function of the climbing fibres and the type of stimulus substitution we discussed in Section 7.4, one cannot help being struck by the resemblance of this system with the lambda configuration of Figure 7.7. The orderly structures of the parallel fibres, Purkinje cells and the inhibitory basket cells appear to have all the elements postulated in Section 7.4 for a system designed to provide for the adaptive development of adequate stimulus substitution by forced acquisition. The climbing fibres would provide the forcing function, and the basket cells the feedforward inhibition which we took at the time to be an appropriate form of lateral inhibition for systems of this type. This would agree with the suggestion made by Marr and others that the climbing fibres facilitate the granule cell inputs that are concomitantly active, such that they become in the future more effective in discharging the Purkinje cells. It would also agree with Oscarsson's view about the different qualities of mf and cf inputs, since it would provide for the gradual substitution of broad contextual inputs for rather more specialized inputs, a process whose biological value is noted on more than one occasion in this volume.

Marr[160] originally proposed that each Purkinje cell relates to an elemental movement which is triggered when the cell fires. Initially the Purkinje cells are activated by the sensorimotor cortex via the inferior olive and the climbing fibres (cf. Figure 8.3). Simultaneously, however, each cell receives 'context' information by way of the mossy fibres and parallel fibres. In the course of time these contexts come to surrogate as adequate stimuli for firing the cell. Thus ultimately the cell fires whenever the learnt context occurs and the contexts take over the control of movements which the cerebellum was initially 'taught' by the sensorimotor cortex. (Compare my notes on the role of adequate stimulus substitution in the perfection of movements—Section 6.10.) As to the role of the granule cells, Marr suggests that they serve to augment the difference between contexts having similar mossy fibre representations.

In a later paper Blomfield and Marr[22] revised these suggestions in the light of material evidence and proposed instead that the Purkinje cells are 'taught' by superficial pyramidal cells of the sensorimotor cortex and that their outputs *suppress* elemental movements initiated by deep pyramidal cells of the cortex.

Thach's studies of Purkinje cell action have shown that the response of these cells to parallel fibre stimulation can be distinguished from their response to climbing fibre stimulation[242, 243]. The former gives simple spikes whereas the spikes are complex in the latter case. In the awake monkey the responses of the Purkinje cells to parallel fibre inputs in the region examined showed a consistent temporal relationship to rapid arm movements, whereas the responses to climbing fibre action did not. This would be consistent with the hypothesis that in the fully trained cerebellum the mossy fibre inputs have come to substitute as the dominant factor in the control of movement. However, there is as yet no evidence that climbing fibre activity causes such long-term changes in the Purkinje cells and there is some evidence that may be taken to argue against it.

Alternative proposals for climbing fibre action have been advanced by a number of authors. Harmon, Kado and Lewis[101], for example, suggest that the climbing fibre 'resets' all parts of the Purkinje cell to some uniform electrotonical condition that enables the cell to sum future granule cell–basket cell–stellate cell inputs without contamination from the residue of previous inputs.

Meanwhile there is little doubt about one response-characteristic of the Purkinje cells which is suggestive of a lambda system, viz. that stimulation of the same cutaneous nerve causes discharges in some Purkinje cells but inhibition in others. Eccles[58], in particular, has demonstrated the surprising individuality displayed by the Purkinje cells with respect to the inputs each receives from the afferent volleys that may be set up experimentally in an array of cutaneous nerves. To show response individuality despite input sharing is a typical 'lambda' characteristic, as we have seen.

Nothing in the real brain, of course, is likely to be quite as straightforward as in the simple systems we invented in the last chapter. Nor do we possess all the physiological data we would need to test the degree to which the action of the real system matches that postulated for our minimal networks. As has been said, the simple deterministic events in our idealized networks can at best reflect only probabilistic occurrences in real systems composed of large numbers of neurons. The arrangement of the basket (and stellate) cells is suitable for controlling the thresholds of the Purkinje cells in the manner envisaged in Section 7.4, but only on the basis of a sampling of parallel fibres, for no single basket cell exclusively controls a specific set of Purkinje cells. In his mathematical analysis of the different paths along which a given mossy fibre input can reach a given parallel fibre and of the action of the granule cells, Marr[160] has formulated conditions which the parameters of the system must fulfil if the Purkinje cells are to act upon *learnt* parallel fibre input patterns but ignore *unlearnt* patterns. If these conditions are satisfied, the Purkinje cells can learn to recognize repeatedly experienced mossy fibre contexts and allow these to substitute for the cerebral instructions represented by the climbing fibre inputs.

The inhibitory action of the Golgi cells on the granule cells is well established, but there is as yet no general agreement about the specific function of this negative feedback. Marr suggests that its function is to regulate the number of active parallel fibres and to keep this number low but above a specific lower bound. The need for this negative feedback function would arise from the fact that the Purkinje cell threshold is not set directly from the parallel fibres with which the Purkinje cell synapses, but from the results of the basket cells sampling a number of different but closely related parallel fibres.

From our point of view it is worth noting that the Golgi cells effect a form of recurrent inhibition on the granule cells which, when taken in conjunction with the divergent distribution of mossy fibre inputs over sets of granule cells, suggest the possibility of a lambda-type learning system lying concealed also in the complex structures of the granular layer.

8.3 THE ALLOCORTEX AND LIMBIC SYSTEM

Although the architecture of the cerebral cortex shows a considerable degree of uniformity over the whole area it also represents a very complex organization about the details of which we know very little. In the adult cortex the cells and fibres are unevenly distributed over a number of layers which give a laminar appearance to the region. The most widely used terminology applied to these laminations is that introduced by Brodman who differentiated six layers in the neocortex and numbered these from the surface inwards. Different areas of the cortex are mainly distinguished by variations in the character and relative thickness of these laminations. A number of different cell types may be distinguished, some almost exclusively confined to one or two layers, others varying mainly in their relative distribution over the different layers. Their interconnections are intricate and still largely unknown. However, all this applies to the neocortex only. The phylogenetically older allocortex, which lies covered by the temporal lobes, has a simpler, three-layered, organization and for this reason is the best structure to consider next.

Phylogenetically the allocortex was the first part of the cortex to reach its full development. Although it developed from structures which were predominantly concerned with olfaction, the 'rhinencephalon', it has in time greatly extended its significance, particularly in relation to emotional processes. It does not show the six cell layers that are characteristic of the neocortex and contrary to the neocortex it does not appear to contain an internal positive feedback system. The particular significance of this in the context of the present investigation and its bearing on the simple architecture of the allocortex will become apparent later.

In the temporal lobes the cortex rolls inwards to form a deep depression bounded by the entorhinal area. This ends rostrally in structures which bulge into the ventricle to form a ridge known as the hippocampus (Figure 8.4). The distinctive pattern of neocortical laminations changes as we pass out of the entorhinal area and becomes relatively simple as we reach the hippocampus proper.

Following Broca and MacLean the non-olfactory portions of this system are now generally known as the *limbic system*. This comprises the allocortex as a kind of inner ring and the adjacent cortical areas or 'juxtallocortex' as an outer ring. The main limbic components of the allocortex are the entorhinal area, the hippocampus, the retrosplenial area and prepiriform cortex. Those of the juxtallocortex are the cingulate gyrus, the orbitofrontal and inferotemporal cortices (Figure 8.4).

The limbic system comprises also certain subcortical structures. The most important of these are the nuclear masses of the amygdala and the thin sheet of nuclei of the septum.

Most of the limbic structures are reciprocally connected. There also appears to be a certain degree of overlap and duplication of function. In consequence it is particularly difficult to unravel the detailed functions of the individual structures. There is probably no other region of the brain where experimental lesions or stimulations produce so many inconsistent results. This may also be partly due to the fact that some of these regions can undergo learning changes so that associations which prevail in one subject may not exist in another.

The bulk of the experimental evidence suggests that the main overall function of the limbic system and associated cortical regions is to relate information from the need detectors and drive centres of the organism with information about the external environment (as supplied by other parts of the brain) and information about the internal environment (partly supplied directly and partly from other regions)[202, 228]. All limbic structures stand in some direct or indirect relation to the hypothalamus, where some of the main nuclear masses controlling drive and emotional behaviour are located. The hypothalamus has reciprocal connections with the hippocampus and amygdala. It projects to the frontotemporal and cingulate cortices via the thalamus.

In consequence limbic structures are frequently found to be implicated in emotional reactions. This includes visceral and autonomic as well as behavioural responses. The latter include the overt expression of emotion and such behavioural phenomena as aggression, fighting, fleeing, rage etc. In a general sense we can perhaps say that the limbic regions form an area in which the current drive state of the organisms comes to give emotional tone to what the senses perceive and where 'drives', therefore, become 'motivations'. In conjunction with the hypothalamus and reticular formation these regions appear to predispose the organism towards certain basic programmes and attitudes in relation to the general complexion of the external situation

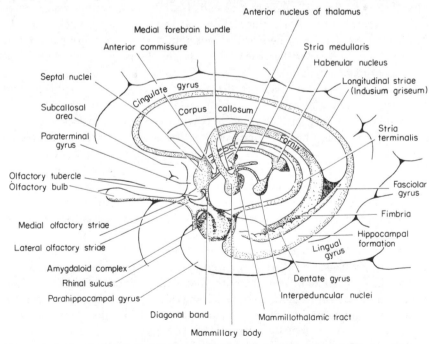

Figure 8.4. Semischematic drawing of rhinencephalic structural relationships as seen in medial view of the right hemisphere. Both deep and superficial structures are indicated (From Truex and Carpenter[256]) See also Figure 6.3

and the organism's current needs and innate tendencies. The control of attention and of the level of arousal or alertness forms an integral part of these functions.

It is asserted in this volume that the brain forms internal representations or 'models' of external objects or events and of their properties and relations. In addition it forms internal representations of the posture and movement of the body (the 'body schema'). The occipital, parietal and inferior temporal areas appear to be the main cortical sites at which these objective representations are formed, whereas the subjective or 'emotional' evaluation of these representations in relation to the current drive state of the organism appears to occur in the orbito-frontal and anterior temporal regions of the cortex in close association with the limbic system. To some extent this association is one in which broadly parallel functions are performed by cortical and subcortical structures at different levels of sophistication and with different degrees of plasticity. One of the most general categories of subjective evaluation concerns the degree of significance the organism assigns to a stimulus object in the motivational context in which it occurs. This in turn influences the general level of arousal of the organism and its attentional mechanisms. There are indications that these abstract estimates of significance are mainly formed in the fronto-temporal cortices, again in close association with the limbic system. The upper end of the reticular formation in turn is profoundly influenced by the cortex and particularly by the basal occipito-temporal cortex and entorhinal area.

It has been suggested that the hippocampus forms a significant link in mechanisms through which the reticular arousal evoked by novel stimuli habituates and gives way to focused attention if experience proves the stimuli to be significant. Although this process is obviously motivation-dependent it is not included in the category of what are commonly called 'emotional reactions'. Some observers believe that, in contrast with the amygdala, the hippocampus is not involved in this narrower category of reactions. Others claim that certain emotional reactions can be elicited by hippocampal stimulation.

The suggestion that the hippocampus is instrumental in suppressing reactions to stimuli that are insignificant in respect of the goals currently dictated by the motivational state of the animal is supported by a number of observations. Animals with hippocampal lesions, for example, are generally known to be hyperreactive (though not necessarily hyperactive). Thus the attention of a hippocampal animal may remain riveted on an object when it should be moving on and dismiss the object as irrelevant in the circumstances. Conversely Grastyan[90] has shown that stimulation of the hippocampus with implanted electrodes produces desynchronization of the contralateral hippocampus and inhibits orienting reactions, conditioned reactions and any behaviour in progress. Adey, Merrillees and Sunderland[2] have shown that stimulation of the hippocampus reduces the activating effects of the reticular formation for a period of two seconds. Livingstone[149] has shown that barbiturates dampen the hippocampus quickly, lessening its tonic inhibitory influence and enhancing reticular evoked potentials for a brief period. Redding[206] found that in the *encéphale isolé* preparation of the cat hippocampal stimulation caused a decrease in the amplitudes of all components of the visual and auditory potentials. This was the opposite of the effect of reticular formation stimulation.

Douglas and Pribram[54] believe that the function of the hippocampus is slightly more specific, viz. that it inhibits awareness of stimuli as a function of the probability of non-reinforcement. By contrast, they believe, the amygdala heightens awareness of stimuli as a function of previous reinforcement.

Hippocampal animals also frequently appear to be unable to inhibit or give up previously learned responses. Warrington[269] believes that this is the consequence of a failure to inhibit or dissipate irrelevant stored information and that this failure may also account for the deficit in long-term memory often observed in patients with hippocampal lesions. On this account, therefore, the hippocampus would also be instrumental in suppressing the effect of irrelevant memories and the apparent memory deficits are not due to failure of registration or consolidation but to failure of proper retrieval owing to the intrusion of irrelevant material (previous events being reported out of context).

Any neural system concerned in the subjective evaluation of a situation must be able to produce or trigger reactions which outlast the duration of the stimuli that aroused them. Some stimuli, such as the continuous rattle of a bedside alarm, are enduring stimuli which can guide behaviour right through to its proper conclusion. But explosive noises, bright flashes, transient pains and things seen in a fleeting glance are not of this kind. Hence it is important for the subjective evaluating systems of the brain to generate changes of the central state of the organism, or to cause the reverberation of images in the representational systems of the brain, which outlast the original sensory stimuli. It is widely held that the limbic system plays a vital part in mediating and controlling such lasting changes of state. Various suggestions have been made about the mechanisms which can produce the required tonic changes or reverberations. Essentially they must be mechanisms based on positive feedback loops. We have met small local feedback loops in the network paradigms given in the last chapter. But here we must look for larger and partly subcortical loops. In 1937 Papez[189] made the first concrete suggestion in this respect. The positive feedback circuit he proposed followed the loop: hippocampus—fornix—hypothalamus (mamillary bodies)—anterior nucleus of the thalamus—cingulate gyrus—hippocampus. Other circuits have been suggested since. Most of these include the reticular formation.

There is no reason to suppose, of course, that only one particular feed-back loop can be involved. It will be suggested in Section 10.3 that there may exist a more comprehensive and 'natural' system of loops which are based on the mechanisms of attention. These loops would run from the cortical areas in which the representation of an event is set up to the regions in which the significance of the event is evaluated and then back to the representational regions where they would potentiate the sustained representation of events which the brain treats as significant in relation to the current drive state of the organism. If it is true that the consolidation of the memory of events depends on the degree of attention given to the event and on the subsequent internal 'replay', any damage to essential links in these loops would tend to interfere with memory consolidation. The fact that lesions in the limbic system, especially in the hippocampus, frequently appear to interfere with the consolidation of learning would support the idea that these structures are implicated in the wider loops we have in mind at the moment.

After ablation of the hippocampus monkeys can still learn new tasks involving delays between significant stimuli, but only if the meaning of the first stimulus does not have to be compared with the meaning of the later stimulus. The close relationship between learning and the attentional functions of the hippocampus is illustrated by the fact that in these animals the impact of distracting stimuli between relevant stimuli is particularly marked. Stimulation of the hippocampus, on the other hand, may cause a fixation of attention[163]. However, our knowledge of many of these effects is still scant and some of the evidence is controversial. We shall return to these questions in Chapter 10.

An interesting analysis recently published by O'Keefe and Dostrovsky[184] suggests that the hippocampus is also closely involved in the representational functions of the brain, possibly owing to its inputs from the temporal lobes. Of the 76 cells they examined in the hippocampus of the rat, 14 units showed activity related to arousal and attention; 21 cells were 'movement units' which fired briskly during sniffing, orienting or bar-pressing movements, but infrequently or not at all during eating, drinking or quiet sitting; 2 units fired only if the rat sniffed at its own but not at another water dish. A further 8 units had distinctly representational properties: they responded solely when the rat was in a particular part of the testing platform to which it was confined and faced in a particular direction. The activity of the remaining 31 cells could not be interpreted.

The hippocampus is sometimes called the hub of the limbic system. The variety of activities in which it seems to be involved certainly appears to bear this out. From our present point of view, however, the main interest lies in its orderly anatomical organization and in the fact that its internal networks show some of the main features which were spotlighted by the theoretical analysis of our last chapter.

8.4 LAMBDA CONFIGURATIONS IN THE HIPPOCAMPUS

The anatomy of the hippocampus shows a ring of large pyramidal cells with dendritic trees facing inwards and axons facing outwards. The dendritic trees have long spical shafts, similar to those of the pyramidal cells of the neo-cortex (see below). Parallel systems of afferent fibres distribute over rows of pyramidal neurons, just as we would expect to find if these were the inputs to a lambda configuration.

Since the pyramidal cells are lying parallel to each other and at the same depth, each cell is impinged upon by different sets of afferent fibres over different stretches of its apical shafts. The main inputs to these apical dendrites come from the entorhinal area which relays impulses from the temporal, orbitofrontal and cingulate cortices. Further inputs come from the septal areas which may also relay impulses of visceral origin. Figure 8.5 illustrates some of the main afferents to hippocampal pyramids taken from two different regions (CA1 and CA3). Gergen and MacLean[75] have suggested that this

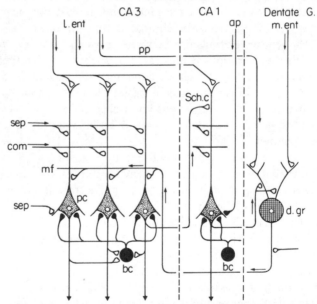

Figure 8.5. Suggested connections of the hippocampus (Adapted from Raisman, Cowan and Powell[204]; Smythies *Brain Mechanisms and Behaviour*[228]. (Reproduced by permission of Blackwell Scientific Publications Ltd.); van Hoesen, Pandya and Butters[112]) Key: ap, alvear path (possibly from medial entorhinal area); bc, basket cells (inhibitory interneurons); com, commissural fibres (from other hemisphere); d. gr, dentate granule cell; 1. ent, inputs from lateral entorhinal area (possible pathway from frontal cortex); m. ent, inputs from medial entorhinal area (possible pathway from ventral temporal cortex); mf, mossy fibres; pc, pyramidal cell; pp, perforant pathway; Sch. c, Schaeffer collaterals; sep, inputs from septal area, hypothalamus and midbrain (via fornix)

looks like a conditioning mechanism in which the fate of a volley in the afferent sensory path from the entorhinal area is determined by the visceral input from the septum. The main efferent connections are via the fornix to the septal region and hypothalamus. There are also diffuse two-way pathways to the amygdala. Other efferent pathways reach the basal ganglia, epithalamus and reticular formation.

The resemblance of the pyramidal layers to the basic lambda systems discussed in Section 7.2 is enhanced by the powerful system of recurrent inhibition acting through the so called 'basket cells' (bc). Each basket cell may cover a territory of 200–500 pyramidal cells. The axon collaterals of the basket cells terminate on the soma of the pyramidal cells and are the only fibres to do so. Historically this was the first example of a recurrent inhibitory system in mammals in which the synapses and the pathways were histologically identifiable. Whether this distinctly 'lambda' type configuration has the adaptive plasticity and discharges the type of functions which I reviewed in the last chapter I cannot say. Anatomically, the resemblance is there and in view of the·fact that· the hippocampus probably represents the highest level of integration within the rhinencephalon it is not unreasonable to assume that it is capable of some degree of adaptive plasticity in the exercise of its functions. Evidence of plastic changes in the hippocampal area has been produced by experiments demonstrating frequency potentiation[151], but this does not, of course, necessarily mean that these changes are adaptive in the sense of the term that concerns us here.

Microelectrode penetrations into the hippocampus have shown that the afferent systems produce long-lasting IPSPs of the type characteristic of recurrent inhibition. Intracellular records obtained by Andersen and others of pyramidal responses to stimulation of the Schaffer collaterals often showed inhibition as the only response to such stimulation. This would be the most common response to be expected if the 'lambda systems' of the hippocampus were to function according to our Model I (Section 7.2). On the other hand, the results of observations on the number of cells in the hippocampus which respond to septal stimulation with spike discharges and inhibition respectively are more suggestive of Model II.

The reader will recall that in the operational mode of Model I there is a negative correlation between the activities of adjacent or proximate neurons, whereas in Model II there is complete decorrelation. In the absence of effective inhibition the correlation would be positive. Noda, Manohar and Adey[182] have examined this correlation in the hippocampus of the cat. Pairs of closely spaced cells were recorded simultaneously by a single microelectrode. These studies showed that during deep sleep and intermediate sleep there was a positive correlation, but during wakefulness and REM (rapid eye movement) sleep there was an almost complete decorrelation (Figure 8.6). During intermediate and deep sleep there was also a coincidence of the long periods of silence which frequently followed a burst of discharges. The authors explain this synchrony in terms of inadequate afferent stimulation.

At low input levels basket cell excitation must first build up until it is strong enough to send inhibitory volleys capable of overriding the excitatory volleys on the pyramidal cells. At the end of hyperpolarization occurring synchronously in many pyramidal cells their excitability will be considerably increased due to what is known as 'postinhibitory rebound'. This enhances the tendency for correlated discharges of pyramidal cells which would then be followed by another cycle of basket cell activation. We can imagine that with higher input activities the basket cell action becomes instantly effective and by suppressing the less excited cells makes the cell discharges contingent on differentials in the selective responsiveness of the cells to the input patterns of the moment—thus producing the observed decorrelation (cf. Model II).

These observations suggest an interesting interpretation of the 'facilitation from below' which we envisaged in the paradigms of Figures 7.5 and 7.6, for example. According to this interpretation the critical effect of these facilitations is not that they decide the level of activity of the lambda systems they

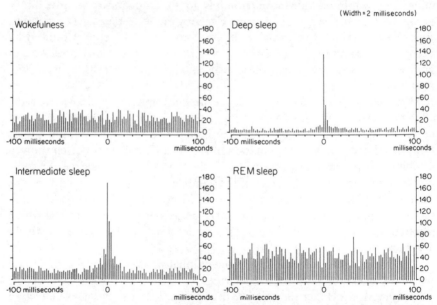

Figure 8.6. Cross correlation histogram of a pair of hippocampal neurons in the cat for four behavioural states. The histogram provides a measure of the probability of encountering a spike in the spike train of one neuron as a function of time before (left half of histogram) or after (right half) a spike in the simultaneously recorded spike train of a second neuron. Samples were taken of spike trains over an epoch of 60 seconds for each behavioural state (From Noda, Manohar and Adey, *Exp. Neurology*, **24**, 232–47, 1969[182]. Reproduced by permission of Academic Press Inc.)

control, but that they switch them from an uninformative mode of operation (highly correlated and synchronized outputs) to an informative mode (decorrelated and desynchronized outputs).

In view of the extreme simplicity of our lambda models and of the assumptions on which they were based we cannot, of course, expect more than broad analogies between model and reality. Even so these analogies may help us to see the realities in a better perspective. There are, of course, considerable differences in many points of detail. For example, the lambda neurons of our models are neatly parcelled into groups ('modules') each of which is controlled by a single inhibitory neuron. In the hippocampus on the other hand, there appears to be no such neat division and each pyramidal cell is impinged upon by axon collaterals of more than one basket cell. Instead of a sharp division between 'modules', therefore, we merely have a progressive shift (as we move along the line of pyramidals) in the constitution of the set of basket cells whose axon collaterals impinge upon the pyramidals.

8.5   THE NEOCORTEX

Although the neocortex is highly structured it has none of the transparent geometrical order of the cerebellar cortex and allocortex and our knowledge of its internal organization is very scanty. The thin convoluted sheet of the neocortex in man comprises something of the order of 7×10^9 neurons. It varies in thickness from about 2 mm in the visual cortex to 4·5 mm in the motor areas. Fibres enter or leave all regions of the inner surfaces. In many areas there is a two-way communication with subcortical centres, particularly with the thalamus. In addition each cortical region communicates with other cortical regions and with its mirror points in the opposite hemisphere. Whereas the cytoarchitectonic structure of the neocortex follows tangential laminations, its functional organization appears to be based on a mosaic of vertical columns. In the primary receiving areas these columns specialize in respect of modalities and submodalities of receptive inputs. In the visual cortex of the monkey, for example, the columns measure about 0·5 mm in diameter and contain about 50 000 neurons. Typically they specialize in the orientation, form and movement of the contour elements of the images projected on the retina. Although this columnar organization has been conclusively demonstrated only for the visual and somaesthetic areas, the architectonic similarity of other parts of the neocortex suggests that a similar columnar organization exists throughout. Although learning as such is not a prerogative of cortical circuits, learning without the participation of the cerebral cortex is limited to simple reactions only. The general nature of cortical involvement in learning first became the subject of lively controversies when Lashley[145] published his well known experiments on the effect of cortical ablations on the learning ability and retention in rats. The most controversial result of these experiments was his theory of 'mass action'. Fundamentally this states that

   (i) for some activities the cortex functions as a whole and the degree of slowing down of retention in these activities is proportional to the amount of cortex removed;

  (ii) each sensory area in the cortex exerts a similar mass action with regard to the retention of learnt habits in that sensory modality;

 (iii) the more difficult the problem to be solved, the greater the effect of any lesion.

Lashley's experiments have been confirmed for the dog and the cat in respect of activities of the same order of complexity as those involved in the maze-learning tasks to which Lashley had subjected his rats. This was of a kind that was bound to involve very extensive cortical areas in any theory. Seen in this light, his laws of mass action essentially boil down to the assertion that if the cortex is involved on a global scale the pathways that become critical in the acquisition and retention of the learnt behaviour patterns are evenly distributed over the cortical surface. This is now generally regarded as too sweeping an assertion.

In fact, how localized learnt habits may be if they involve only a single modality was convincingly shown by Sperry[232]. In 'split-brain' experiments with cats in which all communication between the hemispheres was severed, Sperry showed that if an island consisting of sensorimotor cortex is retained while the rest of the hemisphere is decorticated, tactile discriminations trained in the corresponding forepaw are retained. But they are lost if the island is removed. On the other hand it would be a mistake to conclude from these experiments that the integration of sensory inputs and motor outputs involved in the respective tasks happens solely, or even mainly, within the cortex. In the organization of complex movements the subcortical structures are found to be closely involved. Other experiments in Sperry's laboratory have shown that split-brain animals in which there is no communication between the hemispheres can learn complex tasks in which visual inputs to one hemisphere have to be integrated with tactile inputs to the other. We must conclude that integration was effected at subcortical levels. The giant cortico–cerebellar–cortical loop mentioned in Section 8.1 no doubt also has a part to play in this integration.

In vertebrates the relative proportion of primary (sensory) areas of the cortex compared with 'association' areas decreases significantly as one moves up the biological scale. Whereas the former occupy approximately 90% of the cortex in the cat, they occupy only 35% in the monkey and 15% in man.

For the monkey Pribram has found in a number of studies that removal of a great many regions had no effect on a variety of test situations. However:

1. Removal of the posterior inferotemporal region resulted in loss of learnt visual discriminations.
2. Removal of occipito-parietal region interfered with the learning of habits based upon somaesthetic stimuli.
3. Removal of anterotemporal region reduced the monkey's ability to learn olfactory and gustatory stimuli.
4. Removal of part of the frontal region reduced the ability to perform time discriminations irrespective of sensory modality. He also found that ablations in the frontal regions interfered with intentional behaviour, the differentiation of discrete preferences in choice situations, the ability to direct attention to relevant environmental cues and the evaluation of the success or failure of an action.

These are only a few examples of the many ablation experiments that have been carried out on the cortex. Most of these confirm the notion that the more complex a function, the less localized it is in the cortex.

Although in points of detail the number of cell types that have been described in the neocortex is very considerable, some broad categories of cells are characteristic of the cortex as a whole. The most prominent cell types are the pyramidal and stellate cells. Others are the horizontal cells of Cajal, the basket cells, the cells of Martinotti and the so-called polymorph or multiform cells (Figure 8.7[45, 48, 84, 221, 224]).

The pyramidal cells (pc) are distributed over all the six recognizable layers of the cortex except the uppermost (layer I). Layers II and III tend to contain only small and medium pyramidal cells, whereas the larger cells are found in layers V and VI. In layer IV the pyramidals are outnumbered by stellate cells (st). This layer has a granular appearance and in the visual cortex widens into a broad white band. In the motor cortex, on the other hand it is almost wholly lacking. All but a small fraction of pyramidal cells have apical dendrites reaching into layer I and the majority of pyramidal cells also have recurrent axon collaterals.

Layer I consists largely of horizontal fibres which are axon collaterals of cells in deeper layers. These fibres may spread tangentially up to a distance of several millimetres. This layer also contains the horizontal cells (hc) of Cajal. These have horizontally oriented dendrites and axons which remain confined to the same layer. An important cell type is found in layers III and IV. These are the basket cells (bc). They have a star-shaped dendritic tree and axons which bifurcate into many horizontal and oblique branches which may be of great length. These axon collaterals end in pericellular nests around pyramidal cell bodies and they are generally believed to have inhibitory functions. One distinctive type of stellate cells (fc) has vertically oriented terminal arborizations which break up into end-branches in a 'horsetail' fashion. These branches appear to make multiple synaptic contacts with apical shafts of large and medium-sized pyramidal cells. The polymorph or multiform cells (pm) are most prominent in the deeper cortical layers where their cell bodies take on many different shapes. The dendrites have a wide spread in the overlying cortical strata. Finally, the Martinotti cells (M) are found in all layers. It is held by some investigators that their axons or axon collaterals reach layer I.

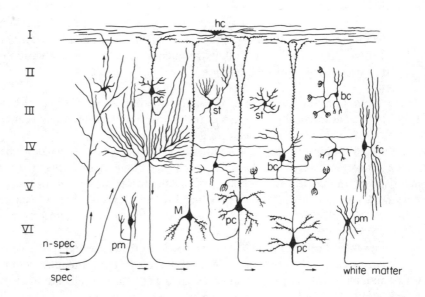

Figure 8.7. Schematic representation of some cortical cell types demonstrable in Golgi preparations (Compiled from various sources) Key: bc, basket cells; fc, fusiform stellate cells; hc, horizontal cells; M, Martinotti cells; pc, pyramidal cells; pm, polymorph cells; st, stellate cells; n-spec, non-specific afferent fibres; spec, specific afferent fibres. Roman numerals at the side of the figure indicate the cortical layers

The efferent fibres of the cortex are formed mainly by the axons of pyramidal and polymorph cells. Some of the efferent fibres, the 'U' fibres, terminate as afferents in neighbouring cortical areas.

The afferent fibres of the cortex, both specific and non-specific, enter each region in a characteristically oblique course (Figure 8.5). On reaching layer IV this course flattens to the horizontal and forms a dense plexus of relatively coarse fibres from which fine branches mainly ascend into layer III and in the case of the non-specific afferents also the higher layers. The specific afferents probably synapse directly with dendrites of pyramidal cells, whereas the non-specific pathways to the pyramidal cells may be polysynaptic.

8.6   LAMBDA ELEMENTS IN THE NEOCORTEX

The point has come to examine to what extent these broad features of the cytoarchitectonics of the neocortex incorporate elements of the type highlighted by the models developed in Chapter 7. In view of the immense complexity of the neocortex it is likely that many of the events occurring here are totally unrelated to the particular functions with which our 'lambda' models were concerned. But we must ask to what extent it is conceivable that embedded in this tangle of organizational relationship there exist the basic elements and connectivities which these models assume.

All the basic lambda elements appear to be present, indeed within each of the radial columns in which the cortex appears to be organized. The function of lambda neurons could be fulfilled by pyramidal cells, at any rate by those of the lower layers. A common requirement of all our models is that the lambda neurons belonging to the same lambda system share the same afferents. The afferent fibres to the cortical columns arborize with a tangential spread of up to 0·6 mm, although the majority probably have a span of only half this value. Still, this is of the same order of magnitude as the diameter of a radial column. It has been estimated that each column receives something like 6000 afferent fibres and contributes 18 000 efferents to the white matter, i.e. to the general pathway of cortical efferents below layer VI. Each afferent fibre may contact up to 5000 cells. This would be compatible with the idea that each radial column comprises complete lambda systems within its organization. The next requirement would be that the pyramidals participating in these structures should be subject to local systems of lateral inhibition. This requirement could be met by the inhibitory basket cells. The pericellular nest of the terminal arborization of these cells would provide the overriding control which this inhibition must exercise to satisfy the lambda hypothesis.

The experimental evidence suggests that the basket cell inhibition is a recurrent inhibition. Although there is no anatomical evidence to show that the basket cells are excited by recurrent collaterals of pyramidal cells, there is physiological evidence that the discharges of the pyramidals are subject to recurrent inhibition and that this is the main form of inhibition in the cortex.

As has been said, every lambda matrix must be followed up by networks which have some degree of convergence or exercise some kind of sampling function. Conceivably this could be the function of the polymorph cells of the lower layers.

This leaves the additional networks to be considered which we found to be essential for the capacity of the cortex to recognize temporal as well as spatial patterns of inputs. The essential step was to convert temporal patterns of excitation into unique spatial patterns. We saw in Chapter 7 that this calls for a positive feedback network which has to code the outputs of axon collaterals of the lambda neurons in the manner discussed at the time. It then has to distribute this information to the dendrites of the associative lambda system (cf. Figure 7.10).

In this respect suggestive evidence comes from the studies of Burns and Grafstein[35] on the tangential spread of excitation within isolated slabs of cortex by means of (probably) random networks based on positive feedback elements. In fact their results point to the existence of just the type of tangential and distributive network which the hypothesis would demand. The point of working with isolated (undercut) slabs of cortex is to prevent a spread of excitation via the white matter of the cortex. In the intact cortex Smith and Burns found that weak electrical stimulation of one point on the cortical surface could affect the firing probability of cortical neurons several centimetres away. The changes are delayed and can be measured only statistically, but they are capable of modifying natural responses.

Nissl[178] first expressed the belief that the upper layers of the cortex are concerned with intracortical association. Sperry found that excitation from the precentral motor area to the adjacent motor areas spread by superficial intracortical fibres.

The horizontal plexus of layer I is the obvious candidate for the tangential spread of positive feedback information as required by lambda systems capable of discerning temporal patterns of inputs. However, according to Burns and Grafstein layer I plays only an intermediate part in the tangential spread of excitation. Their microelectrode records, taken at various depths of the cortex, suggest that the main tangential spread of excitation is multi-synaptic and is mediated by a sheet of interconnected neurons which lie about 1 mm below the surface and derive their excitation from the fibres in layer I above. The same observers believe that this sheet consists largely of small pyramidals in layers II, III and IV and they show that it is capable of conducting excitation over unlimited distances across the surface of the brain. The presence of positive feedback elements in this system is shown by the persistence of activity up to 5 seconds after application of a strong stimulus. They also regard it as probable that in the intact cortex the horizontal spread of excitation is further assisted (and accelerated) by cortico-cortical fibres passing through the white matter.

These results suggest that the tangential spread proceeds at three levels: over short distances in layer I, over longer distances in the middle sheet of interconnected cells and over still larger distances through the U fibres of the white matter.

The only remaining elements which have appeared in the lambda configurations modelled in Chapter 7 are the 'forcing contacts' which are needed for systems relying on forced alignment and adequate stimulus substitution (Section 7.4). The 'horsetail'-shaped axonal arborizations of certain stellate cells are known to make climbing contacts with apical shafts of pyramidal cells. All the same they do not really fit the picture. What we are looking for in the present context is a relatively small number of afferent fibres making either climbing contacts with apical dendrites or grasping the postsynaptic neuron in any other commanding fashion. Globus and Scheibel[84] found such elements in 1967 in the form of ascending non-specific afferents making climbing contacts with apical dendrites of pyramidal cells.

There are four main sources of afferent fibres in the primary cortices: the specific and non-specific afferents already mentioned, the 'association' fibres from other cortical regions and the callosal fibres from the opposite hemisphere. According to Scheibel all extracortical afferents go to the dendrites of the vertical shafts of the pyramidal cells and all intracortical fibres to the basal dendrites or the arches of the shafts. Some workers believe that the specific afferents terminate closer to the cell body than the non-specific.

The main source of the non-specific fibres must be sought in the non-specific (extralemniscal) afferent pathways and in the subcortical regions which participate in the arousal of the cortex, such as the reticular nucleus and intralaminar nuclei of the thalamus. This arousal must not be thought of as a uniform depression of thresholds. It is a patterned activation, not a volume control. Klee[135], for example, found that in the cat motor cortex 12% of the cells examined with microelectrodes were facilitated by RF stimulation and 88% were inhibited. Complete suppression of spontaneous discharges occurred in 20% of the cells. If arousal took the form of a general sensitization of the cortex one would expect all spontaneous activity of cortical cells to be facilitated. Such facilitation is only rarely observed.

As in the hippocampus the recurrent inhibition in the cortex is strong and prolonged. The effectiveness of this inhibition is assured by the intimate somatic contacts of the basket cell terminals on the pyramidal cells. The power and spread of the inhibitory mechanisms of the cortex is illustrated by the observation of Krnjević, Randić and Straughan[143], that if cortical neurons are electrically stimulated at suprathreshold strength they may inhibit neighbouring neurons within 1 cm radius and for periods up to 200 milliseconds.

It has been suggested that such lasting inhibition may promote temporal integration. It is also known that the cortical neurons have a long time constant, as indicated by the long duration of EPSPs, compared with other neurons such as the motoneurons. This, too, facilitates temporal integration. Another property promoting integrative functions is the lack of 'accommodation' (rise of threshold with stimulus strength) in cortical neurons. This allows summation of subthreshold depolarizations without considerable change of threshold. Dendritic conduction is not of the all-or-nothing type characteristic of conduction in axons and the apical dendrites have no refractory period. This also assists summation, as later activation sums with first. Clare and Bishop[43] conclude from their extensive investigation of dendritic conduction that the role of the dendrites is to raise the level of excitation of the cell body and thereby lower its threshold to influences arising via axons impinging nearer the soma. This would tally with the observation that the non-specific afferents penetrate to higher layers in the cortex than the specific and with the 'rising facilitations' we have envisaged in a number of our elementary lambda models.

The importance of temporal summation in systems concerned with the recognition of temporal sequences was stressed in Sections 7.4 and 7.6. In the lambda configurations of Figure 7.10, for example, the function of the *B* neurons is to convert temporal patterns of excitation into characteristic spatial patterns. But, unless we assume that the *B* neurons maintain a particular pattern of activity through self-excitation (as in re-productive memory functions), the spatial pattern of their activities still has a temporal spread. To recognize such a spatial pattern as a whole the recognition system (*RC*, Figure 7.10) would have to rely on fairly extensive temporal summations in its dendritic apparatus.

However, one must not drive the comparisons too far. The elementary lambda configurations of Chapter 7 were never intended as final hypotheses. They were merely designed to help us see more clearly how the known properties of neurons may generate the postulated molar and functional properties of large systems of neurons. That the real systems of the brain are unlikely to follow these idealized simple systems other than in a broad and probabilistic fashion has been stressed more than once. To illustrate a typical discrepancy which shows that the truth cannot be as simple as our Model I, for example. According to Eccles[57] it appears that the production of the recurrent IPSP requires more than a single stimulus. It needs some form of synaptic facilitation produced by repetitive stimulation. The latency of action of these recurrent IPSPs is 4–7 milliseconds for simple volleys, but shortens with repetitive stimulation to 2–3 milliseconds.

Recurrent inhibition can be verified experimentally by applying electrical stimuli to the axons of pyramidal cells (e.g. in the pyramidal tract). Since this 'antidromic' excitation cannot pass beyond the cell body, all observed effect of the stimulation in the cortex must be due to recurrent axon collaterals. This is one method in which the results are illuminating despite the artificiality of the applied stimulus. But in other respects artificial stimulation can tell us little about the natural action of the neurons examined. We cannot test by these methods to what degree the action of cortical systems resembles that of the lambda configurations considered in Chapter 7 simply because we cannot artificially create an input volley which both has a spatial pattern or distribution of the kind we assumed for the inputs to these systems and also maintains a natural level of intensity.

The hypothesis that some cortical systems function in a manner analogous to these lambda systems demands that there exist cortical neurons with highly selective input preferences and that when the stimulus situation changes some of these neurons are silenced while others, previously silent, are activated.

Evidence of highly individualized unit activities interspersed with long inactive periods is found in the association areas. Noda and Adey[179,180] have noted this as a common phenomenon in the middle suprasylvian gyrus of the cat. Their investigations were concerned with the degree of correlation which could be detected in the activity of pairs of neurons within the same domain. The technique was similar to that employed in the hippocampus (see above), and the results are equally suggestive. Once again it was found that highly individualized unit activity (decorrelation) occurs only in behavioural arousal and paradoxical sleep. In intermediate and deep sleep the activities of pairs of proximate neuron become highly correlated. This correlation is also greatly affected by depth of anaesthesia, as shown by Holmes and Houchin[113] in rat cortical neurons. With anaesthesia light enough for a withdrawal reflex no correlation was observed. With deeper anaesthesia the correlation returned. Adrian and Matthews[5] in 1934 were already suggesting that cortical structures tended to discharge synchronously unless afferent bombardment was present. Single unit studies have now supported this prediction. The simplest hypothesis to explain this effect would be to assume that only a sufficient level of afferent input can activate the recurrent inhibition which decorrelates the activities of the neurons within its domain. This hypothesis agrees with the observations by Eccles about the minimal stimulation required to activate the recurrent IPSPs (see above).

Creutzfeldt, Luk and Watanabe[46] have noted in the motor cortex of the cat that a certain degree of summation of recurrent activity may also be necessary to make IPSPs possible. Spontaneous EPSPs in their experiments rarely reached firing level, hence no spontaneous IPSPs were observed. Weak stimuli applied to the thalamic projection nuclei evoked a slowly rising EPSP, on which steps indicating temporal summation of several EPSPs could be recognized, and some firing occurred. Only with increasing stimulus strength did an IPSP follow the primary excitation. This had a long duration (80–150 milliseconds) and was followed by rhythmically appearing summated EPSPs, the afterdischarge. The IPSPs decreased during anaesthesia.

The inhibitory potentials observed in the cortex following stimulation of the reticular formation suggest that the type of cortical activation which occurs during arousal consists largely of a decorrelation of unit activity through the intervention of recurrent inhibition. In other words, arousal mobilizes the cortex for the type of binary information processing we have envisaged in our lambda models—once again Model II being the most appropriate one. Thus, as has been noted before, the final effect of reticular arousal, therefore, is not a uniformly facilitating one. Through the inhibitory processes which are brought into action a sizeable proportion of neurons may become inhibited during alertness and spontaneous activity is suppressed accordingly. (Jung, Kornhuber and Da Fonseca[130] have pointed out that strictly speaking one should only speak of 'arousal' when the spontaneous activity of the neurons increases as well—which rarely is the case. However, for convenience I shall continue to use this term in the broader sense.)

It is evident that these processes increase the signal-to-noise ratio in the cortex. Evarts[62] has described an increase in signal-to-noise ratio as characteristic of the effects of general alertness upon the responses of units in the visual cortex of the cat. It was also found that more units in this region are inhibited than excited when the animal is aroused from natural sleep. Various observers have noted that in the motor cortex the number of inhibited units may exceed the number of facilitated ones during reticular stimulation. Others have remarked upon the pronounced individuality of the responses of cortical neurons in the alert state of the animal.

The desynchronization of neural activity which EEG recordings show at the onset of intensive sensory processing may also be interpreted as an indication of the type of decorrelation and diversification of cellular firing patterns with which we have here been concerned.

The question of the areas of the brain in which the internal representations are formed of the external world and of the body image draws our attention to the non-primary areas of the cortex, the 'association' areas. They are often called the 'silent' areas because in EEG recordings they appear to show no response to peripheral stimuli except in small limited regions. This apparent silence does not, of course, mean inactivity or lack of participation in processing the new information.

The 'silence' of these areas is evidence for rather than against their representational functions. EEG recordings relate to summated shifts in dendritic potential over large populations of neurons. If the activity of these neurons is highly individualized (as it would be in an ensemble of representational lambda systems) the mere *redistribution* of active neurons that would occur as one dispersive representation succeeds another would not show in these records.

Even when there is a noticeable EEG response as in the primary areas, the relation of the evoked (EEG) potential to the firing pattern of the individual neurons in the population below the surface electrodes is not at all straightforward. It differs, for example, between rapidly changing potentials and slower changing ones. Characteristic patterns of normal EEG activity were shown in Figure 6.12.

An idealized example of a typical EEG response in a primary receiving area to a single stimulus is shown in Figure 8.8. This consists of a short-latency, diphasic (positive–negative) response which is attributed to the specific afferents from the corresponding relay nucleus of the thalamus. The diphasic response is followed by slower components with longer latencies, the *late components*. In general a slow negative wave indicates depolarization (EPSPs) in the apical dendrites of the cell population or hyperpolarization (IPSPs) in the deeper neurons. A slow positive wave indicates the converse.

The late components are believed to represent mainly the effects of the non-specific inputs which rise from the reticular formation and non-specific thalamus. This input is not to be thought of as the mere tardy arrival of sensory excitations along slow, polysynaptic and highly convergent pathways. Rather, it represents (at least in part) the ascending output of subcortical mechanisms concerned in the evaluation of the significance of the stimulus in relation to the drive state of the organism. This includes the mechanisms of arousal and attention. Some of the late components appear only when the stimulus has significance as a cue for performance (cf. Section 10.3). In the case of novel stimuli they disappear if the stimuli fail to prove significant and the brain habituates to them.

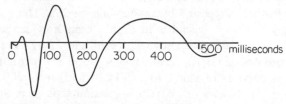

Figure 8.8. Idealized example of a typical EEG response to a single stimulus as it might be recorded in the primary cortical receiving area of the stimulus modality (negative recorded upwards). The short-latency positive–negative response is followed by slower components with longer latencies

In the responsive regions of the association areas the observed EEG responses to single stimuli belong mainly to three different types. The first type is a positive–negative diphasic wave, very similar to the one evoked in the primary cortex but of slightly longer latency. The second is the most common type and consists of a mainly positive slow wave with longer latency. The third type is a long latency wave with ill-defined features and latencies 20%–100% longer than those of primary responses.

The full significance of these various waveforms is extremely difficult to interpret in functional terms. Evoked responses in the responsive regions of the association areas commonly relate to more than one modality. However, this convergence may occur at a variety of different levels. Some may be due to intracortical connections, some to convergence in the thalamic association nuclei and some to convergence in the ascending reticular system. Convergent sensory information may also reach the cortex from limbic structures through their projection to the non-specific thalamus. Nor does this list exhaust all possibilities.

Some of the sensory inputs converging in subcortical structures may themselves be of primary cortical origin. In some cases in which it could be shown by cooling a primary area or by applying strychnine that the area exercised control over the convergent response in an association area, the latency of these responses was such that a cortical-subcortical pathway seemed the most reasonable hypothesis [37].

Neurophysiology still has some way to go before these and other factors can be completely analysed and cortical waveforms given an exhaustive interpretation. For the time being the information we can extract from EEG recordings in respect of the particular problems dealt with in this volume is likely to remain very limited. But the possible significance of some of these phenomena will become clearer as we go along (cf. Chapter 10).

8.7 CONCLUDING REMARKS

In this chapter I have tried to fill in some of the background of fact and theory relating to a number of important structures in the brain, keeping in mind the particular features suggested by the lambda models. These models were designed mainly to help us visualize in simple terms how certain properties of neurons and certain types of network organization may yield the kind of system properties we are interested in. In view of the abstract nature of these relations it would be extravagant to expect to find neat replicas of these models in the brain. Even so it may be significant that there are structures whose fine anatomy exhibits particular traits of the lambda models, such as input sharing and lateral inhibition, and that there are others which at least contain the basic elements required by the lambda systems.

The relationships discussed in Chapter 7 are very general ones and for the purpose of this work it is important to remain at a high level of generality lest we lose sight of the overall picture. Our aim is to map out the logical relations that can help us to see, if only dimly, how one thing may be connected with another, rather than to frame detailed hypotheses about limited functions. In our present state of knowledge detailed hypotheses require the addition of many special assumptions and this must remain the province of the specialist in each of the fields concerned. However, in his search for fruitful hypotheses the specialist, too, depends on general suppositions of how one thing may ultimately be related to another. What can usefully be said at a general level is not wasted in the search for detailed explanations. Thus for the specialist, too, it may be valuable to have at the back of the mind the knowledge that the combination of input sharing and lateral inhibition may signify special learning capacities or that forcing inputs acting on such a system may serve important functions of stimulus substitution. Both are notions that have been used in Marr's theory of cerebellar function, for example.

Again, it may prove fruitful to realize that the results of the correlation studies of Noda and coworkers[179, 182] may indicate underlying functions of the type explicated in the lambda models.

In the next chapter we shall follow up some of these functions. In particular we shall try to form a clearer idea of how the representational functions envisaged in the lambda system of Figure 7.12 may in fact be applied by the brain in the construction of internal models of the physical world.

CHAPTER 9

Shape Recognition and Internal Models

9.1 PERCEPTION AND MOVEMENT

In this chapter we return to the internal models which the brain forms of the outer world. To see the world in terms of these models is in effect to order the perceptive data by imposing on them 'templates' or 'schemata' which have formed in the course of prolonged and active experience. The recognition of patterns briefly exposed as in the tachistoscope illustrates the decisive influence of the viewer's stock of templates. Shape recognition under these conditions is generally defective except with simple familiar patterns. The process has been aptly characterized by Woodworth as 'schema with correction'. The pattern is interpreted in terms of familiar patterns with something missing or something added which, in turn, is familiar. Typically the subject's reaction is of the kind: 'triangle with a crooked bottom', 'square with a rounded corner', etc. According to our analysis movements of the eyes, head or body are essential in the early formative stages of model building but not in the final application of the models to the visual inputs. The tachistoscope shows that whereas this is true for simple shapes, complex shapes may require active visual exploration even at the later stages of development.

The ordering of perceptive data by the imposition of templates based on experience conveys many biological advantages. As already mentioned in Chapter 2 it facilitates the development of appropriate responses to the objective properties of the environment and the positive transfer of training. It also enables complex data to be apprehended as unitary wholes and increases the discriminability of patterns from background 'noise'[244]. Gregory[94] has pointed out a number of other advantages. For instance, since the perception of objects now requires identification of only certain key features of the objects, high performance can be achieved with a limited rate of information transmission. Since the models are essentially predictive, performance can be further improved by a reduction in reaction time. The use of internal models also enables the system to carry on during temporary absence of input, as when blinking or sneezing while driving, or when inputs change in kind. Thus in maze-learning a rat can continue to run a maze once learned though it is denied each sensory input—vision, smell, kinaesthesis etc.—in turn.

261

Of course, there are also disadvantages. Thus on the strength of certain salient similarities the wrong model may be called up and systematic errors may occur. A plausible case can be made out for the view that a number of optical illusions are based on errors of this kind.

According to our analysis,

    (i) internal models may be interpreted as aggregates of conditional expectations about the way the sensory inputs transform in response to self-produced movements of eyes, head or body;

   (ii) the concept of directive correlation enables us to interpret 'expectation' in a precise and objective sense as a state of adaptedness which matches the way in which particular sensory input variables (s) depend on particular movement variables (m);

  (iii) this state of adaptedness calls for neural representations of the character of the functions $s=f(m)$ concerned;

  (iv) at the simplest theoretical level the character of such a function may be registered in neural terms if there exists a set of neurons which respond to specific combinations of s and m and if, during learning, (a) those neurons of the set become sensitized which respond to the particular combinations of s and m that the function specifies and (b) during prolonged training these neurons become associated with each other and conditioned in a manner which enables them to be jointly triggered by appropriate input configurations, thus providing a pattern of outputs which maps on the aggregate of expectations of how s transforms as a function of m; thus, after adequate training, the model can be triggered without participation of the movements to which it relates;

   (v) even comparatively simple combinations of certain neural operations (OR functions, AND functions, adequate stimulus substitution, positive feedback) permit such prepresentations to be formed (Section 7.8.).

According to the same analysis not only figural properties but all objective properties of the environment are wholly or partly represented in the brain in terms of particular aggregates of conditional expectations. Thus the distance of an object would be partly represented by expectations of how the apparent size of the object will transform as we approach or retreat. During training such expectations come to be triggered by appropriate cues, e.g. ocular accommodation and convergence. If the elicited expectations are subsequently falsified by experience, either the cell assemblies that constitute the respective expectations or the conditions that trigger them must be restructured. For example, false expectations may be induced experimentally if the subject is made to wear glasses that change the accommodation and convergence. In this particular case the evidence suggests that the subject gradually adapts to this situation by altering the relation between the accommodation and convergence on the one hand and the class of elicited expectations (i.e. registered distance) on the other[264]. In other words the changes occur in the triggering mechanisms.

The notion of groups of cells which become associated during learning such that they can briefly come to act as a closed system, was first introduced by Hebb[104] in 1949. Hebb also propounded the view that 'receptor adjustment' (head- and eye-movements) is the most prominent feature of visual perception, whether in rat, chimpanzee or man—except after prolonged training. But the 'cell assemblies' he envisaged formed mainly in consequence of two or more cells being repeatedly active at the same time, and 'expectancy' for Hebb was no more than a central facilitation of cell discharges which preceded their sensory facilitation.

Expectations can function at very different levels. At a low level they may relate to no more than the transformation of primary sensory inputs in response to simple movements. Expectations at this level play a crucial role in the basic processes of perception and in the formation of cell organizations which represent the salient features of the figures and shapes we see in the visual plane. At a higher level there are expectations which relate to the manner in which these projected shapes or figures transform as we advance or retreat in the environment, move to the right or to the left etc. These play a critical part in the perception of solid objects and of their relations in space. At yet another level we have expectations concerning the consequences of manipulating objects in one way or another. All these expectations are conditional since they relate to the consequences of movements which may or may not be executed, and all are applications of the reafference principle.

Since objects can also move or change independently, without interference on our part, the brain obviously must also be able to form (unconditional) expectations about how some observed change or movement is likely to continue. However, since in the visual, tactile and proprioceptive sphere these expectations are only relevant at a level which presupposes the cognitive faculties we have considered above, they are of secondary importance in the present context. This does not apply to the sense of hearing. Auditory inputs do not transform in response to self-produced movements except in their directional qualities. The most significant expectations in this sphere probably relate to the sequence of coming auditory inputs as a function of the auditory inputs that went before and the context in which they occurred. At any rate it seems to me that our ability to recognize melodies and other acoustic forms regardless of their pitch can only be explained in terms of the expectations that the sounds we have heard elicit about the sounds we are about to hear. However, this subject lies outside the scope of this volume. It may be noted in passing, though, that the theoretical networks we considered in Chapter 7 are also capable of registering expectations of this type.

The importance of self-produced movements in the developmental stages of visual form perception has been demonstrated in a number of experiments performed by Held, Hein and others. Held and Hein[107] have shown that if two kittens are brought up in conditions in which both animals experience moving patterns of visual inputs, but one kitten merely passively whereas the other induced movements of the shapes by its own activities, only the second kitten develops visually guided behaviour. Similarly, rats placed in environments in which bodily movement was restricted were found to be significantly inferior in maze-learning capacity than animals raised in an environment which provided adequate opportunities for free movement[276]. Studies relating both to the effects of early deprivation and to the effects of early enrichment confirm that motility is as important as the richness of the visual stimuli in the development of perceptual faculties, and that the experience of visual forms in the early stages of development is effective only to the extent to which the visual forms can act as cues for attentional processes and/or overt activity. Thus Gibson, Walk and Tighe[79] found in rats that the early experience of different figures or shapes only facilitates their subsequent discriminability if the figures or shapes are three-dimensional objects or reliefs which can be singled out from the background and to which the animal can respond as articulated signals or cues. No comparable effects were obtained with two-dimensional figures.*

In the primate infant the development of the visual powers shows a number of features which we can only understand if we realize that the eye is a reaching, grasping and prehensile organ and that the ability to see develops as an integral part of the development of total behaviour[78]. Here, too, it has been found that motility as well as enriched stimulation is needed to facilitate progress[272].

In the adult there is less opportunity to study the formation of basic perceptual schemata but we can study the adaptations and compensations the brain has to make when the subject is confronted with special sensory rearrangements. In these cases stimulation dependent on natural movement has been shown to be essential for the achievement of full and accurate compensation[105, 106]. Movement and active exploration (contour following, counting of corners etc.) has also been found to be essential for the development of the visual faculties in subjects who were blind from birth but recovered their sight later in life[217].

Much research done during recent years has shown that throughout adult life vision remains guided by behaviour as well as behaviour being obviously guided by vision. As Smith[227] has put it, it seems 'that we see and do and in so doing see anew and differently'. In many ways it seems that the interaction between movement and perception remains reciprocal and that the sensory

---

* See also the work of Riesen, Kurke and Mellinger on interocular transfer in visually naive and visually experienced cats[207] and of Chow and Nissen on interocular transfer in infant chimpanzees[42].

effects of behaviour modify or modulate the perceived characteristics of the visual environment[139]. Sometimes, too, the neural state which initiates movement appears to determine, at least partially, the conscious experience of perception[65, 262].

According to the present account the main element in the perception of objects consists of the selective activation of internal models or schemata which have formed as the result of previous experience. Although these models may be triggered exclusively by visual data they generally include also expectations which extend over the non-visual features of the object which in the past have proved to be significant in relation to the subject's goals. In this sense perception is a reading of general object characteristics from visual images.

One of the most difficult problems posed by shape recognition concerns the mechanisms that cause specific responses to become attached to specific *classes* of shapes or figures irrespective of the size, position and orientation of the object in the visual field. It does not particularly matter in this respect whether the response is an overt one or the kind of internal response which we mean by the *recognition* of a shape or object as being one of a particular kind. The problem is a challenging one because the phenomenon suggests that during training the brain can learn to attach appropriate responses to stimulus configurations which in terms of actual retinal inputs it has never experienced before. Having learnt to discriminate between particular sets of squares and triangles in the size, position and orientation in which they were represented during training, the brain appears to be able to generalize this information and extend the discrimination to triangles and squares in any position, size or orientation. Within certain limits, at any rate, the resulting discriminations appear to be invariant to scale, translation or rotation of the figure. This contrasts with machines that can learn to discriminate between particular patterns of inputs repeatedly presented to them, but fail to cope with projections they have not experienced before. The brain differs from these machines in that it has the power to extract particular properties from the figures or shapes and, as we have suggested, it does so mainly on the reafference principle. There are also machines that achieve pattern recognition by compiling property lists and these, too, tend to use simple forms of the re-afference principle, e.g. scanning and contour-following.

9.2   SHAPE RECOGNITION AND CONTOUR-FOLLOWING

The problem of shape recognition has remained unsolved despite the discovery of receptive cells in the visual cortex which respond selectively to the movement of straight-line stimuli and angles whose orientation in the visual field is characteristic and constant (Section 6.4). Hubel and Wiesel themselves recognize that specialized as the cells are that they discovered in the cortex 'they nevertheless represent a very elementary stage in the handling of complex forms, occupied as they are with a relatively simple region-by-region analysis of retinal contours. How this information is used at the later stages in the visual path is far from clear and represents one of the most tantalizing problems of the future'[119]. From the elementary ability to respond to specific contour elements it is still a far cry to mechanisms that can learn to classify shapes such as chairs and tables according to complex properties for which we cannot expect innate detectors to have developed during evolution.

The main fact that emerges from the discovery of these specialized cells in the visual cortex is the profound preoccupation of the visual system with the contours of visual shapes. This suggests that contours play a special part in shape recognition.

The tracking of contours generally relies on central vision. This is directed by the fovea, a densely innervated depression of about 2 mm diameter close to the centre of the retina. Whereas up to 100 rods of the outer retina may be represented by no more than a single fibre in the optic tract, each cone of the fovea contributes a single fibre to this tract. However, none of these channels is isolated. Already at the retinal level each is subject to lateral influences from neighbouring channels.

Although the fixation of visual objects is normally controlled by the fovea, neighbouring regions may substitute if the fovea is damaged[48]. Patients with occipital lesions which result in a central island of blindness tend to develop a vicarious fovea in the margin of the scotoma, i.e. of the obscured portion of the visual field.

An interesting observation made on patients with central scotoma is that after the injury they can promptly discriminate and name any contoured figure that is circumscribed around the scotoma, such as large outlined triangles, squares or circles. This shows that the shape recognition does not rely on processes within the boundaries of a figure seen.

The primary perception of contours depends on the sharp gradient in brightness between the object and its background. The retinal cells most immediately concerned in this are probably the cells which respond maximally to changes in illumination. They can act as gradient detectors because of the small jerky movements which the perceiving eye is known to execute even while it is anchored to the object of attention. These movements are accompanied by a high frequency tremor of about 20 or more cycles per second. The brightness contrast detected by this mechanism may be further enhanced by lateral inhibition. Systems of lateral inhibition may also account for the signals which enable the subject to know which side of a boundary is the dark one. At any rate there is convincing evidence that this knowledge is not derived from knowledge of the oculomotor response occurring at the time. However, the overall importance of movement is shown by the fact that vision proves impossible when optical atachments are fitted to the eye which result in images that are completely stationary relative to the retina.

To pass from knowledge of the salient contour features or elements of a shape to knowledge of the shape as such we need knowledge of the spatial relation between these features or elements. On the reafference principle the brain can factor out information regarding the spatial relation between particular contour elements by moving the eyes from contour element to contour element while registering at the same time the nature of the movements required. It can do so either by scanning the contour elements in their proper serial order (contour-following), or by jumping haphazardly from salient element to salient element. Either method could yield the required information. In the first case the contour elements need not necessarily be individually identified and labelled by the brain. In theory the brain would have to do no more than to register the nature and sequence of the movements which the optical pursuit of the contour permits. In the second case, however, the individual elements (lines, angles, terminations etc.) must be identified. Apart from this difference, the formal network requirements are similar to those we discussed in Chapter 7 in connection with the reafference principle.

In continuous contour-following the characteristics of the contour are represented by the family of permitted movements. This representation is invariant in respect of the translation of the object within the field. If only the *relative* directions and *relative* magnitudes of the movements were registered by the brain the resulting representation would also be invariant to the size and orientation of the image. In this process the primary function of the 'simple', 'complex' and 'hypercomplex' cells in the visual cortex would be to guide the eye in the execution of the contour-locked movements. We shall see that the actual events in shape recognition are unlikely to be as simple as this. But the paradigm is nevertheless a useful one to bear in mind.

Although the idea of contour-following suggests a continuous movement of the eye along the contour, in fact the eye proceeds by discrete jumps. When the eyes scan the visual field they move in brief jerks or 'saccades'. As they move from one target to the next they carry out a rapid 'preset' flick of approximately the correct amplitude, followed by a final drift which brings the fixation target to the fovea. During the saccades the visual inputs are suppressed. Reading a normal line of 114 mm a skilled reader will make about six fixation pauses depending on the difficulty of the material or interest in it.*

Only as a first approximation, therefore, can we think of contour-following as sequences of discrete movements which take the eye from one salient feature to the next. Nor do these discrete movements invariably adhere strictly to the contour. Stratton[238] showed many years ago that in tracing the contour of circles the saccades do not follow the appropriate curvilinear paths but form straight lines. And there are other inaccuracies, such as a preference

---

* For a comprehensive review of research on eye movements (1932–1962) the reader may consult Scott's annotated bibliography[215].

for horizontal and vertical movements. However, since the visual inputs are suppressed during the saccades their precise course is not strictly relevant in the present context, the main consideration being that statistically their terminal points should cluster around the actual contours.

During infancy, developments in the accuracy of shape perception proceed in close conjunction with tactual exploration[1]. Throughout the first few months the major visuomotor activities primarily consist of internal ocular adjustments of accommodation and position, convergence and pursuit, coupled with rotations of the head and movements of arms, hands and fingers within the visual field[261]. At about three months the infant stretches out his hand towards an object he sees. At this stage he still glances repeatedly to and fro between his hand and the object. A month or so later he may grasp the object and cease to look at his hand[272]. Now, too, he begins to explore the object with his fingers, comparing the shape he feels with the shape he sees[196]. Significantly, pictures of solid objects are still ignored.

Not until 8 or 9 months does the infant grasp fully that as an object is turned round in space the visual pattern changes regularly but the object as felt remains the same. Until that age, for example, he will make no attempt to grasp a baby's bottle if it is presented with the nipple turned away from him[260]. Only gradually does he begin to realize that objects have a permanent identity and that when they pass behind a screen they do not cease to exist but may reappear[197]. In all this we witness clearly the gradual development of ever more comprehensive expectancies. For a long time, though, the child fails to realize which characteristics of objects are essential for classifying or naming them and recognition may occur only when the object appears in familiar settings. By the age of 4 the infant can match tactually objects perceived visually and match visually objects perceived tactually.

Complex shapes and the interrelationships of their parts are not perceived with complete accuracy until the age of 5 or 6. According to Piaget this is

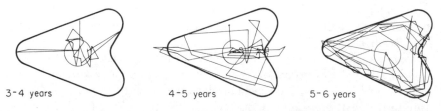

3-4 years   4-5 years   5-6 years

Figure 9.1. Saccadic eye-movements of children of different ages when looking at a shape. The development of contour-following is evident (From A. V. Zaporozhets, *The development of perception in the preschool child*, in *European Research in Cognitive Development* (ed. Mussen). © 1965 by The Society for Research in Child Development, Inc. Reproduced by permission of The Society for Research in Child Development, Inc.)

because only at this age does perceptual exploration become systematic and does the child learn to direct his attention and his gaze regularly and successively from one part of the field or complex shape to another, thus comparing all aspects effectively. Comparative records of actual eye-movements executed by a child gazing at a shape show that this is also the age at which contour-following movements predominate (Figure 9.1). These movements are saccadic and they remain so even if the child is instructed to trace the lines smoothly with the eyes (Figure 9.2). During the earlier stages of perceptual learning the infant appears to depend more on registering salient features other than contours. If presented with a large black triangle, for example, the neonate will direct the eyes at the vertices of the triangle, typically remaining on a single vertex in a given session.

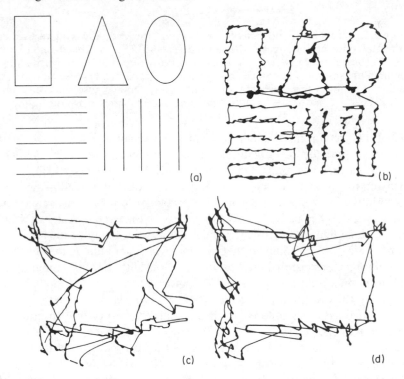

Figure 9.2. Saccadic eye-movements used in examining geometrical figures (a); trying to trace the figures (b); looking without instruction (c); looking after the instruction 'look at the figures and count the number of straight lines' (d). After a shape has been learned by laboriously outlining it, it is not necessary to scan it precisely with saccadic eye-movements; it can be perceived with a fleeting glance. Looking without special instruction (c) the subject seems to be able to take in the patterns without outlining them (From Abercrombie[1] after A. L. Yarbus, *Eye Movements and Vision*[275], 1967. Reproduced by permission of Plenum Publishing Corp.)

One of the factors that appear to hold up contour-following at the early stage is the difficulty the child has with oblique eye-movements. Yarbus[275], for example, has shown that the records of the saccadic movements used in looking at horizontal and vertical contours are straight, but those used for oblique contours are curved (Figure 9.3). Oblique lines are also more difficult to draw. A child can copy a square adequately at the age of 5 but may fail dismally in trying to copy a diamond.

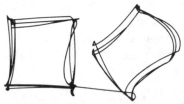

Figure 9.3. Saccadic eye-movements used in outlining a square with vertical and horizontal sides and a square with all sides at 45° (From Abercrombie[1] after A. L. Yarbus, *Eye Movements and Vision*[275], 1967. Reproduced by permission of Plenum Publishing Corp.) Since the eye has six pairs of muscles, two of them oblique, it is not at first clear why the oblique line should cause such difficulties. Yarbus believes that it may result from non-simultaneous working of the different muscles

Contours retain their importance in the recognition of novel shapes throughout adult life. Investigations with eye-marker cameras show that when the adult meets a new shape like an irregular inkblot, the eye's fixations fall chiefly on the blot's contours[150]. The importance of contour-following is also shown in the behaviour of patients with particular lesions in the visual areas of the cortex. When in one of Adler's patients with cerebral lesions recognition of whole figures was lost, it required contour training to reconstitute it again[3, 4]. Similarly it is known that in people who were blind from birth but to whom sight was restored later on in life, the faculty of shape recognition is contingent on a transitory period in which the patient develops the technique of running the eyes round the boundary and counting the corners[217].

The visual system is tailored to throw contours into prominence and the 'tractive' influence of a contour on the eyes once they have locked on the contour is well known. A brain that can register the sequence of movements resulting when this tractive influence asserts itself, has a record available of the properties of the contour which lends itself for categorizing reactions related to these properties and hence to the shape. It is difficult to see why the brain should not avail itself of such records. Zaporozhets[278] has pointed out how the attentional responses with which we inspect one portion of a stimulus object after another must take a form which corresponds to the shape and other attributes of the object. Internalized versions of these responses could therefore serve as bases for the internal representation of the objects, particularly in the absence of the objects.

All the same, an account of shape recognition solely in terms of contour-following is likely to miss the mark. The hypothesis is not seriously threatened by the observation that contour-following takes time whereas we know that we can recognize at any rate simple shapes at a glance (or almost at a glance: the exposure required even for these may be 100 milliseconds or more). It would be reasonable to assume that contour-following enters only into particular developmental states of shape recognition and that we develop instant recognition later through the process of adequate stimulus substitution illustrated in Section 7.8. This would enable frequently experienced retinal projections in due course to become direct releasers of classifying responses which were originally based on the characteristic sequence of eye-movements involved in following the contour. Thus the shape can now be perceived at a glance.

We must reject explanations exclusively relying on contour-following for different reasons, quite apart from the fact that it is demonstrably absent in the first years of life. In a narrow sense, of course, it might be argued that by definition the properties of a shape are the properties of its outlines. On this narrow view logic dictates that to discover the properties of outlines the brain must begin by following the outlines. But this is too narrow a view. In a wider sense the properties of a shape extend over the total effects produced by the outlines. These include such relations as symmetry, asymmetry, regularity or irregularity, roundness, squatness, jaggedness and other features[6]. It would be unrealistic to assume that the brain cannot be aware of some of these features from the start, particularly since they include the sort of features which appear to control shape discrimination in the lower species. The studies of J. Z. Young[277] and his collaborators on learning in the octopus, for example, provide a wealth of information on the faculty of shape recognition in the lower species. Given suitable training schedules the octopus can be taught to discriminate between (say) a vertical and horizontal rectangle, or between a diamond shape and a square. Sutherland[240] has proposed that these discriminations are performed on the basis of simple dimensional comparisons between these projections. Other investigators, too, have concluded that the animal relies on elementary dimensional comparisons for which it has 'wired-in' detectors. Animals like rats and chicken seem to discriminate shapes mainly in terms of salient parts of the figure. In rats this tends to be the base line. Animals at this level readily transfer to figures of different size but have difficulty with rotated figures.

The only wired-in detectors we can identify in the visual apparatus of the higher vertebrates are the simple, complex, and hypercomplex cells of Hubel and Wiesel. But this does not rule out that there may also be wired-in detectors for other types of elementary features.

Studies of the interest shown by very young infants in different shapes introduced into their field of vision show that they are more strongly attracted by patterned shapes such as a chequer-board than by plain shapes of the same size. Among patterned shapes they appear to prefer a bull's eye pattern to a striped pattern, but they are indifferent to crosses compared with circles, for example. However it is clear that the infant's initial powers of actual synthesis must be very limited. In view of the importance of people in the life of the infant and the fact that the facial pattern is the most consistently distinctive aspect of a person, the observation that infants initially show little if any preference for face-like patterns over other patterns of similar complexity (e.g. 'scrambled faces') indeed suggests that the organization of form perception must be very rudimentary at birth. But even if we were to assume that the newborn infant has wired-in detectors for contour elements only and that the recognition of other elementary features is initially acquired only on this basis, more elaborate features could soon come to be recognized as composites of elementary features standing in particular spatial relations to one another. It seems reasonable to assume that the visual exploration and assimilation of novel shapes takes the form of the eye darting from recognizable feature to recognizable feature and assimilating their mutual spatial relations, as well as running around the contours and taking in the landmarks it meets on the way.

To factor out spatial relations, e.g. the distance between two points on the retina, the reafference principle provides a more economical method than, for example, a system of wired-in detectors capable of signalling the distance between any possible pair of stimuli on the retina. To detect that the retinal distance between projections *A* and *B* is the same as between *C* and *D* the visual system has to do no more than discover that the eye movement required to shift fixation from *A* to *B* is the same as that for *C* and *D*. Even on the simple view that the movement executed in shifting fixation from *A* to *B* is physiologically recorded by innate detectors reporting the distance of *B* from the fovea when *A* is fixated, it is clear that the only innate distance detectors required would be for the distances of stimulated retinal points from the fovea.

In Section 7.8 we have seen in what manner the reafference principle and networks of the type illustrated in Figure 7.12 might enable the brain to assimilate elementary spatial relations in the visual plane. Given the capacity to recognize any set of elementary shapes of figural elements and the spatial relations of their retinal projections, complex shapes or figures may subsequently come to be recognized as particular arrangements or juxtapositions of such elements. Supporting evidence that this may be the case, even in the recognition of such simple figures as triangles, comes from the study of the fragmentation of after-images. The after-images of compound figures do not fade away evenly. Frequently different components of the figure suddenly vanish in their entirety and at different intervals. Thus in the after-image of a triangular figure an entire side may suddenly disappear, leaving a clearly perceptible V-shape. This suggests that a triangle is perceived as a particular arrangement of individually recognized lines rather than as a stimulus configuration which has become an adequate stimulus substitute for a classification originally based on the characteristic movement sequence involved in tracing its contour. However the evidence is equally compatible with the theory that the triangle is recognized as a fusion of three V-shapes. Indeed, there is no reason to assume that the mechanisms of shape recognition are limited to any one single process. Possibly the triangle is recognized as being all of these things. The burden of proof must rest on the shoulders of anyone who postulates that the brain uses only one operative principle in developing the faculty of shape recognition. The danger of monolithic explanations was mentioned in Chapter 1. It seems more reasonable to assume that the visual apparatus exploits all the modes of shape exploration that are open to it and that it achieves much of its final powers of discrimination through the resulting overlap and overdetermination. This would offer the particular advantage that owing to the general restraint of compatibility and continuity each operational method could afford to function at a lower level of accuracy than would otherwise be the case.

The value of this type of restraint is quite general. As Marr[161] has pointed out, in shape recognition it is only necessary to localize the components of any image to an extent that will prevent confusion with other images. The exact position of edges, corners and other recognizable features of a complex shape need not be retained, because the general restraint of continuity of form will mean that the exact relative positions can always be recovered from a knowledge of the approximate positions, the number of terminations and the approximate length of the segments of a figure.

9.3 SHAPE RECOGNITION IN CENTRAL AND PERIPHERAL VISION

Three points stand out from what has gone before:

(i) the importance of the reafference principle in the exploration of the visual scene particularly during the ontogenetic development of the faculty of shape recognition;

(ii) the importance of central vision and of the mechanism of fixation in this visual exploration;

(iii) the importance of some mechanism of adequate stimulus substitution which enables simple features originally classified in terms of the outcomes of active visual explorations subsequently to be recognized at a glance.

Regardless of whether the eye explores a novel shape by moving around its contours or by darting haphazardly from one salient feature to another, we cannot dispense with the process of active visual exploration as such in the assimilation of novel shapes. And in the first instance exploration means the exploitation of the principle of reafference. The basic principles of the type of neural networks that could effect this exploitation were illustrated in Sections 7.8–7.10.

The early development of vision and shape recognition must be seen against the background of the general behavioural development of the infant. In the young infant the exploration of the visual scene is no isolated event. It is part of a general process in which the infant develops its behavioural equipment, even though it is true that in this development nature has given priority to the sense of sight.

In the newborn infant the eyes move in unison and it can fixate only momentarily and monocularly. At a later stage monocular fixation alternates between the two eyes and after about eight weeks this alternation has resulted in a teaming of the eyes which enables them to converge simultaneously on an object of interest. Ocular prehension precedes manual prehension: at about 20 weeks the infant can pick up a small object on the table with the eyes but only after another 20 weeks or so can he pick the object up with his fingers[78]. Then begins a period of intensive development of hand–eye coordination and the active manipulation of objects. The subsequent development of the faculty of vision is dominated by such object-oriented manipulations. The solid shape of objects, therefore, comes to be recognized before the geometric shapes of their projections in the visual plane. It is objects that are handled, not abstract shapes. In consequence infant vision is faithful to objects rather than their retinal projections. Tilted plates are seen as tilted plates and not as ellipses. If geometric shapes such as circles are shown at that stage the infant sees them as suggesting real objects such as balls. It is not surprising that under the age of 6–7 years perception is 'synchretic': wholes emerge as more readily distinguishable than what later in life we learn to recognize as significant details[260].

However, it is important not to be confused by this observation. The fact that wholes are more readily distinguished than details does not imply that at this stage the brain fails to learn to factor out more and more significant details and geometric properties of retinal images. It does not mean that at this stage the brain fails to expand its faculties of feature detection. All it means is that the particular category of new information resulting from this expansion initially remains pooled with all sorts of information from other sources in determining the infant's developing responses and his classifications of the objects he sees. Only at a later stage does the child learn to separate this category of information from the others and produce responses specifically related to it.

Similarly, the child learns to abstract colour information only at a comparatively late stage despite the fact that sensory awareness of colour differences exists already soon after birth. Even children as young as fifteen days can follow a spot of coloured light which is moved to and fro on a background of different colour but equal brightness. But for a long time the child regards colour as an inherent characteristic of certain particular objects. Only after two or three years does it develop responses which are exclusively related to colour information.

The eye is a prehensile organ. This means that the preeminent process in visual exploration is the process of fixation, the process of shifting images from the periphery to the area of central vision and of holding them there. Centralization is the fundamental response of the visual system. We know that stimulation of any part of the primary visual cortex triggers oculomotor responses which direct the eye to the respective point of the visual field. Cells which respond to particular contour elements like edges and angles have an obvious part to play in any mechanism seeking the centralization of such elements as in contour-following. But it is also evident that the process of centralization must function at several distinct levels. Shapes near the periphery of the visual field appear as no more than blurred patches and it is unlikely that any narrowly definable class of cells controls the centralization of such a shape in the first instance. Only when this initial process has brought (say) the centroid of this shape into an approximately central position can the details of the shape, e.g. particular contour elements, assume control over subsequent fixations and the detailed exploration of the shape. This must be a competitive process. For although we have loosely spoken of exploratory movements as self-induced movements, in strictly causal terms, of course, each such movement must be induced by some sensory stimulus gaining ascendancy over others. The detailed visual exploration of the now broadly centralized shape must therefore be conceived as a sequence of fixations in which one visual detail after another gains control over the mechanism of centralization.

According to the expectancy thesis a shape originally learnt through visual exploration later comes to be recognized instantly in terms of the expectations it elicits about what the eye would meet in successive fixations if it were to explore the shape. Assuming the primacy of central vision this means in the first instance what the fovea would meet in successive fixations by way of features recognizable by the wired-in central analysers. The mutual relations of these features in the visual field are characterized by the direction and magnitude of the eye-movements that link the successive fixations.

The following is an outline of the type of mechanisms this suggests for shape recognition through central vision.

I. At the lowest level we have the 'primary analysers', the wired-in detectors for particular contour features such as for bars in particular orientations, bars stopped at one end, angles etc. We cannot assume, of course, that the wired-in detectors discovered by Hubel and Wiesel are the only ones. There may be more complex analysers not yet discovered. However, at some level of complexity we must reach a point at which a particular feature is no longer 'innately' detectable but requires visual exploration and learning. Are there wired-in detectors for T-shapes? We do not know. Perhaps there are for T-shapes but not for H-shapes. At this general level of discussion it does not matter. What matters is the nature of the supplementary mechanisms that come into action when the level of complexity exceeds what can be detected by the existing analysers.*

II. For these higher levels of complexity learning processes are required which, initially at any rate, depend on the outcomes of exploratory activities such as contour-following. This is because we cannot regard a complex shape or figural element in this context as the mere sum of simpler shapes or figural elements. For the purpose of factoring out its distinctive characteristics the H-shape cannot be regarded as the mere sum of three recognizable bars. The whole is more than the sum of its parts: it is the sum of its parts plus the relations between them. These relations are reflected in the outcomes of exploratory activities: such and such movements of the eye result in such and such sequences of salient contour elements striking the fovea. To register these outcomes is in effect to compile a characteristic property list of the contour in question. In neural terms this means registering the direction and amplitude of the movements that take the fovea from one salient contour element to another and registering simultaneously the character of each element on which the eye comes to rest during the exploration. A high degree of generalization of the contour's properties would result if the movements are classified according to relative amplitudes and changes of direction rather than absolute amplitudes and absolute directions (taking the head as frame of reference).

In this particular application the movement information could be derived either from the oculomotor apparatus or from the internal attentional processes which cause each of the relevant contour elements in turn to attract the eye, i.e. to gain control over the oculomotor apparatus.

III. Assuming the primacy of central vision this means that during the exploration the brain must register what sets of activated analysers (X) relating to what retinal locations (P_x), are consistently followed by what recognizable contour elements (Y) arriving at the fovea in consequence of what movements (M) of the eye. (Merely to assume that the brain registers the succession of contour elements arriving at the fovea as a function of eye-movement would give us no more than a keyhole type of exploration in which instant recognition of the shape could not develop—see below.) Given a sufficiently comprehensive exploration of the shape, the aggregate of these registrations forms an adequate neural basis for categorizing the shape accord-

---

* Although one tends to think of the Hubel and Wiesel analysers as innate equipment, this is not strictly true since they depend for their normal development on early visual experience.

ing to the mutual relations between the centrally recognizable elements (lines, curves, angles, terminations etc.)

IV. If, as learning progresses, a sufficient sample of these classifying outputs can become conditioned to any particular projection of the shape, then the mere occurrence of that projection in due course permits instant recognition of the shape, i.e. recognition without prior exploration. The system thus calls for two basic networks: one for combining movement information with foveal input information, and one for permitting the adequate stimulus substitution required by this conditioning.

V. The most elementary network configuration that could perform these twin operations is that symbolized in Figure 7.12. In this application the received value of Y at the fovea would be represented by specific e inputs and a record of the last eye-movement by specific a inputs (or vice versa), while the horizontal inputs to the B system would represent the analysers at other retinal locations (X at P_x) which the image of the shape activated just prior to the movement. Naturally one would have to think of the B system as a vastly expanded one, possibly comprising a considerable number of parallel systems.

VI. The system as it stands eventually permits the shape in any projection experienced during learning to trigger a characteristic set of expectations about what the fovea will receive following any one of a number of possible movements of the eye. These expectations can be extended to cover also the sensory consequences of a *succession* of steps if the horizontal inputs to the B system are preceded by a system in which any one visual input configuration can trigger outputs representing the visual input configurations to be expected from particular movements of the eye. We shall meet a system of this type in Section 9.4 (Figure 9.4). When learning is complete the shape can then instantly be recognized in any one of the projections experienced during the exploratory phase in terms of the comprehensive expectations it now elicits. These expectations now cover the alternative projections in which the shape was encountered during the visual exploration as well as the succession of events at the fovea following particular eye-movements. The complete set of these expectations constitutes the 'model' that is activated in the separation of the figure from the ground and the act of recognition.

VII. So far we have considered only projections of the shape during the exploratory phase in which at any one time some part of the shape is fixated, i.e. caused to fall on the fovea. However, it is easy to see that peripheral projections of the shape can also be covered by the proposed system if the centralization of the peripheral projection is treated as part of the exploratory process. In other words, given the primacy of central vision, peripheral projections of shapes can be recognized in terms of expectations about what the eye will meet when the images are centralized. It should be noted though that these expectations are formed at a somewhat different level, viz. at the level at which whole images compete for central attention rather than the salient elements of a given image. This difference is highlighted in the syndrome of Balint. In this syndrome the patient can perceive whatever he fixates on, but nothing else.

A few observations must be added to this outline.

(1) The mechanism appears to permit the instant recognition only of images occurring in projections on the retina that have been experienced before. This, however, is not true. It permits the recognition of shapes occurring in projections never experienced before on condition only that each of their essential elements has previously been experienced at the respective retinal location. For, the virtue of networks of the type suggested in Figure 7.12 is that the outputs are line-labelled both according to the recognized feature and its position in the visual field, so that place information can be separated from quality information and learnt relational responses formed on the basis of the place information can generalize to inputs of different quality appearing in the same locations. Hence the system can learn to recognize instantly mutual relations between figural elements never before experienced in that relation, provided only that other elements standing in the same relation have been experienced at the respective retinal locations. Thus the system could instantly recognize the compound shape EH in a projection never experienced before provided only that (a) the E and the H (or the elements of any other resolution of the compound shape) are separately recognizable at the retinal locations at which their projections appear and (b) on other elements (say X and Y) appearing in the same locations the system had previously learnt appropriate relational responses on the basis of place information only, so that, for example, the response 'X *to the left of* Y' could automatically generalize to 'E *to the left of* H'.

(2) The mechanism permits a high degree of overdetermination of the received shape. A triangle may be recognized as three lines in a particular relation, as three vertices in a particular relation, as the superposition of three V-shapes or as closed figure with three singularities (often the way in which young children will draw it). And in so far as the brain is able to recognize all of these features there is no reason to assume that it will go exclusively by just some of them.

Such overdetermination permits a low degree of resolution in the inputs and outputs of the mechanisms we have considered. This in turn permits a significant degree of generalization from experienced shapes to similar but not previously experienced ones. Additional degrees of generalization result if the movement information specifies relative amplitudes rather than absolute ones and changes of direction rather than absolute directions. This would give scale and rotational invariance. (Translational invariance has already been covered under the heading of peripheral projections.) Since the nervous system is known to be often more efficient in computing relative magnitudes rather than absolute ones, this is not wholly inconceivable. However, it may be rash to rely mainly on this hypothesis. The difficulty we have in recognizing inverted photographs (of people for example) shows that rotational invariance is not as perfect as the above hypothesis would lead us to' expect.

The brain has additional means available for achieving a certain degree of scale and rotational invariance, viz. in the expectations that develop in the course of our experience of changes in image scale as we advance towards an object or retreat from it and of rotational changes when we manipulate the object. Thus an inverted figure may be recognized in terms of what we expect to see when we turn it upright. This may be the more realistic hypothesis. However, as I have stressed before, in the field of shape recognition it is almost certainly a mistake to search for singular solutions to explain the capabilities of the visual system.

(3) We note that in the mechanism outlined above the position in the visual field of a recognized shape is a *computed* function. The same applies to its position relative to any given visual frame of reference. Being a computed function it is one on which the brain may become confused. This accords with the phenomenon of preservation. Patients suffering from this defect may see the pattern of a person's dress extended right across the wearer's face, or they may see a person walk right through the table. Shape discrimination has remained intact but the allocation of position has failed.

(4) At a first reading it may seem wasteful to provide the system with sets of input fibres which make separate provision for every possible combination of eye movement and figural information. The reasons which recommend consideration of this hypothesis are twofold. In the first place the outputs can be segregated in a way which makes it possible subsequently again to separate the place information from the shape information. This is of obvious importance for the mechanisms of attention. Frequently these mechanisms are more concerned with the 'what' rather than the 'where'. Secondly it meets a well known difficulty which confronts all shape recognizing mechanisms: to be able to do what the eye can do they must be able to respond appropriate to a field which contains a large number of identical objects. In many of the models which have been proposed for shape recognition the output channels occupied by a given shape left no room for more than one instance of that shape being present in the field at any one time.

It follows from the postulated properties of lambda systems that once the visual system has assimilated a number of frequently occurring shapes, the first reaction to the presentation of a novel figure must be expected to trigger the shape recognizing neurons whose existing alignments most closely match the new input configurations. As these alignments are the result of past experience, it follows that one must expect novel objects to be perceived in terms of previously experienced and familiar objects.

Another consequence of this property of lambda systems to respond according to the nearest input configuration on which any of their neurons have come to align would be the following. If, after the eye has been trained on a figure, part of the figure projected onto the retina is blotted out through lesions in the afferent pathways to the cortex or in the primary receptive areas of the cortex, so that the number of sensory input channels is diminished, the visual system may still respond as if the figure were complete. For the lambda neurons that receive the maximum synaptic drive from the diminished number of input channels when the figure is presented after the lesions occurred are still likely to be the same as those that received maximum drive from the complete set of input channels when the figure was presented before the lesion. They still are the ones with maximum alignment on the figural inputs that are left. Hence the pattern of outputs from the shape detecting system may remain the same and complete perception results despite the lesion. (This would *not* be the case if part of the figure were merely painted over with the colour of the background.) This could account for the completion of figures across scotomata, i.e. across blind spots produced by cerebral lesions. Under a variety of conditions projected images are known to be completed across such regions, so that there is no gap in perception although part of the stimulus falls into areas of blindness. In patients in whom, for example, half the visual field of the examined eye is blind, a figure H may be projected on the retina so that one leg falls into the blind half. In a number of such cases patients have reported seeing a complete H: the missing leg had been filled in by the brain. Even in the transient scotomata of migraine or of 'visual fits' completion is frequently observed.

Unless one realizes that conscious perception resides in the activation of representations which consist of aggregates of transformation expectations, the phenomena of completion are hard to understand. This includes completion across the blind spot of the normal eye. Patients with scotomata which obliterate sizeable portions of the field are only conscious of their defects when the scotomata are new. Clearly their new experiences now clash with expectations still carried over from experiences incurred before the injury. This is borne out by the fact that the patient does not see gaps or blank patches in the field when the scotomata occur. Conscious awareness of gaps or blank patches itself implies aggregates of particular expectations of how sensory inputs transform (or fail to) as the result of movement. Instead the patient notices experiences incongruent with his expectations: objects appear to be displaced in homonymous quadrants or sectors of quadrants. Sometimes these distortions take the form of reduplication or further multiplication of contours. There may also be perversions in the perception of motion. A patient might complain, for example, that in part of the field he sees a passing motor cycle as a 'string of motor cycles standing still'[241].

These distortions and perversions tend to disappear after a few weeks or months following injury, presumably as old expectations are corrected or obliterated and new ones take their place.

The fact that perception consists of the triggering of organized representations relating *en bloc* to the individual objects seen is also illustrated by phenomena of omission. Lashley[146] has reported that once when he travelled along a Florida highway a migraine attack set in with a small paracentral scotoma. While this lasted an appropriate shift of gaze would make a pursuing patrol car disappear while the road itself and the rest of the landscape remained subjectively continuous.

9.4   THE STABILITY OF THE VISUAL SCENE

The processes we have considered so far contain nothing to account for the stability of the visual scene which is maintained as the eyes move and the retinal projections of the scene run across the retinal receptors. Whenever we move our eyes the retinal images sweep across the receptors. Yet we do not experience movement if the environment itself is static. The world does not spin around us as the eyes rotate in their sockets. Another aspect of the same question relates to the identity of visual objects: how do we know that the green patch appearing at retinal location Y now is a projection of the same object as the green patch that appeared at location X a moment ago? A third aspect relates to the detection of objective movements: how do we know that a particular shift of the projection was due to a movement of the eye and not a movement of the object?

All this calls for a mechanism which can tell the brain that if the projection of an object appears at retinal position P at one moment it must be expected at position P' when the eye moves through an angle x', at P'' when the eye moves through an angle x'' etc. Then if the image fails to appear at the expected position the amount of mismatch can serve as an indication of the degree of movement inherent in the object itself.

The objective sense in which the term 'expectation' may be interpreted was analysed in Chapters 5 and 7. It means here that during the formative stages of perception (and in the course of whatever adjustments must be made later to correct for changes in our optical system) the brain must build up a set of connectivities which is adapted to a state of affairs in which a projection at P will be followed by one at P', P'', $\ldots$, if the eyes move through angles x', x'', $\ldots$ respectively. In other words, the brain must build up a set of connectivities which uniquely represents the way in which images transform in response to the different movements of which the eye is capable.

Of course, compensation for eye movements is only part of what is involved in the stability of the visual scene. In the wider sense in which 'stability' means a stable representation of the three-dimensional world we perceive around us, head and body movements must be taken into account as well. I shall treat this aspect of the matter as a separate problem. We shall turn to it when we take up the question of internal representations of solid objects and three-dimensional space. In the present section the question is solely how the brain constructs stable representations from the succession of projections which cross the retina as we move our eyes. The head is assumed to be stationary and questions of depth are left out of account. We can therefore also confine ourselves to monocular vision.

It is not difficult to conceive of lambda systems that could perform this stabilizing function. The demands are similar to those that were met in the system of Figure 7.12. If we treat the retinal position of an image as a function of eye-position only, as would be the case when the eye is being trained on stationary objects, it is easy to see that it would suffice to have a system which enables the brain to learn that an image I now located at P_0 when the eye is in position X must be expected at P_1 when the eye is in position Y, at P_2 when the eye moves to position Z etc.

Once again, therefore, we require a neural system which in a given context can elicit an aggregate of expectations in the objective sense in which 'expectation' was dealt with in Section 7.8.

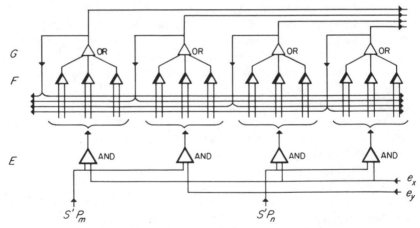

Figure 9.4. Segment of supplementary network for stable-image formation

We may assume that the system concerned derives its basic information from the output channels of the system discussed in the last section. We may start, therefore, with a set of afferent channels in which the current pattern of excitation represents what images are present at what retinal location. Figure 9.4 shows a representative segment of the type of lambda network that could meet the case. The input fibres $S'P_n$ and $S'P_m$ are members of a set in which excitation is specific to particular combinations of shape and position. Fibres e_x, e_y . . . , inform about the current position of the eye. (The human brain has knowledge of current eye position accurate to about 2°.) The rest of the system follows now familiar principles. The pattern of outputs from the AND gates represents what images are where on the retina in a given orientation of the eye.

Row F again forms a system for adequate stimulus substitution functioning in the now familiar manner. The dendritic inputs of this row are taken from feedback fibres as shown in the illustration. The excitations or traces present in this dendritic system therefore relate to the last activated combination of SP and e.

During learning any F neuron consistently responding to this pattern in a facilitated module aligns its synaptic potencies on the pattern. Again it is assumed that when learning is complete such a neuron can be fired by the dendritic input pattern even in absence of facilitation from below. Hence when learning is complete the appearance of an image I at any retinal site when the eye is in a given position comes to activate an aggregate of G neurons which represents the aggregate of alternative combinations of image location and eye-position which can be expected if the eyes move to a new position. This aggregate (as represented by the outputs from the OR gates in row G) is a stable pattern which will be re-excited every time the eye moves to a new position and its expectations are confirmed. If the expectations are not confirmed, this would appear as discrepancies between the firing pattern of row E and row G. This would then indicate that the object itself had moved.

This simple model covers only expectations in respect of stationary objects. To extend the systems to cover also expectations relating to a moving object, we would have to add movement detectors (which is based on the class of discrepancies mentioned above). But as I am here only concerned to indicate in broad outline the type of networks that could achieve the basic capabilities of the visual system, I shall leave such complications aside. The main point is to appreciate the general manner in which a stable image may be generated from the fleeting projections on the retina.

9.5   INTERNAL MODELS OF THE OUTSIDE WORLD

The last section dealt with the question of stable-images of a visual scene. The real problem of stability goes deeper than this. We do not merely possess stable-images of a two-dimensional field; we also have stable conceptions of the three-dimensional world in which we move, stable representation of an environment in which objects are allocated their proper positions in space and the subject sees himself in a proper relation to these objects. As I tilt my head the verticals in the room remain vertical even though their orientation has changed on the retina. As I move my eyes, head or body the physical world stands still. However, I am aware not only of the space in front of my eyes but also of the space beyond my field of vision and to some extent even of the room behind me. This awareness of absent space illustrates particularly well the general nature of our internal representations. It is difficult to see how this awareness could be other than a set of expectations about the things I shall see when I turn my head. The aggregate of these expectations constitutes my internal model of the room.

Again, an object comes to be perceived as permanent even when it is partly or wholly hidden by another object. Infants soon learn that an object has not gone out of existence when a screen is slowly drawn over it and to expect its reappearance when the screen is withdrawn.

We can all continue to walk or drive through gaps in the sensory data— and not only inertially, for we can make appropriate decisions or adjustments during the data gaps. Behaviour may continue through quite long gaps in the sensory data and remain appropriate despite the absence of relevant sensory data. We must then be relying on internal data, viz. on internal models of the external reality. One can imagine intermittent sense data maintaining and updating these models rather in the way in which the revolving beam of a radar screen maintains and updates the radar presentation of the surrounding world.

Seeing, in fact, means relating a complex of constantly changing patterns of light, shade and colour registering on our retinas to an equally complex store of 'memories' of previous experiences about tables and chairs, distances, sizes and movement etc, which express themselves in the expectations the visual scene elicits in the beholder. In this sense, perception goes beyond the evidence of the senses. In this sense, too, perception is both inferential and predictive. Much of this was already understood in the nineteenth century by von Helmholtz when he described perception as a process of 'unconscious inferences'.

There are psychologists who appear to believe in a rather more passive theory of perception and who would deny that perception presupposes inference and that previous knowledge is used to supplement or interpret current sensations. Beginning as an infant, they would say, the human being learns the distinctive features of objects, the layout of places in the environment and the invariant features of events, without the addition of cognitive elements. But these theories overlook that you cannot discover the invariance of a feature or relation except by introducing variation and then drawing inferences from the experienced results. Thus the interpretation of current experiences *must* draw upon previous experience (i.e. the use of some previous knowledge) and upon some process of inference. As MacKay[155] has pointed out, rather than thinking in terms of filtering the input to extract invariants, we must think in terms of the brain organizing an invariant response to the input. (In our language: a unique internal representation.)

The idea that the brain builds up a small-scale model of the outside world has frequently been mooted since the 1930s and is now widely accepted. In this country Craik was the first to champion this view[220]. However, the physiological form these internal representations take now looks very different from what the original supporters of the idea seem to have had in mind. It is not a form to which we can apply the concept of 'scale', for example. The results of our analysis make it quite clear that these 'models' do not consist of facilitated neural pathways whose geometrical relations mimic those of the objects we see.

Introspection makes it seem almost a truism that the human brain forms internal models of external realities, but the examples given in Section 2.2 suggest that infrahuman species, too, may form internal connectivities or patterns of excitation which serve as broad representations of the three-dimensional space surrounding the animal. At any rate this appears to be true in the higher orders.

What an organism omits to do may be as revealing in this respect as what it does. As has been mentioned, the occurrence of an unexpected event in a given situation commonly elicits an alerting reaction and orienting response. The organism turns towards the source of the unexpected stimulus. If the event recurs frequently in the same circumstances habituation results and the orienting response extinguishes (Section 6.6). Working on habituation to tones of different durations, Sokolov observed that if the subject is habituated to a long tone and then a short tone is substituted the orienting reaction again takes place but this time to the unexpected silence following the short tone. The reactions depend, therefore, on what is expected in the circumstances. Similar observations have been made in respect of orienting or 'surprise' reactions elicited by far more complex stimulus situations. Sokolov[229] rightly stressed that these phenomena are hard to explain except on the assumption that a neural model of the environment is produced in the nervous system, an expectancy as to what is where, what leads to what, what follows what etc.

The very fact that we interpret sensory patterns in terms of discrete and identity-maintaining objects supports the notion of the brain forming internal models of the external world. Much of this faculty can be acquired only by learning. Until about four months of age the infant appears to live largely in a world in which places and movements predominate. An object moved to another place may still become a different object. From this age onwards, too, the child appears to expand rapidly the range of expectations which make the phenomena it meets unsurprising. The image of his mother in a mirror ceases to be a surprising (and to that extent frightening) appearance of a second mother. The child is formulating an internal model of the outside world which develops constantly and steadily, provided the gap between the current model and what the child is currently experiencing is not too large. If the gap cannot be bridged, fear may be produced.

The synthesis of neural representations of spatial relations in a three-dimensional world requires information about the orientation and movements not only of the eyes but also of the head and body. When learning is complete and the internal models can be formed, the visual images of a given scene must be able to arouse a set of expectations which covers not only how the scene will transform when I move the eyes but also how it will transform in response to movements of head and body. As sources for this movement information the brain has available the proprioceptors and tactile receptors, the gravity detectors of the vestibular apparatus and any awareness it may possess about the movement of the visual frame of reference.

As a suitable mechanism for accomplishing these internal representations we might think of a simple system like that of Figure 9.4, except that information from these various sources would now be added to the information relating to the orientation of the eyes in their sockets. However, it is probably more realistic to think of the mechanism for constructing a stable model of the three-dimensional world as a separate system. This system would draw its visual inputs from the outputs of the mechanism for stabilizing the retinal image. If we were to assume a single comprehensive system, expectations relating to the effect of eye movements would not be independent of expectations relating to the effect of head and body movements. So if I were to attach to the head an optical instrument which affects the latter expectations but not the former (e.g. binoculars), all expectations would be confounded. This is not the case. If we look through binoculars the image remains stable as regards eye movements and the world we see dances about only in consequence of head, or body, movements. (Optical instruments, of course, do not affect expectations relating to the effect of eye movements, because the same eye movement continues to effect the same shift of retinal images.)

The notion of separate systems is also supported by reports of patients with parietal lesions who confuse real solid objects with coloured pictures of objects, suggesting that the stable-retinal-image mechanism remained functional while the three-dimensional-modelling system was incapacitated[47]. Similar perceptual confusions may be shown by animals and young children.

The three-dimensional system (or set of systems) could function in much the same manner as that envisaged for the stable-retinal-image system. Network configurations of the general type illustrated in Figure 9.4 could accomplish the required operations provided we assume that the *e* inputs now relate to information about head and body position and the *SP* inputs are replaced by the outputs of the mechanism which provides image-stability in respect of eye movements, i.e. by the outputs of the original mechanism to which the diagram refers.

In theory the movement information this mechanism requires could reach it straight from the sources I have listed, i.e. in an undigested form. This may well be true for the vestibular inputs. Alternatively or additionally, however, this information could first be digested elsewhere and used to compute the net movement of the head in relation to some frame of reference such as the floor (a tactile and gravitational frame of reference), or the walls of the room (a visual frame of reference). In this case the brain may also be relying on an internal representation of body posture and body movement which is constructed from the internal 'feel', as it were, and which is known as the 'body schema'. It is generally accepted that the parietal lobes are most closely concerned in the syntheses of such body representations. Dependence on the body schema in the brain's synthesis of internal models of the visual world may account for the unilateral *visual* neglect which in Man is often a prominent manifestation of unilateral parietal disease or damage. This effect is not found in the monkey[55].

The two mechanisms considered above, i.e. the one for stabilizing the retinal image and the other for stabilizing the three-dimensional scene, between them allow the formation of neural connections which represent an aggregate of expectations of how the retinal images will transform in response to movements of eyes, head or body. In so far as these expectations are correct, they define the true relative positions of the perceived objects, the perceiving subject and the frame of reference. This seems to me the only general and truly valid sense in which we can say that the brain constructs an internal model (visual in this case) of the three-dimensional world enveloping and surrounding the body-mass of the subject.

Similarly, if tactile information is suitably integrated with proprioceptive and/or motor reflux information we can arrive at internal representations and aggregates of expectations which relate to what tactile stimuli will be met if the subject moves in this way or that.

Such internal models based on tactile information, of course, cannot extend beyond the behaviour space of the subject. They may also be subdivided into functional areas. For the blind person there may be central space concerned only with his own body. This may be surrounded by a space represented in terms of expectations about things that can be touched or grasped. This space, in turn, may form the inner shell of a wider space which comprises the objects that can be reached by moving a few steps in one direction or another and so on (cf. Birkmayer's *Raumschalen*[20]).

In the seeing person the visual, proprioceptive and tactile expectancies come to be extensively integrated. Thus while the eye is distracted by one object the proprioceptive and tactile representations often enable the subject to carry on with the manipulation of another object. In the manipulation of all objects, as in the development of particular behaviour strategies, the current neuronal model of the environment substitutes for the peripheral stimulation produced by the environment.

However, the degree of integration of the visual and tactile models of the outer world appears to differ greatly between the species. The ability to recognize or match in one sensory modality (say by touch) what has earlier only been experienced in another (say by sight) is highly developed in humans. We find it easy to select the right change in our pockets without having to look at the coins and to make the same kind of comparison even with objects which have only been seen before but never felt. But this type of 'cross-modal' integration is virtually unknown in the infrahuman species, although it has been demonstrated for the chimpanzee and the orang-utan[55].

Since we have seen that the internal models must be interpreted as aggregates of *expectancies*, there is a genuine sense in which we can say that the brain generally acts upon *hypotheses* or '*unconscious inferences*' rather than direct stimulations. In an equally valid sense we may say that it acts upon *cognitive maps*. All these expressions, and others commonly found in the literature, fall into place as soon as we know how to interpret these aggregates of expectancies in terms of specific patterns of neural excitation generated by particular network configurations in the general manner outlined above.

Experiments with inverting prisms, worn by subjects over long periods of time, throw an interesting sidelight on the structure of the networks engaged in producing neural representations of external spatial relationships.

The most thorough studies with inverting prisms are probably those undertaken by Kohler[137, 138] and Erismann over many years at Innsbruck. The devices they employed provided either up–down or right–left reversals. It is clear from their reports that, in subjects wearing such devices over long periods of time, motor readjustment precedes 'perceptual' readjustment by days or weeks. That is to say, expectations of what the hand or foot will meet when the subject moves adjust more quickly than the expectations of what the eye will see. After two weeks or more subjects could engage in fencing, skiing or riding a bicycle in heavy traffic, although there remained a permanent tendency to make false starts. Of special interest, however, was the apparent piecemeal nature of the perceptual readjustments. With left–right reversing prisms subjects may report at some stage that they 'see' a car on the correct side of the street and facing in the correct direction yet the car bears a licence plate in mirror writing. With up–down reversal subjects might note that snow falls steadily downwards past trees that are seen upside-down. This confirms what we had to assume for quite different reasons, viz. that the networks concerned in the construction of internal models of the outside world have feature-specific inputs and are departmentalized according to the schemata they process (compare inputs to system of Figure 9.4). It cannot surprise if this departmentalization breaks through in the profound adjustments we have to make in exceptionally artificial situations.

9.6   MODELS AND MEMORIES IN THE TEMPORAL LOBES

The main cortical areas in which the integration of visual information and the formation of (sight-oriented) internal models of the external world appears to take place comprise the association areas surrounding the occipital pole, the lateral surface of the *inferior* temporal lobe and the hidden cortex of the floor of the superior temporal sulcus. The occipital pole contains the primary visual receiving area (area 17). This projects to the surrounding association areas 18 and 19 (Figure 6.5). The second of these borders on the inferior temporal gyrus. (The *superior* temporal lobe, on the other hand, contains the primary receiving area for auditory signals (areas 41 and 42) and the auditory association area (22). In the dominant hemisphere this area plays an essential part in the comprehension of speech. Patients with lesions in this region can hear what one is saying but cannot interpret the sounds. Adjacent to the primary auditory area lies the primary receiving area for peripheral vestibular stimuli.)

In monkeys trained in visual form discrimination removal of areas 18 and 19 leads to permanent loss of this discrimination. In Man lesions in this area produce severe impairment of object recognition. Stimulation of the same areas produces sensations like flashes, stars, stripes, wheels, but not complete images of the type sometimes resulting from stimulation of the temporal lobes. Some observers believe that the representations in areas 18 and 19 relate to brightness, colour, movement and outlines and are mainly confined to the significant elements that go to make up the final image. Irritative and destructive lesions that cause visual hallucinations, visual aphasias and visual perseverations tend to involve not only the occipital areas but also adjacent temporal and parietal fields. Lesions in these areas may also produce psychic blindness (visual agnosia): the patient can see the object but can attach no meaning to it. He may walk around a ladder (thus showing that he sees it) but may be unable to name the object or recognize its purpose. Studying a series of patients with *right* temporal lobe damage, Milner, for example, found striking and consistent impairment of complex visual discrimination tasks, particularly those in which attention has to be given to many aspects of a complex picture[167, 168].

Complex visual representations, especially learnt representations, appear to be more specifically related to the inferior temporal lobe. In the monkey lesions in this region severely impair learning and retention of visual problems involving discrimination of complex forms, the encoding of visual stimuli, size constancy etc[21, 87, 123, 201]. Bilateral removal of inferotemporal cortex severely affects visually guided behaviour and discrimination learning, but discrimination in other modalities (auditory, tactile etc.) remains unimpaired. Despite these visual learning deficits, other, more 'basic' visual functions remain intact. Visual acuity, critical flicker frequency and the threshold for detecting brief stimuli remain unaffected and no scotomata result from partial lesions in these regions. This contrasts with the primary visual (striate) cortex where lesions produce scotomata and visual threshold changes but have relatively little effect on visual learning.

The discoveries of Hubel and Wiesel have shown that the retina and visual pathways do not simply transmit a mosaic of light and dark to some central sensorium. Rather, from the retina upwards specific features of visual stimuli are abstracted and their presence communicated to the next higher level. Thus at each successive level of these processing mechanisms we find single neurons which respond to increasingly more specific features of the visual stimuli and which have progressively greater receptive fields. More than a dozen areas on the way from the visual to the inferotemporal cortex have been found that yield more or less specific responses to visual stimuli. Thus while the cells of one area might respond best to moving objects regardless of orientation or shape, those of another region might respond best to objects of a particular colour or to objects presented at a particular distance from the eyes. Recent studies by Gross, Bender and Rocha-Miranda[96, 97] have shown in the monkey that to some extent this progression is continued right into the inferotemporal cortices. The response to a variety of visual stimuli was examined for several hundred individual neurons in the cortex of the inferior convexity of the temporal lobe. With the standard background illumination used all neurons encountered were spontaneously active with discharge rates varying from 1–30 per second. The activity of over 80% of the neurons was altered by visual stimuli such as light or dark slits. The majority of these responded by increases rather than decreases in firing rate and almost all responded more vigorously to a moving stimulus than to a stationary one. Significant features were the magnitude of the receptive fields of the responding neurons and the fact that this invariably included the fovea.

As regards the specificity of the adequate stimuli these studies produced some remarkable results. A few inferotemporal neurons had more specific trigger features than have been reported for the complex and hypercomplex cells discovered in the striate and parastriate cortices by Hubel and Wiesel. Some neurons preferred a 3° diameter circle or a 5° × 5° square to a standard 1° slit. Many cells however appeared to be less sensitive to such stimulus parameters as orientation, length or width than cells in the striate or parastriate cortex. This apparent lack of specificity could mean that these cells had complex and specific trigger features which the investigators never found. This probability was suggested to the authors by the extraordinary complex trigger features which were accidentally found for some of these cells. One cell, for example, consistently gave optimal responses only to shapes resembling a monkey's hand held upright or sideways. Other cells were found to respond much more strongly to three-dimensional objects than any two-dimensional stimulus shape. As I have already mentioned elsewhere, observations of this kind have suggested to the authors that stimulus adequacy in the inferotemporal cortex may depend on more than retinal inputs, e.g. also on tectofugal inputs relating to the orientation of the eyes or head.

Another significant result was that the recorded neurons yield their specific responses to particular stimulus features only if the cortex was maintained in an active state as indicated by low voltage, fast (i.e. desynchronized) EEG activity. In the experimental arrangements used this condition was maintained by means of acoustic, somaesthetic or olfactory, 'arousing' stimuli.

From our present point of view these results are especially interesting because this is the first known instance of neurons in the neocortex which appear to be selectively responsive to complex three-dimensional relations in conditions in which the preliminary evidence also suggests that we are on the track of representational functions acquired by learning.

No doubt these results are only the beginning of new investigations of unit activities in the temporal lobes. However, already at this stage it is evident that this search will not be an easy one. The effect of movement and postural factors may have to be taken into account in addition to the effect of visual stimulation. And a great deal of attention will have to be given to the question of long-term changes in the systems investigated.

It is also important to realize that the assumption that the brain forms neural representations of external objects does not necessarily imply that there must be neurons which only respond when an object of a particular kind is presented to the senses. It merely implies that there must be an aggregate of neurons in which there is a unique pattern of distribution of responses (comparable, for example to the binary pattern 0101100) when an object of that kind is perceived. And if this is the case, it is obviously exceedingly difficult to detect.

At first sight it may seem an attractive idea that there should exist a hierarchy of cells which are responsive to increasingly complex objects, beginning with cells in the visual cortex detecting simple things like the edges of objects in front of our eyes and ascending to cells in the temporal lobes which respond to such complex objects as the shape of a hand. But on closer inspection this hypothesis loses much of its appeal. The controversy has come to be known as the question of the 'grandmother cell'. Do we really have individual detector cells for every conceivable object we can recognize, e.g. a cell for recognizing the concatenation of features representing our grandmother? It is clear that the general results of our analysis argue against this notion on *a priori* grounds. The evidence of brain lesions also argues against it on empirical grounds. Brain injury hardly ever causes a specific failure to recognize certain objects but not others. It seems likely therefore that the 'hand-detector' reported by Gross, Bender and Rocha-Miranda was a freak result and that further investigations will show that apparently selective cells of this type may also be triggered by one or more dissimilar objects. At any rate, our analysis suggests that rather than employing unique detectors for complex objects the brain breaks down the visual message separately into a variety of fundamental characteristics.

Iversen and Weiskrantz have suggested that the effects of inferotemporal lesions are less due to memory deficits than to changes in the way in which component parts of complex stimuli are attended to and categorized.

Selective attention is bound to play a crucial role in the discrimination of complex shapes. Although it will be suggested in the next chapter that the controlling mechanisms for selective attention are centred more rostrally, viz. in the anterior temporal and frontal cortices, lesions in the posterior representational areas may affect the attentional processes in two ways, first because they are a source of inputs to the attentional systems and, secondly, because the decisions of the attentional mechanism must be implemented *inter alia* in the posterior areas (Chapter 10). Hence there must be some feedback loop to these areas.

Complete removal of the temporal lobes in the monkey yields both representational and attentional deficits. The ablation results both in psychic blindness and in disturbances of the processes of attention. The animal now tends to shift attention mechanically from object to object—indifferent to the significance of the object unless it is brought home to it in some direct way. Thus there may be a tendency to mouth everything, but the object is instantly rejected if it proves inedible. Additional effects of this syndrome—known as the Klüver–Bucy syndrome—include tameness and hypersexuality[228].

Similarly, in Man removal of temporal lobes causes loss of recognition of complex shapes, letters, words, faces, people. There is severe impairment of visuomotor tasks and also loss of all interest except in relation to immediate needs. There is poverty of expression and loss of all emotional and aggressive behaviour. There is also loss of recent memory.

Loss of memory function is a frequently recurring theme in these lesions. The temporal cortex appears to act as an important element in the detailed memory store in which a continuous record of our experiences can be stored and present experiences can be compared with past experiences. Without temporal lobes monkeys do not form a learning set on object discrimination problems. Each new problem is a new experience. Pribram has found that some inferotemporal lesioned animals may still perform simultaneous visual discriminations as well as the controls, but they fail on successive discriminations. (On the simultaneous discriminations they sometimes even perform better since they may sample more freely, their sampling not being biased or restrained by memories of past experiences.)

The evocation of sequential experiences which Penfield has obtained by temporal lobe stimulation was mentioned in Section 7.6. Other observers have obtained a variety of interpretative illusions from similar stimulations: objects may seem larger than they are, or nearer, or they may appear to be receding when they are not. Again, they may seem familiar (or strange) when they should not. In the dominant hemisphere (see below) stimulations may lead to utterances of an uncharacteristic type resembling psychotic or paranoid delusions. Sem-Jacobson and Torkildsen[216] report two types of memory recall following temporal lobe stimulation: precise coherent recalls from the mesial regions and hallucinatory fragments from the more posterior regions. Stimulation may also cause temporary amnesias. In these cases the retrograde period and the recovery time depend on the strength of the stimulus.

The temporal lobes also appear to be involved in the recognition and registration of temporal sequences of events, quite apart from serial factors involved in shape recognition and other applications of the reafference principle. In Man the ability to judge temporal order may be severely impaired by temporal lesions. If a patient is asked to count and a stimulus is applied to the temporal lobe for a few seconds while he is counting, he will pause and then continue again. If he is now asked why he stopped he will deny stopping. For the stimulus period no time passed for him. Walter, who reports these findings[166], believes that the brain's clocks may lie below the temporal artery. He reminds us that this artery owes its name to the fact that the ancients sometimes used its pulsations to measure time.

The empirical evidence, therefore, points to the posterior association areas and inferior temporal lobe as the probable sites at which the cortical components of sight-oriented internal representations of external objects or events, and their properties or relations, are formed and stored. In Chapter 7 we arrived at some general ideas of how this storage may occur. In the simple network paradigms we studied at the time the synaptic alignments which constitute what we have called the 'latent representations' form the permanent memory store. The recognition of an object (event or situation) consists of the activation of the multifarious latent representations that characterize the familiar elements in the perceived object or situation, including those of familiar properties and relations. The uniqueness of the object or situation lies mainly in the uniqueness of the particular combination of familiar elements which it contains. Its novelty lies in the presence of unfamiliar elements and novel combinations of familiar elements. We have seen how the proposed network configurations could detect this novelty and mismatch. Recent (unconsolidated) memory would consist of the maintenance of the relevant excitations through the self-reexcitement made possible through positive feedback loops. This could yield processes of reverberation which greatly exceed the duration of the original stimuli. Consolidation of the memories would take the form of further synaptic alignments and structural or biochemical changes which transform unstable alignments into more stable forms. This would depend on the period over which the reverberation is maintained, which in turn must depend on facilitations controlled by extraneous factors connected with the processes of attention and the frontal, limbic and reticular structures involved in these processes. The temporal lobes have rich connections with the limbic system, especially the hippocampal gyrus, uncus and amygdaloid areas. Via the temporal pole they also maintain powerful reciprocal connections with the frontal cortex.

Our earlier discussions have suggested that the internal representation of an object is not a single compact organization but an aggregate of diffuse organizations with multiple read-outs which come to be activated in the perception of the object. As already mentioned, we believe that through processes of convergence the different characteristics of an object that come to be represented in the cortex increase in the level of abstraction as we move from the posterior to the more anterior areas. This particularly concerns the projections from the temporal lobes to the frontal association areas and the particular contributions made by these areas. We shall see in Section 10.1 that place information is perhaps one of the most important categories of information that is lost in this progression of analytical-synthetic processes. By contrast it has a crucial part to play in the spatial guidance functions which are based on the posterior cortical areas.

Since the body functions as an important frame of reference in the perception of spatial relations, the brain's internal representations of the external world can be complete only to the extent to which they are integrated with the internal representation of body posture and movement. This subject will be taken up in the next section.

9.7   THE PARIETAL LOBES AND THE BODY SCHEMA

As we turn from the neural representation of the environment to the 'body schema', i.e. to internal representations of the body, its postures and movements, the emphasis shifts to the parietal lobes. This particularly concerns the somatic association areas 5 and 7 (Figure 6.5) and their relation to the primary somatosensory cortex (areas 1, 2, 3). But the parieto-temporo-occipital junction which centres around the suprasylvian gyrus and angular gyrus (areas 39 and 40) and the visual association areas also enter the picture. First, however, a word must be said about certain differences between the dominant and non-dominant (minor) hemisphere.

Brain hemisection shows that the organization of language and verbal reactions is mainly (though not exclusively) a function of the dominant hemisphere (commonly the left), and that non-verbal reactions are correspondingly more important in the minor hemisphere. The latter also has better perception and better awareness of spatial relations. According to the findings of Sperry's team at Caltech the right hemisphere can comprehend nouns and can recognize the concept of negativity; but it cannot grasp verbs, nor can it pluralize or recognize the difference between active and passive constructions.

Some of these differences are already noticeable in lesions of the temporal lobes. Thus the minor hemisphere is superior in visual constructional tasks and temporal lobe lesions on this side produce greater deficits in patterned visual recognition whereas temporal lesions in the dominant hemisphere produce greater deficits in verbal memory tasks, particularly in learning verbal material in excess of the immediate memory span. This memory deficit is even greater if the hippocampus is removed. The minor hemisphere can draw the picture of a cube and form simple associations like going from 'sock' to 'shoe' whereas the dominant hemisphere cannot.

Similar differences exist in relation to the body schema, although these phenomena are complicated by the fact that extensive lesions in the dominant hemisphere may also affect the patient's ability to express his complaints and a misleading picture of the extent of disorders in the body schema (somatognostic disorders) may result. Disorders in accomplishing constructive tasks are more frequent and severe with lesions in the minor hemisphere, whereas ideational and ideokinetic disorders are more closely associated with lesions on the dominant side. The kinaesthetic factor is less important in the latter.

The same considerations that argue for the existence in the brain of neural representations of the outside world in the sense in which we have understood this phrase, also argue for the existence of internal representations of the body, its postures and movements.

The term 'body schema' was first introduced around the turn of the century by Bonnier who argued that awareness of the body as based on diffuse sensory impressions from muscles, joints, skin or viscera is not sufficient. In addition there must be some spatial quality in the awareness of the body. At about the same time Wernicke argued that the brain must build stable spatial images corresponding to the distribution of receptor elements in the sense organs. The totality of these stable images constitutes 'body consciousness' as opposed to 'consciousness of the external world'. The importance of the integrity of the body schema for motor behaviour was first elaborated by Head[102].

Today we know that our tactile capabilities as well as motor skills depend on our general ability to handle spatial relationships and that our knowledge of external space is mainly constructed on a frame of reference provided by the body.

We owe to Schilder[214] the first accurate description of the extent to which the body schema relies on proprioceptive, labyrinthine, tactile and also visual impressions. The whole parietal lobe appears to be related to proprioceptive stimuli and here is also an extensive reactivity to vestibular inputs. Although the apprehension of spatial data is more occipital than parietal, the parietal lobe plays an important part in these proceedings.

Lesions in these regions may result in failure to recognize shape, size, structure, weight, consistency and, in the final synthesis, the identity of an object (astereognosis). The patient may detect the parts of an object only, or can add the parts together only by tracing around the contours. Similarly he may have difficulties in putting together one-dimensional units so as to form a two-dimensional figure or pattern (constructional apraxia). Sometimes movements can only be executed if they are part of a semi-automatic sequence but not voluntarily (which illustrates again the importance of intact neural 'models' in voluntary movement). When damage is more particularly parietal, knowledge of body, writing and arithmetic seem more specially affected[47].

The hands are the main organs that link the personal space with the extra-personal space and this is an important aspect of parietal functions. This concerns not only the detailed control of fingers and hand but also such strategic decisions as to whether to carry on a given task with one hand or to bring in the other hand too. Such decisions depend on a fully integrated perceptual apparatus and on the experience incurred in voluntary exercise of practical skills. In patients with parietal lesions the integrated perceptions may be lacking: the patient may feel a key placed on his hand, he may know it to be heavy, cold etc., but he cannot bring these and other facts together and arrive at the concept of a key in the absence of visual stimuli[48].

Another aspect of the body schema relates to knowledge of the topography of the body and of the identity of its separate parts. With major parietal lesions a patient may fail to recognize parts of his body as belonging to himself, although there is no sensory loss (Gerstmann's syndrome)[188]. In rare cases the patient believes that the limb is missing or that the perceived limb is not part of his body. If asked to touch the limb he may touch the corresponding limb of the examiner instead. Instructed to touch all limbs of a doll in turn, he may fail to touch the one he believes to be missing in his own case. In severe cases the patient may disown all of the one side of his body. It would seem then that internal representation of the physical self and the distinction between the physical ego and other objects depends on the harmonious integration of this proprioceptive body image with the visual representations we have of our body and of the objects that are foreign to it.

We must expect the general principles concerned in the formation of the body schema to be broadly the same as those we met in connection with the formation of internal representations of extra-personal objects, events or situations and their relations or properties. For, once again we are dealing with the representations of relations and properties. The body schema must be thought of as an aggregate of expectations concerning the manner in which somatic sensory inputs transform as the result of movement. These expectations, once again, relate to functional relationships of the type $s=f(m)$ and, as before, we imagine such relationships to be represented by cell assemblies whose patterns of outputs can be mapped on samples of ordered pairs of the variables concerned in the represented functions (Sections 2.2 and 7.8).

9.8 SUMMARY

Throughout the preceding chapters we have dealt only with broad principles and with formal operations which I have tried to illustrate with the aid of simple models. As much as possible I have avoided tying ourselves down to hypotheses which might be more detailed than the analytical results of our investigations would warrant. During the analytical stages of any investigation it is important to leave as many alternatives open as possible. It must be left to the weight of the empirical evidence to narrow these down step by step as investigations progress.

The naive picture of the brain is one in which activity in afferent sensory pathways (some more specific than others) controls activity in the efferent pathways through vaguely defined intermediate systems of an associative nature whose function is to mediate appropriate stimulus–response associations.

By way of pulling together some of the threads of our analysis up to this point it is worth recalling again what the idea of the brain forming internal models of external realities adds to the naive idea of the functions of these associative systems. For the present we are concerned only with the internal representation of objective realities. The picture that has emerged in this respect is broadly the following:

(1) The internal representations which the brain forms of the environment, of the body posture and of the relation of the body to the environment take the form of aggregates of expectations. These expectations relate to the sensory inputs that occur in consequence of particular movements of our eyes, head, body or limbs. The stable retinal image, for example, consists of a set of expectations which are triggered by the stimulations the eye receives when it looks in one direction and which relate to the stimulations the eye will receive if it turns to any other direction. The stable concept or 'cognitive map' of the three-dimensional environment is based on a similar set of expectations except that these now also include the anticipated effects of head- and body-movements.

(2) The neural correlate of these aggregates of expectations must take the form of spatial patterns of neural excitations which can be mapped on samples of consistently experienced combinations of movements (or movement sequences) and resultant sensory transformations (or sequences of transformations). In the first instance this calls for networks which have a built-in capacity to register an adequate variety of possible combinations of this type. These

networks, therefore, must contain units which are selectively responsive to specific combinations of such inputs, i.e. units which function in the manner of logical AND gates.

(3) The visual inputs to these AND gates relate to specific aspects of the total visual information. In the first instance this means specific aspects of the primary sensory inflow (e.g. contour elements). But we must assume that there are also systems which function at a higher level of abstraction and which derive their inputs from the outputs of the lower-level systems. These inputs, therefore, would already represent aggregates of expectations of a more elementary kind. For example the system concerned in the synthesis of a stable representation of the three-dimensional environment may draw its inputs from the outputs of a lower-level system which synthesizes a stable retinal image from the fleeting stimuli that cross the retinal receptors as the eyes scan the scene.

(4) The movement information which the AND gates need may be derived from a variety of sources, depending on the level of abstraction at which the system functions. Thus in the stable-retinal-image system it may be derived from corollary discharges of the oculomotor system. At the higher levels of abstraction the relevant movement information regarding the orientation of eyes, head or body may also reach the cortex from the pulvinar, the vestibular apparatus and, at a higher level of abstraction, from the body schema in the parietal lobes.

(5) The patterns of conditional excitations specified under (3) above must be expected to feed into associative networks in which more 'global' or 'contextual' aspects of the sensory inputs come to be accepted (on the basis of consistently experienced combinations) as adequate stimuli for the release of the respective final outputs of the system (Figure 9.5). This conditioning may be effected in arrays of neurons which in the untrained state can fire only if facilitated by the outputs of the respective AND gates. When learning is complete, however, these neurons can come to be fired *en bloc* by the appropriate contextual inputs. In these networks the contextual inputs, as it were, become grafted on the output arcs of a whole set of pertinent AND gates. In this manner the appropriate contextual inputs eventually come to trigger outputs representing aggregates of relevant expectations (as was first explained in Section 7.8). The synaptic alignments which mediate this conditioning process amount to a latent representation of the environmental feature (e.g. set of spatial relationships) which the triggered set of expectations defines. They constitute the stored representation of the feature. The feature is *recognized* in a perceived object if the perception of the object (acting through the 'global' inputs) triggers discharges in the appropriate set organizations of the associational system.

(6) The evidence suggests that the cortical components of the aggregates of visual expectations that form the mainstay of our internal representation of

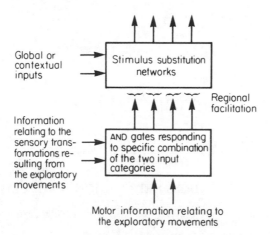

Figure 9.5. General neural organization suggested for the factoring out of object
properties on the reafference principle

the external world are mainly stored in the inferior temporal lobes whereas the
proprioceptive and tactile expectations that constitute the body schema are
mainly based on the parietal lobes.

(7) At the lower levels of abstraction these associative systems may be
coupled with positive feedback circuits of the associative type. This enables
activity to be sustained in these systems beyond the duration of the sensory
stimuli. Systems of this feedback type could furnish that substrate of sustained
activity which our conscious awareness of the environment (and of our relation to the environment) demands. Awareness of our environment does not
cease the moment we shut our eyes. Nor does awareness of an object entirely
cease when the eyes dart to another. Positive feedback circuits of the associational type may also exist on the input side of these representational systems,
thus permitting the formation of expectations which relate, not to singular
sensory events and singular movements, but to temporal sequences of sensory
events and/or temporal sequences of movements.

(8) The outputs from these systems are of the nature of categorizing reactions.
When the outputs of one such system supply the inputs to another we have a
step leading to a higher level of abstraction. The intervention of convergent
systems would raise the level of abstraction still further. The sum total of the
outputs of these representational systems constitutes the core of the neural
events that give objective meaning to the stimuli that impinge on the senses.
Overt behaviour based on conscious awareness of the environment results
from integrating networks in which the output of these representational
systems is integrated with signals representing the internal environment and
the motivational state of the organism. This is one of the questions we have
to take up next.

CHAPTER 10

Central Organizational Relationships

10.1 WHAT–WHERE SEPARATION AND ATTENTION

The two key concepts our analysis has brought to the fore are:

1. The concept of directive correlation. This concept enables us to express in precise terms the type of correlations that characterize goal-directed activities and it permits an objective and precise interpretation of 'goals': they are the terminal events referred to in the definition of the directive correlations.
2. The notion of expectations as the fundamental ingredients of the internal representations the brain forms of the physical world. We have seen in what manner such expectations can be registered in neural terms and how they can form the basis of classifying reactions which permit the recognition of an object as being one of a certain kind.

The last chapter was exclusively devoted to internal representations. In the present chapter it is again the turn of the directive correlations. In particular we must consider how appropriate responses or internal reactions come to be attached to the internal models (and thus particular directive correlations come to build up), how goals are represented in neural terms and how they come to be created by the impact of sensory information on drive information. We must also consider the character of the internal processes that result in the organism switching from the pursuit of one goal to the pursuit of another. Above all, we must try and relate all this to the general organization of the brain so far as that seems possible in the present state of knowledge. The reader must be warned, however, that at this point our enterprise is bound to become distinctly speculative.

First I must return to the subject of attention and, since attention is often controlled by quality information rather than place information, we must also consider how the one may be separated from the other.

To this end let us start with a simple theoretical model of an elementary activity projected into space, such as reaching out and grasping some desirable object lying within reach of the organism. The desirability of the object is determined by the drive state of the organism. For simplicity we assume

that there is only one relevant cue dimension in this respect, viz. the colour of
the target object. Finally we assume that the movements are controlled visually in that this control presupposes fixation of the eyes on the target.

We may then begin by distinguishing three basic systems which we can
expect to be anatomically distinct, partly on account of their different input
sources and output destinations and partly on grounds which will become
evident presently.

1. The 'fixation system'. This, we assume, deals solely with the head- and
   eye-movements required for optical fixation of the chosen target.
2. The 'attention system'. This controls the fixation system and, when a
   suitable object has been spotted, gives the 'go-ahead' signal to 3.
3. The 'telekinetic system'. This deals with the movements projected into
   space, in this case reaching out for and grasping the fixated object.

The fixation system must clearly operate under control of the attention
system. The telekinetic system, in turn, depends importantly on the fixation
system as a source of information about target position (either directly or,
indirectly, via the internal models of the external world which the fixation
system has helped to build up during the preliminary exploration of the scene).
For heuristic reasons we shall assume that all three systems are learning
systems.

The only information about the outside world that is relevant for the fixation system and telekinetic system concerns the position of the chosen target.
(The retinal location of the target image for the fixation system and the real-
space location of the target for the telekinetic system.) The criteria for the
choice of target (target quality, here conveyed by target colour) are irrelevant.
The attention system, on the other hand, is not concerned with the position
of the targets, only with their quality. In other words, the fixation and telekinetic systems are only interested in data relating to the 'where', the attention
system only in data relating to the 'what'. Since the outputs of the visual system
report what is where, the model suggests the desirability of intermediate networks which separate the 'what' from the 'where', i.e. quality information from
place information. How this separation might be accomplished is illustrated
in Figure 10.1 in a simple paradigm in which we assume that there are only
two relevant target qualities (conveyed by the colours red and blue respectively) and three relevant spatial positions (P_1, P_2 and P_3). For the fixation
system P_1, P_2, P_3 must be interpreted as retinal locations of the target image,
for the telekinetic system as target positions in real space as represented in the
internal modelling systems discussed in Chapter 9. Only three pairs of input
fibres from the visual system are shown. R_1 is active if a red target appears in a
position P_1, B_1 if a blue target appears in position P_1. The other input fibres
relate to red and blue targets in positions P_2 and P_3 respectively. The initial
OR gates (top left) destroy the position information and thus report to the

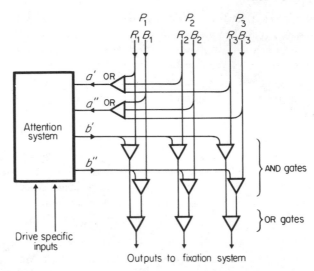

Figure 10.1. Example of circuitry separating quality information from place information ('what–where separation'). The 'attention system' shown on the left receives only information relating to the colour of the perceived stimulus. If the colour is significant in relation to the current drive state of the organism it activates the position information relating to the stimulus for use by the optical fixation system

attention system, i.e. target selector, solely what object colours are being perceived.

The function of the outputs of the attention system is to potentiate the position information relating to the chosen stimulus object so that this information comes to assume control over the motor apparatus either of the fixation or of the telekinetic system. By implication it blocks excitation to these motor systems from unattended stimuli. It is easy to see how these functions are accomplished by the remaining gates shown in the diagram.

Despite the simplifying assumptions on which it is based, the model illustrates the main types of connectivities required for effective 'what–where separation' as a precondition for the selection of targets by one system and their optical fixation or physical manipulation by another. The reader may also note in this connection that the visual processing and modelling systems suggested in Chapter 9 are all of a kind which permits quality information to be separated from place information in the general manner illustrated above.

Now on purely logical grounds there is no need to employ separate machinery for target selection as distinct from optical target fixation (or pursuit) by the fixation system or target manipulation by the telekinetic system. We need not necessarily have separate coding for quality and position. All outputs of the visual system could be fed straight to the fixation (or telekinetic) system together with the 'demand' signals issuing from the drive centres.

These systems would then have to learn simply to produce the correct action in response to the various possible combinations of visual, drive and proprioceptive signals. But our model also illustrates that there are powerful reasons for having separate machinery for dealing with quality and place.

The first reason is that of economy in the number of pathways required when many decisions depend only on quality and many others only on place. The second reason for a separate attention system is even more fundamental and concerns the transfer of learning: having learnt to fixate and reach out for one target the fixation and telekinetic systems at once know how to fixate and reach out for any other. Without the 'what–where' separation assumed above, they would not know how to deal with a blue target if they had only been trained on a red one. Thus, only by assuming that there are separate organizational systems for the evaluation of 'what' information and 'where' information can we explain the ready transfer of motor skills from target objects on which we have learnt the skills to target objects not met before.

So far we have assumed that there is only one type of action and that this action goes ahead automatically as soon as an appropriate object has been located. Let us now expand the model and assume that there are two alternative activities, e.g. grasping and striking, the appropriateness of either depending on the drive state of the organism and the nature of the object. Clearly the quality of the object must now control not only the attentional functions considered above but also an additional decision function which results in the chosen object being either grasped or struck depending on the nature of the target and the current drive state of the organism. By our assumptions both these functions depend solely on the drive state of the organism and the quality (rather than spatial position) of the target objects. It is therefore plausible to lump these two functions together as a single system which we may call the *what-evaluation system*, and for the same reasons as those given above it is also plausible to think of this system again as a separate neural organization. Thus the what-evaluation system would receive inputs relating both to the drive state of the organism and to the quality (but not place) of the perceived objects. Its outputs would divide into two distinct segments:

1. One set of outputs would go to the what–where separation system associated with the fixation system and there potentiate the (retinal) place information relating to the chosen target object, thus establishing the control of this information over the head- and eye-movements concerned in the optical fixation (or pursuit) of the target. Either directly, or via the fixation system the same type of output would also potentiate the (real space) place information on which the telekinetic system depends in its dealings with the target object. Direct potentiation would be required if the fixation system is merely used to build up and maintain the brain's internal model of the environment.

2. The second set of outputs, decision outputs, go to the telekinetic system and, when learning is complete, result in grasping or striking. In a sense, therefore, these outputs have the character of a programming function.

Thus the what-evaluation system has to learn to select specific outputs of category 1 and 2 depending on the drive state of the organism and the reported quality of the perceived objects. The fixation system has to learn the correct head- and eye-movements in response to the retinal place-information potentiated by outputs of type 1 from the evaluation system. Finally, the telekinetic system has to learn the correct body- and limb-movements in response to the current combination of programming inputs (type 2) entering from the evaluation system and potentiated (real-space) place-information entering from the (real-space) what–where separation system.

Both the fixation system and the telekinetic system, of course, also need a certain amount of proprioceptive and/or motor command reflux information to discharge the particular functions we have allocated to them.

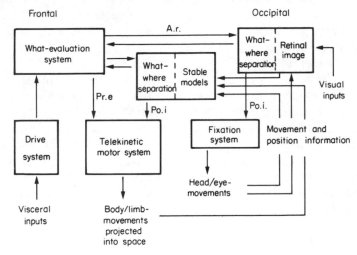

Figure 10.2. Organizational model assuming that the evaluation of object-qualities and object-place proceeds in separate networks. A.r., attentional reflux; Pr.e., programming excitations; Po.i., positional information

Figure 10.2 gives a schematic representation of the main functional systems and their interrelations which our model suggests on the assumption that the evaluation of object-quality and object-place proceed in separate neural organizations. I have indicated above some *a priori* reasons which argue separate neural machinery in this respect. We shall see presently that there is also a considerable amount of empirical evidence which suggests that this separation is carried out in practice and that, broadly speaking, the evaluation of place-information mainly proceeds in the posterior cortex whereas the evaluation of quality-information is the concern of rather more frontal areas.

The importance of the primitive schema of Figure 10.2 is that it can serve as a nucleus for understanding a much wider range of functional relationships than might appear at first sight. I shall attempt to arrive at an outline of some of these relationships by advancing stepwise from this elementary model.

As a first step we can imagine an extension of the system's power to factor out specific object qualities and relations. In the above model we thought only in terms of one single cue dimension, viz. the colour of the target objects. But, as we know, the brain learns to abstract from its representations of the outer world a great variety of object qualities and relations. The type of networks that can achieve this factoring out have been discussed in earlier chapters. To move one step further, therefore, we must imagine the what-information to be based on inputs from the whole gamut of networks used for factoring out significant properties and relations of external objects.

We have also seen that to reach the required levels of abstraction these analysing networks must be cascaded to some extent—the outputs of the one feature extracting network feeding into the next (Section 7.9). The outputs of the system forming stable (two-dimensional) images of the visual scene, for example, must be expected to feed into networks for constructing the three-dimensional models of the outer world. We shall see in Section 10.3 that the anatomy of the primate cortex indeed shows staggered systems of local projection in the parietal and temporal areas, each of these being coupled with reciprocal connections to the frontal cortex in a manner suggestive of the reciprocal connections of the what-evaluation system of Figure 10.2. Parallel systems of this type are found in the visual, somatic and association areas.

If the analysed features of the external world are to be evaluated in accordance with the drive state of the organism, the feature information must impact with drive information. The evidence suggests that at the cortical level this impact occurs mainly in the orbitofrontal–insulotemporal areas (Section 10.3) and that these areas, therefore, incorporate the basic what-evaluating functions of the cortex. At the subcortical level the limbic system appears to be implicated in a similar manner and at the lowest level also the reticular formation—another example of the degree of parallel processing that permeates the nervous system. For the time being, however, we shall concentrate mainly on the cortical level.

The above considerations apply to all voluntary activities in which place-information is relevant in the execution of the action but not in deciding the significance of the target object. However, reflux from the what-evaluating areas to the where-evaluating areas is only essential in activities in which the exact position of the object matters. This is the case in approach and attack behaviour, but only to a lesser extent in avoidance and flight behaviour (when only the general direction of the offending object is relevant). It follows that we can expect the former type of activity to be supported mainly by the posterior cortical areas and the latter by the frontal areas. This indeed appears to be the case. The basal ganglia, for instance, appear to be partly concerned with balancing avoidance reactions supported by discharges from the frontal cortex against grasping reactions supported by the posterior cortex[51].

The same argument applies even more forcefully to object-induced activities whose implementation requires no external place-information at all. Typical examples are visceral activities, fear reactions and the movements concerned in the expression of object-induced emotions. In these cases we can expect the efferent pathways from the cortical what-evaluating systems to proceed straight to the lower executive centres (unless the required movements call for additional elaboration and refinement in the precentral motor cortex).

In addition, of course, there are drive-related activities which are neither object-directed nor object-induced, such as the emotional expression of hunger, pain, anxiety, joy etc. It is clear that these expressive activities can be released by the respective drive centres without necessary reference to the representational cortex or the what-evaluation systems. Thus whereas the evaluation centres would elicit object-attached fear, the drive centres acting in isolation would elicit blind alarm reactions only.

We have now distinguished between three main categories of activity:

(i) activities which are object-induced and object-directed;
(ii) activities which are object-induced but not object-directed;
(iii) activities which are neither object-induced nor object-directed.

The origin of the respective motor excitations in the functional units we have mentioned up to this point may then be broadly represented as in the schema of Figure 10.3. (For simplicity the fixation system has been omitted.) However, this simple schema must be qualified by the observation that in general the 'blind' reactions of the drive system are held in check by the better informed ones of the evaluation centres. This is a common relationship between higher and lower centres: the higher centre inhibits the lower, with selective release when called for. But if the restraining influence of the higher centres is removed the lower centres reveal their native tendencies. A well known case in point is the 'sham rage' in decorticate preparations.

Before I conclude this section I must add a footnote about the attentional excitations and some brief comments on the optical fixation system.

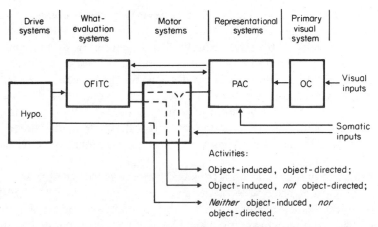

Figure 10.3. Synthesis of three distinct categories of activity. Key: OC, occipital cortex; OFITC, orbitofrontal–insulotemporal cortex; PAC, posterior 'association' cortex; Hypo., hypothalamus

Attentional excitations

Our model has shown that the flow of neural excitations which constitutes the process of focused attention may be viewed as a particular output segment of the what-evaluation centres of the brain, viz. the output segment that projects back to the representational areas and there fulfils the kind of potentiating functions we assigned to the attentional signals in our model. 'Potentiation' is here to be understood in a relative sense. The question is left open whether it takes the form of facilitating the selected pathways or of inhibiting the others.

In our simple model the need for this reflux segment from the evaluation system to the representational system arose from the assumption of what–where separation. However, it is easy to see that similar reflux projections must be expected even if this particular form of abstraction is not assumed. So long as there exist different levels of abstraction there must be a similar reflux segment if the evaluation system decides cue values on the basis of more abstract features of the environment than those which have to be taken into account in implementing the behavioural decisions of the system.

The optical fixation system

Since the optical fixation or pursuit of selected targets plays only a subordinate role in the very broad organizational functions with which I am concerned in this chapter, I propose to deal with the oculomotor apparatus only in a cursory fashion and to confine myself to one or two salient points.

In simple terms the central problem is the nature of the mechanism that makes the eyes lock on the sight of food when I am hungry, on the sight of a glass of water when I am thirsty or on a pencil when I want to write.

We have seen that in terms of neural pathways the process of selecting a visual target really means a process in which the neural patterns of excitation which contain the relevant place-information are put into effective control of the head/eye system. This is tantamount to a process of potentiating the respective pathways from the position analysing mechanisms to the respective motor centres.

According to the above account the significance of perceived objects in relation to the current drive state of the organism is determined by the what-evaluation centres of the orbitofrontal–insulotemporal cortex. These are supplied with quality-information which we assume to be separated from the place-information by systems of the type illustrated in Figure 10.1. In the concrete examples given above the fibres a', a'' (Figure 10.1) would take the form of sets of forward projecting fibres whose excitation signals the presence of an apple (glass of water, pencil) in the visual field. Fibres b', b'' would take the form of reflux projections from the frontal evaluation areas to systems which would perform the function of the AND gates shown in the diagram. These potentiating AND gates must lie either in the areas in which the what–where separation takes place (hence in the representational areas of the cortex) or in areas to which these regions project and which in turn project (directly or indirectly) to the oculomotor centres in the brainstem.

In this connection the *frontal eye fields* assume particular significance. The movements of the eyes are controlled from three main sources:

   (i) the primary *visual cortex* and adjacent areas (18, 19);
  (ii) the *vestibular apparatus* acting partly through the cerebellum and reticular formation;
 (iii) the *frontal eye fields* which lie in the frontal lobe rostral to the primary motor cortex; stimulation in these areas elicits conjugate eye movements.

Although the posterior eye fields must be credited with a certain primacy in the control of eye-movements in the sense that they supply the processed information on which the fine control of the eye/head system essentially depends, the frontal eye fields dominate over the posterior fields in the sense that they are essential for voluntary eye movements. Destruction of the frontal eye fields increases optokinetic responses, but voluntary eye movements in response to visual stimuli are now impossible—and so is the voluntary release of an object from fixation (although the subject can still turn the eyes towards a sound). In man it is also known that the intracortical occipito-frontal projections (occipito-frontal fasciculus) are essential for voluntary eye-movements. The frontal eye fields are closely related to the frontal associations areas and the temporal lobe. These regions in turn function in close association with the limbic system and hypothalamus.

The suggestion lies close at hand that the frontal eye fields are part of the effector arc of a 'what-evaluation' system which draws its inputs from the occipital and inferotemporal areas concerned in constructing and analysing our internal models of the outside world. The suggestion implies that 'voluntary' movements are essentially movements based on our internal models of the outside world (and our total evaluation of these models), as distinct from movements elicited by more primitive exciter arcs.

It is still uncertain where this effector arc achieves its final controlling influences over the oculomotor system. It seems plausible to assume that it acts by potentiating pathways originating either in the visual cortex or in the nuclear regions of the superior colliculus. Projections are known to exist from the frontal eye fields to both these regions.

10.2   THE INTERNAL REPRESENTATION OF GOALS

At more than one occasion we have come up against the question of the neural representation of goals. The term 'goal' is here, of course, to be understood in the objective sense in which we have learnt to formulate it in Chapter 4 and in which it denotes one of the defining variables of a specific directive correlation or set of correlations. 'Goals' in this objective sense are not, of course, to be confused with 'goals' in the subjective, psychological sense in which they relate to imaginative processes in which we visualize the desired outcome of particular activities as a guide to action. 'Goals' in this sense are consciously imagined situations which we compare in our thoughts with the anticipated outcomes of different courses of action open to us. Their neural substrate lies in the respective internal representations, whereas the neural substrate of 'goals' in the objective sense is formed by the neural conditions that result in the respective directive correlations.

In the elementary machine model introduced in Section 5.6 we have a simple paradigm which illustrates how a set of reactions formed to a set of inputs consisting of certain drive inputs (D_2), certain episodic sensory inputs (L') and a range of contingent sensory inputs (H', I', J', K') may result in directive correlations between the outputs and the environmental conditions represented by the contingent sensory inputs whose goal (SG) is determined by the combination of the drive inputs and constant sensory inputs. A system which has acquired the respective input–output associations is in a state of conditional readiness to meet certain contingencies in certain ways conducive to the same end-result. This is the hallmark of directive correlation. The directive correlations build up as in a variety of experiences appropriate reactions are strengthened and inappropriate ones extinguished. (The introduction of expectancies as special ontogenetic mechanisms does not, of course, diminish the importance of reinforcing what is appropriate and discarding what is inappropriate.) In neural terms, the goals are *represented* by the acquired directive correlations, but they are *determined* by combinations of drive (or motivational) inputs and particular episodic sensory inputs or input conditions, in the sense that any switching of goals is produced through changes in such combinations.

The simple model of telekinetic activity introduced in Section 10.1 exhibits these relationships in a rudimentary hierarchical organization. The what-evaluation system is responsible for matching choice of target and choice of action programme to the environmental circumstances on which the appropriateness of either choice depends (given the drive state of the organism). Meanwhile the telekinetic and fixation systems are jointly responsible for matching the implementation of the programme to the current position of the target. To that extent, therefore, the respective goals may be said to be 'represented' in the directive correlations (acquired during learning) that mark the activities of these functional units. However, the example also illustrates that the organizational units of the brain cannot in general be mapped on the categories of goals that we may detect in a particular behaviour pattern. Thus the goal that may be defined as 'grasping object X in location Y' is not represented within any one particular unit of the basic schemas of Figures 10.2 and 10.3. The reader will recall in this connection that we cannot on *a priori* grounds expect the structuring of goals and subgoals to be mirrored in the structure of the neural networks that produce the appropriate behaviour (Section 5.2).

One is bound to ask, what are the likely functional components of a system for which learnt goals are created by the combination of drive and sensory inputs? Our analysis shows that there is no simple answer to this question. The system needs plastic networks capable of learning to produce appropriate outputs in response to particular input configurations. But the optimal partitioning of these networks into separate units specializing in particular input and output categories, and possibly the implementation of specific subgoals, depends on pragmatic factors. The most important of these concerns the transfer of learning. When a particular subgoal, such as fixating an optical target, or grasping a fixated target, regularly appears in a large variety of contexts and as a means to a large variety of ulterior goals, it pays to have a separate system which specializes in the implementation of this subgoal. Having learnt to grasp one fixated target our model system could grasp any other without further learning. *Thus the systematic study of learning transfer holds the main key to unravelling the functional organization of the brain.* Our model has also shown how such a specialized subsystem may be related to a higher system so that the subgoals it has learnt to implement can be activated or switched by the higher system as the occasion requires.

When a specialized subsystem depends on only a relatively small number of input variables, such as the optical tracking system, one may study its dynamic characteristics and possibly arrive at a predictive model (sometimes with help from engineering theory). But when the number of input variables is large, or the system is only semi-independent, this procedure is hampered by the difficulty of adequately specifying or controlling the initial state of the system (as required by predictive models). The potential contribution of those procedures is therefore bound to remain limited.

What, then, does the neurophysiologist gain from knowledge of the goals and subgoals that punctuate a given behaviour pattern? To so general a question only a general answer can be given. He gains little from knowledge of the goals or subgoals as such, but a great deal from knowledge of the directive correlations that are made manifest in the organism's pursuit of these goals. For, to know the range and extent of the directive correlations is to know the informational requirements the neural pathways must satisfy. And to know the pathways that satisfy these requirements is to know the functional significance of these pathways. The informational requirements are those that permit the directively correlated variables to become appropriate functions of the coenetic variables (Chapter 4). Thus the directive correlation symbolized in the upper diagram of Figure 4.7 requires that the mechanisms producing A_t have adequate information about B_0. (It may be noted in passing that if B is generally affected by A the channel $B_0 \rightarrow A_t$ will be of the nature of a feedback loop. In these conditions, therefore, a structured set of directive correlations implies a corresponding set of feedback loops.)

Directive correlations, of course, cannot be directly observed. They are mainly inferred from the results of experimental psychology. The executive directive correlations are inferred from observation of behaviour under systematically varied conditions, whereas the ontogenetic directive correlations are inferred from the observed behaviour changes under constant conditions. Either type of correlation may include not only observable variables but also hypothetical intermediate variables such as those we have defined in terms of internal representations of the outer world.

10.3   THE EVALUATING FUNCTIONS OF THE FRONTOTEMPORAL SYSTEM

The evidence reviewed in Chapter 9 suggests that the visual representational systems of the cortex lie in the occipital and inferotemporal regions whereas the representational systems for body posture and movement lie in the parietal regions. One of the major functions of the occipital and inferotemporal cortices thus would be to code and store expectations of how our visual inputs transform in a given situation as a function of self-induced movements. Similarly one of the major functions of the parietal cortex is to code and store expectations of how the proprioceptive and kinaesthetic inputs transform as a function of self-induced movements (Chapter 9). The reader will recall that what we have called 'internal models' or 'representations' of external objects or of the body scheme consist essentially of the activation of aggregates of organized cell assemblies, each of which has come to represent a specific set of expectations regarding the sensory consequences of possible movements. The neural form in which expectations of this type may be coded and stored was discussed in Chapters 7 and 9.

By contrast the 'what-evaluating' systems of the brain deal with a third major class of expectancies, viz. expectancies relating to the ultimate physiological consequences of an action and the ultimate satisfaction of the needs of the organism. In other words, the evaluating systems of the brain deal with the *subjective* estimation of a situation. At the most sophisticated level this includes weighing the anticipated outcomes of actions in terms of the total set of possible outcomes that are available. Thus the main concern of these systems is with the *significance* or *meaningfulness* of stimuli in relation to the overall drive state of the organism. A stimulus is 'significant' in this context if it has cue value, that is to say if the stimulus event is such that an appropriate reaction to it would promote the degree of *executive* directive correlation of the organism's behaviour in respect of its current goals. (The process of learning to treat a stimulus as significant, on the other hand, constitutes the development of an *ontogenetic* directive correlation, for it is an enduring adaptive change in the organism which matches the given circumstances in some particular respect.)

In the sequel I shall refer to the 'what-evaluation systems' of the brain simply as *evaluating systems*. The main inputs to these systems must be derived from two sources: the drive centres or visceral sensibilities and the representational systems of the brain. They are systems in which sensory information from the representational systems impacts with information derived from the drive system. By this I mean that the outputs of the evaluating system are formed as appropriate functions of the combined information content of these two categories of input.

We have also seen that the evaluating centres have two main categories of outputs: they project general programming signals to the executive (motor) systems and more or less selective potentiating signals ('attentional signals') to the representational systems. Thus the mechanisms of attention form part of the subjective evaluating systems of the brain. They comprise the segment that deals with the obligatory reflux projections from the evaluating systems to the representational systems (Section 10.2). The biological value of systems deciding cue values (attentional systems) lies in the fact that informational overloading is prevented by adaptive and selective filtering of inputs. This filtering may be effected in part at the peripheral receptors or afferent pathways (we know that corticofugal influences of this type exist) and in part at the representational systems of the brain. The former, of course, can only select modalities and peripheral locations, whereas the latter can select external objects, events or situations.

As we know, the brain operates in broadly parallel ways at several levels. When a particular function is performed at more than one level we must expect to find reciprocal connections between the structures performing this function at the several levels, since each centre may have to be informed about the decisions of the others. Thus we must expect to find additional pathways to and from the cortical evaluation centres, viz. those which reciprocally link them with their subcortical counterparts.

The balance of the evidence suggests that at the cortical level the subjective evaluating systems are localized in the frontotemporal and limbic cortices which receive projections from the hypothalamic drive systems via the anterior and dorsomedial nuclei of the thalamus [199]. At the subcortical level rather more primitive evaluating functions appear to be performed by certain limbic structures, certain non-specific thalamic nuclei and, in a broad sense, also by the reticular formation. Reciprocal connections are known to exist between all these regions.

It is reasonable to assume that the more abstract and complex the environmental factors that have to be taken into account, the more they are a matter for the frontotemporal cortices to deal with rather than the limbic system or the reticular formation. However, the results of lesions and ablation often so closely affect both the cortical and limbic systems that it is often difficult, if not impossible, to isolate their separate contributions.

The frontal lobe of the cortex includes a wide range of areas. Here lie the precentral motor area (area 4) and the supplementary motor areas (6, 8), the frontal eye fields (mainly area 46), Broca's motor speech area (44, 45), the frontal pole (9, 10) and the orbital cortex (11, 12); see Figure 6.5.

The frontotemporal complex which concerns us in this section mainly consists of the frontal pole, the orbital cortex, the insula and the anterior areas of the temporal lobe. These frontal and temporal complexes are closely related. The dorsomedial nucleus of the thalamus projects to the frontal pole, the orbital cortex and to the temporal operculum. This nucleus forms an important ascending link from the hypothalamic drive centres and appears to relay (as well as integrate) many of the excitations which lend affective tone to the objects or events we perceive. Its functions appear to be paralleled to some extent by the anterior nucleus of the thalamus which projects to the cingulate gyrus and the nucleus ventralis anterior which projects to the insula.

These close relationships with the major drive centres of the brain, as well as the fact that the frontotemporal complex is a region of convergence for different sensory modalities, support the suggestion that this region is a major evaluating area.

The main descending connections from this complex to the subcortical

structures of the limbic system and hypothalamus are formed via the entorhinal area, the hippocampus and the amygdala (Figure 8.5). The frontal
cortex also projects to the septal areas which in turn project to the hypothalamus, both directly and via the preoptic area. The basal ganglia form an
important link in the motor-efferent pathways from the frontotemporal and
limbic evaluation systems. The presumptive 'programming' character of these
discharges was mentioned in Section 10.1.

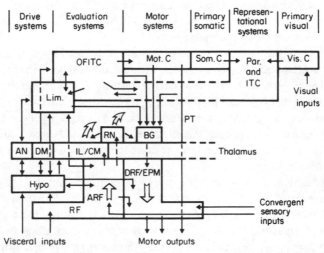

Figure 10.4. Expansion of the schema of Figure 10.3 and interpretation in terms
of known cerebral structures and projections. The structures shown have been
positioned according to vertical columns designating their main function. Key:
AN, anterior nucleus of thalamus; ARF, ascending reticular formation; BG, basal
ganglia; CM, centromedian nucleus; DM, dorsomedial nucleus; DRF, descending
reticular formation; EPM, extra-pyramidal motor system; Hypo., hypothalamus;
IL, intralaminar nuclei; ITC, inferotemporal cortex; Lim, limbic system; Mot. C.,
motor cortex; OFITC, orbitofrontal–insulotemporal cortex; Par., parietal cortex;
PT, pyramidal tract; RN, reticular nucleus of thalamus; Som. C., somatic cortex;
Vis. C., visual cortex

Figure 10.4 shows an expansion of the basic schema of Figure 10.3 in
which I have added a number of units involved in subcortical drive and evaluation functions. The representational system of the cortex has been expanded
to cover somatic as well as visual representations and the motor system has
been differentiated into its cortical and subcortical elements.

Reactions to novel stimuli begin with general arousal and general orienting
responses which habituate with repetition, to be replaced by focused attention
if the stimuli prove to be significant. Novelty is detected in the representational
areas and it is plausible therefore to expect these areas to be a source of arousal
excitations. However, in so far as estimation of significance is a learnt reaction
of the evaluation systems we must expect the inhibition of arousal to be

controlled from the evaluating centres. A number of investigations have indeed shown that the habituation of the arousal responses may be mediated by the frontal cortex [83, 109, 158, 202].

The inhibitory influence of the frontal cortex appears to be fairly extensive. Stimulation of some regions in the orbitofrontal cortex may produce drowsiness or even sleep. At the subcortical level the hippocampus appears to be especially implicated in these inhibitory processes [91, 200]. Possibly some of the cortical influences are channelled through this organ to the reticular activating system. Bilateral ablations of the hippocampus have been found to reduce habituation in the rat. The hyper-reactivity of hippocampal animals has already been mentioned. Bilateral amygdalectomy has also been found to produce less rapid habituation to novel stimuli. However, the influence of the hippocampus appears to be dominant in this respect. Thus Pribram mentions that electrical charges recorded in the amygdaloid complex whenever the animal is exposed to novel events fail to subside upon repetition of the events if the hippocampus is ablated.

Centres concerned in estimating the significance of stimuli must also be expected to be able to elicit arousal. This effect has been demonstrated for the frontal cortex by a number of investigators. Thompson, Denny and Smith [245] have shown, for example, that stimulation of certain frontal areas in the cat may increase evoked responses in the primary cortical areas while diminishing responses evoked in the associations areas of the cortex—a typical arousal phenomenon (Section 10.8). Cortically induced reactions of fear and apprehension also appear to be frontal phenomena. At the subcortical level stimulation of the amygdala may produce fear reactions and arousal.

As has been mentioned, transient stimuli often call for reactions which outlast the duration of the stimulus. Thus the passing perception of a fearsome object may call for an enduring state of alarm. This suggests a need for reverberatory mechanisms which can sustain both the internal representation of a perceived object and an appropriate state of arousal. I shall return to this subject later, but at this point it is important to note that, since the evaluation centres derive their inputs from the representational centres of the cortex and since both the attentional and arousal excitations which they elicit must eventually project back to the representational centres, we have here a system of natural feedback loops which, in theory at any rate, could mediate the required reverberation. Some of the attentional projections from the evaluation centres to the representational centres may take the form of direct intracortical (frontotemporal and fronto-occipital) projections. Others may project from the evaluation centres to the representational centres via the limbic system and non-specific thalamus (Figure 10.4), while the general arousal loops would also take in the reticular formation. In cortical EEG records the ascending excitations of these loops are probably expressed in the 'late components' which reflect the cue value of the sensory stimuli evoking the recorded potentials (Section 8.6). These positive feedback loops could be sufficient to account for the required reverberation, especially if we assume that their potentiating effect in the representational areas of the brain includes facilitation of the intracortical feedback loops which can sustain the excitation of the respective representational cell-organizations in the cortex and hence sustain the representations of the significant stimulus objects or events beyond the duration of the peripheral stimulation.

These large 'natural' loops are an elaboration of the obligatory reflux from the evaluation system to the representational system which we discussed in Section 10.1. To what extent they do in fact account for observable reverberations we do not know. In addition there may be more localized loops which carry within them the seed of rhythmic activities or reverberation. This has been asserted by a number of investigators and various phenomena have been adduced as evidence. A neat example is the perceptible 'echo' following local stimulation which has been obtained by Parmeggiani, Azzaroni and Lenzi[190] on the graphs of electrical recordings taken around the Papez circuit (Section 8.3).

In Chapter 7 we gained some insight into the kind of neural networks that could register temporal sequences of events and could learn to form adaptive responses to any event that triggers an internal representation of any such registered sequence. In particular we have seen how such networks can mediate anticipations regarding the outcomes of response sequences. The frontal association areas of the cortex show many signs of activities of this kind and calibre. The higher functions of time discrimination, the evaluation of temporal sequences or serial order, the anticipation of outcomes and the organization of temporal sequences appear to belong to the special competences of these cortical regions. Without the frontal lobes the temporal organization so characteristic of normal behaviour appears to be greatly reduced.

The dependence of response pattern on significance, situational context and operant implication, irrespective of modality, is particularly noticeable in electrical recordings taken in the frontal areas. Of special interest in this respect are the 'expectancy waves' which Walter discovered in the EEG of the frontal cortex[266, 267]. Computer analysis of numerous recordings taken in this region shows that the evoked potential following a stimulus may be succeeded by a secondary surface-negative wave which may last for some time if the first event signals that a second event will occur at a definite interval of time after the first. If a series of flashes is presented to a human subject the surface-negative component of the evoked potential shows rapid habituation. If then a click is introduced after each flash and the subject is required to respond to the click by pressing a button, the second negative wave after the flash reappears and now lasts until the click occurs. The flash evidently has become a warning signal to which the subject responds by preparing himself for the response. In other words, the flash has become significant and the negative wave may be interpreted as an expression of the adaptive adjustment the subject makes to the flash–click sequences in a context in which the attainment of his current goals is at stake. This adjustment may be viewed as an ontogenetic directive correlation in a perfectly objective sense, the goal of the correlation here being the sustained absence of behaviour which contravenes the instructions of the experimenter.

The negative wave is known as the *contingent negative variation* (CNV)[268]. It is a non-specific response which illustrates the degree of abstraction attained in the reactions of the frontal cortex. It can hardly be denied that the contingent attribute of 'significance' is an attribute of a high order of abstraction.

The above observations imply that, generally speaking, the responses of the frontal centres must be related to the information content of stimuli rather than their intensity and modality. This is also confirmed by electrical recordings.

The importance of the frontal lobes in the processes of abstraction is further illustrated by the fact that patients with frontal lesions are frequently handicapped in the manipulation of objects in the abstract. For example, the patient may not be able to show you how to handle a hammer without having one in the hand. In these patients, what is out of sight is out of mind. (Abstraction in the above sense is not to be confused with the use of symbols, e.g. mathematical symbols in conceptual processes.) Goldstein and Scheerer[88] have presented many illustrations of concrete (as distinct from abstract) behaviour in patients with frontal pathology. Thus a female patient asked to take a comb to the examiner could not do this without combing her hair. Another patient could not demonstrate how to drink out of an empty glass whereas he could drink out of a full one. Yet another patient could throw balls very accurately into three boxes located at different distances from him. But when asked which box is further and which nearer he was unable to say, nor could he give an account of his procedure in aiming. He was unable to use abstract concepts accurately. Although this shows that the frontal regions are still involved in representational functions (albeit at an abstract level) their role in the subjective evaluation of the content of these representations and in the control of attention or arousal appears to be paramount. If the frontal lobes of a monkey are removed the sight of a snake no longer induces fear reactions. After prefrontal lobectomy a human patient still feels pain but is less harassed by it[163].

The operation of prefrontal lobectomy was first introduced for human patients by Moniz following Jacobson's observations in 1934 on the effect in chimpanzees of lobectomy in experimental neuroses. Following such operations the human patient is less excitable and his neurotic symptoms may be greatly reduced. However, there may also be significant personality changes and intellectual impairment. Some of these illustrate once again the abstract nature of the relationships which are evaluated in the frontal areas. Thus the patient may show symptoms of being 'less well-organized', 'less refined' or 'less altruistic'. Frequently he will appear to be less inhibited by the abstract relationships that are at stake in this context. For example, he may treat all strangers as if they were well known to him[38, 175].

All this, and much other evidence, suggests that the orbitofrontal–insulo-temporal complex performs subjective evaluating functions similar to the 'what-evaluation' I defined in Section 10.1. This evidence includes the pheno-mena of *pain*. The most common sensation we feel is *projected* pain: the pain is specifically localized to the site of injury. This is possible because one path-way followed by the pain fibres in the spinal cord is up to the sensory cortex, relaying in the posterior ventral nucleus of the thalamus. This is the pathway that enables us to localize pain, presumably because it enables the pain signals to be incorporated in the body schema (Section 9.7). But this is not the path-way through which we feel the hurt. If the connection between the thalamus and the sensory cortex is severed the patient can still feel the pain but cannot localize it. The area where the unpleasant nature of pain is experienced is the orbitofrontal cortex, which receives fibres from the posterior ventral nucleus of the thalamus via the medial nucleus. Orbitofrontal lobotomy relieves pain, but the patient still has a localized sensation that something is 'wrong' since the perceptual pathway is still intact.

Pribram, who is well known for his systematic studies of the frontal lobes and insulotemporal system in the monkey, describes the activities of these regions as a *differentiation of discrete preferences*[199]. This description makes two important points. First, that these centres deal with preferences (i.e. subjective evaluations) and, secondly, that under the impact of high-variety inputs of sensory origin they produce high-variety outputs from the (com-paratively) low-variety inputs they receive from the drive centres.

In monkeys with lesions in these areas the outcome of an action fails to terminate or maintain the action effectively. Hence sequences of behaviour which depend on each stage being released by the successful completion of the preceding stages may become disrupted because the component actions are not maintained appropriately. The duration of each action is altered. Conversely, electrical stimulation in these areas may elicit 'arrest', attention and search reactions. The damaged animals also appear to be unconcerned about the positive or negative outcome of the actions. There is an indifference to injury. Monkeys with such lesions may repeatedly grasp a flaming match, for example. Reactions to frustration remain intense but may cease before the cause is removed.

It follows from our analysis that we can expect the connectivities between the frontal evaluation areas and the posterior representational areas of the cortex to be reciprocal and complex. For obvious reasons we must expect to find extensive projections from the posterior areas to the frontal areas and, since we take the representational systems to be staggered systems (with the outputs of one supplying inputs to another), these projections, too, must have a staggered character. For two reasons we can also expect to find reciprocal connections from the frontal areas to the posterior representational areas. In the first place we require the 'attentional' projections from the evaluation areas in the frontal cortex. The function of these projections is to potentiate relevant representations in the posterior areas in accordance with the current drive state of the organism. We have assumed above that this 'attentional' flow mainly sweeps through wide subcortical arcs which take in the limbic system and reticular formation and ascend to the cortex via the reticular nucleus and intralaminar nuclei of the thalamus (Figure 10.4). However, it is also conceivable that some connections serving similar functions pass directly to the posterior cortical areas through intracortical association bundles.

Secondly, the reader will recall that the neural registration of the expectancies on which the whole internal modelling system depends needs a great deal of movement information, since these expectancies mainly relate to the consequences of self-induced movements. A brief review of some possible sources of this category of information was given in Section 7.10. The exact type of information required, of course, must depend on the nature and level of abstraction of the property or relation represented in the respective parts of the representational cortex.

Additional sources of movement information are available in the motor and premotor cortices, possibly also in frontal regions to which the body schema projects and in the frontotemporal evaluation systems in which particular programming signals are initiated (cf. Section 10.1). Also on this score, therefore, we could expect projections from the frontal motor and evaluation areas to the posterior representational areas of the cortex.

The extent to which the anatomy of the primate brain broadly supports these suggestions may be gauged from recent accounts of the anatomical interrelationships between the parietotemporal and frontal cortices in the rhesus monkey[128]. Modern anatomical studies of the pathways involved in the outward progression of information from the main sensory areas of the cerebral cortex have revealed surprisingly similar patterns of staggered local projections coupled with reciprocal projection to the frontal areas and final projections to the limbic system. Figure 10.5 gives a schematic representation of the essential features of these patterns for the visual system. This shows a cascade of local projections from the primary visual areas of the cortex to areas 20 and 21 in the inferior temporal lobe and to the temporal pole. Each local projection is paired with a projection to the areas in the premotor cortex and frontal lobe. Some, in turn, receive reciprocal projections from frontal target areas. The earlier frontal target areas also have reciprocal connections with the primary motor cortex. Finally there exists a complex set of projections to the limbic system from the most rostral of the frontal target areas, from the frontal pole and from the temporal areas. Analogous patterns of

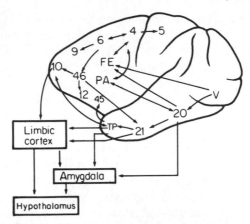

Figure 10.5. Anatomical interrelationships of parietotemporal and frontal cortex relating to the visual system in the rhesus monkey, as revealed by Nauta technique. Virtually parallel relationships exist for the somatic and auditory modalities (Adapted from Jones[128]) Key: FE, frontal eye fields; PA, precentral agranular area; TP, pole of temporal lobe; V, visual cortex

association fibres exist in the somatosensory and auditory modalities (bar differences in localization, of course). There are only two major differences: the somatic receiving areas also project directly to the motor cortex, and neither the somatosensory nor the auditory system has projections paralleling those from area 20 to the amygdala.

For part of the way the three sensory systems remain largely separate except in projecting from their premotor fields to the primary motor cortex. But at the later stages they come together, e.g. at the temporal pole, in parts of the orbitofrontal cortex and at the frontal pole. This suggests that the posterior representational systems initially develop only within their own modality, achieving final synthesis only in the more rostral areas of the cortex. Conceivably the limbic projections of these systems comprise the first descending steps of the subcortical 'attentional' feedback loops mentioned above.

10.4   THE HEDONIC DRIVE SYSTEM

The next block in Figure 10.4 to look at is the 'drive system'. So far it has been tacitly assumed that this consists of simple need detectors which generate appropriate demand signals when a physiological need arises and terminates them when the need is satisfied. This picture is too simple in many respects.

In the first place we must distinguish stimuli which *initiate* behaviour from stimuli which *meter* behaviour and eventually lead to stimuli indicating *satiation*. What may superficially appear as a single biological need, hunger for example, in fact relates to an aggregate of different metabolic requirements. Different systems may be involved both in initiating the required behaviour and in metering its progress. Food intake, for example, may be initiated by stomach contractions and low glucose levels but metered by receptors in the mouth or throat, by gastric osmoreceptors or by stomach distensions.

Secondly, behaviour is not only initiated by metabolic and other deficiencies. It may be initiated by pain, by high intensity stimuli regardless of modality, and by factors quite unrelated to any of these categories, as in play, social behaviour etc. Similarly there are several distinct ways in which behaviour may be monitored as it runs its course (cf. Chapter 6). We also have to take into account that there may be considerable interaction and overlap between different need detecting systems or monitoring systems. Neural circuits regulating hunger and thirst, for example, may overlap so extensively that it is difficult to activate either of them selectively by punctuate electrical stimulations.

For these reasons our efforts to arrive at a broad conception of the basic functional organization of the brain are best served if for the time being we think only in terms of a basic set of fundamental physiological need detectors and satiety centres (such as those of hunger or thirst) and treat these jointly as a single integrated system. For want of a better term I shall call this system the *hedonic drive system*. The 'drive system' entered in Figures 10.3 and 10.4, therefore, is to be understood in this sense. However, in view of the complexity of even this basic system it must be accepted that the logical separation between the hedonic drive system and the evaluation systems is not likely to be matched by clear cut anatomical divisions in the actual brain.

The vertebrate brain monitors the internal environment through units which are mainly concentrated in the hypothalamic area. But there are also important chemoreceptors in the reticular formation.

The hypothalamus lies at the base of the brain below the thalamus, intermediate between the higher regions of the brain and the brainstem. It is in close juxtaposition to the pituitary gland and adjacent to the structures of the limbic system (Figure 8.5). The main afferents come from the limbic system, the prefrontal region and the diffuse thalamic projection system. Its main projections are to the brainstem and spinal cord, to the frontotemporal and cingulate cortices via the dorsomedial and anterior nuclei of the thalamus, and to the pituitary gland. However, the hypothalamic area is also a relay area for a number of fibre tracts, some of which are unrelated to the hypothalamic nuclei. This makes the study of the region particularly difficult.

The hypothalamus is one of the few areas whose stimulation frequently evokes integrated emotional behaviour, though of a primitive type. Electrical stimulation may elicit rage reactions in some regions and fear reactions in others. In the cat typical rage reactions include snarling, biting, spitting, struggling, clawing, tail lashing, rise in blood pressure and heart rate, sweating and other autonomic functions. These occur also if the visual system is removed. Significantly, the rage reactions cease immediately upon termination of the stimulation.

The hypothalamus governs autonomic and somatic functions, via the brain-stem and other regions, and the endocrine functions, via the pituitary gland. Thus, some components of hypothalamically induced behaviour are neurally controlled while others are controlled through the endocrine glands.

The main control functions of the hypothalamus extend over feeding and drinking behaviour, sexual behaviour and certain autonomic functions such as the control of body temperature. Stimulations or lesions in different areas may decisively affect the intake of food or water. Complementary effects of lesions in the lateral and ventromedial hypothalamus suggest that the former is a feeding centre and the latter a satiety centre [191, 228]. Electrical stimulation in the anterior hypothalamus may elicit pronounced sexual behaviour in the male monkey. In the female cat anterior lesions may abolish sexual behaviour even if followed by oestrogen treatment. By contrast, ventromedial lesions may lead to atrophy of the ovaries. This effect is prevented by oestrogen treatment and thus appears to be an endocrine one [246].

The notion of feeding centres and satiety centres arose naturally from the discovery by Anand and Brobeck [9] in 1951 that in the rat small localized lesions in the lateral hypothalamus can abolish food intake and small lesions in the ventromedial hypothalamus produce hyperphagia and eventual obesity. But it soon became clear that hypothalamic 'centres', if they exist, function normally only in conjunction with complex highly encephalized systems broadly coinciding with our 'evaluation centres'. Thus Fonberg found that dorsomedial amygdala lesions in the dog produce a syndrome of aphagia and adipsia that seems identical with the lateral hypothalamic syndrome. The basal ganglia (which we regard as part of the 'programming' effector arc of the higher evaluation centres) also appear to be involved.

The close relationship of specific drive centres to a more generalized drive system has already been mentioned. Thus Fonberg also found that the lateral hypothalamic syndrome showed marked changes in the emotionality and personality of the dog. There is not only a loss of hunger but at the same time a lack of general drive and absence of energy. The dogs were sad and indifferent and did not yap or play.

The formal contributions made by the outputs of the hedonic drive system to the evaluation systems have been outlined previously. They determine the preferences which the evaluation system develops in relation to the information it receives from the analysing and representational systems. They determine dispositions. And in so far as they monitor progress towards need satisfaction, they may influence learning changes through the central reward system (Chapter 6).

Whereas the hedonic drive system integrates the stimuli from need detectors and satiety centres, no such integration would be required for pain. At least there appears to be no formal reason for postulating separate systems for detection of the onset and the cessation of noxious stimuli. We should therefore expect that the pathways of pain ascend directly to the appropriate levels of the evaluation systems.

The ascending pathways of pain project partly to the bulbar reticular formation, partly to the intralaminar nuclei of the thalamus and limbic system and partly to the somatic receiving areas of the cortex after relay in the posterior thalamus[159]. The primary somatic areas of the cortex are not, of course, evaluating areas as we understand this term nor do they function as evaluating areas in the special case of pain. This is shown by the fact that stimulation of these areas does not cause sensations of pain nor pain-specific behaviour. It is plausible to assume that the main function of these cortical pain projections is to assist in the conscious projection of experienced pain in relation to the body schema.

10.5   MAJOR FUNCTIONS OF THE LIMBIC SYSTEM

A brief outline of the limbic system was given in Section 8.3. We are now in a position in which we can see more clearly the logical relationship of some of its functions to the overall organization of the brain.

The three main functions we have attributed to the system are closely related.

1. *The evaluation of information about the state of the external environment in relation to the current drive state of the organism.* This might take the form of direct evaluation of simple stimuli as well as low-level participation in the evaluation of complex stimuli which is performed by the frontotemporal cortices. The subcortical structures of the limbic system probably lack the organization required to evaluate the subjective significance of complex stimulus objects, since at the highest level this calls for the formation of aggregates of expectancies which make particularly complex demands on the organization of the neural networks. But the subcortical limbic structures nevertheless appear to form a vital link in the various reactions, emotional and otherwise, which the expectancies formed in the frontotemporal cortex elicit when particular external events occur. This particularly concerns the level of arousal. The arousal-inhibiting processes which are implied in the habituation of the orienting reactions appear to be mediated largely by structures of the limbic system, especially by the hippocampus. The limbic system also appears to be implicated in the pathways of focused attention.

The close relationship of the hippocampus and amygdala to both the representational cortex and the hypothalamus has been mentioned on more than one occasion. Lesions in either the hippocampus or amygdala have effects which in many respects resemble those resulting from lesions in the cortical evaluation areas. Such lesions may affect motivational or attentional behaviour, the balance between fear and fearlessness, aggression and docility, excitability and placidity etc. Direct stimulation of the hippocampus has little effect on established behaviour. The general effect tends to be inhibitory particularly in respect of orienting and exploring. Stimulation of the amygdala yields more frequent behavioural reactions. The most common reaction in the intact unanaesthetized animal is a 'searching response'. This commences with immediate arrest of on-going activities, followed by an attitude of expectant attention. Other effects mainly relate to the balance between opposing patterns of behaviour ('eat/don't eat', 'attack/retreat' etc.). Amygdaloid lesions may cause indiscriminate fearless approach, indiscriminate ingestions of food, indiscriminate sexual advances and other phenomena showing deficiencies in evaluating functions[86]. In the monkey destruction of the amygdala induces plasticity and reduces the galvanic skin response, for example.

It seems therefore that the hippocampus is more particularly concerned with an object or event having significance regardless of the sign of that significance for good or evil, whereas the amygdala react also according to the sign. Thus the former would have the greater influence on the attentional reactions and the control of reticular arousal, the latter on specific patterns of behaviour and emotional reactions.

2. *Reverberation.* Since it is important that the passing perception of a significant event should be able to effect changes in the central state which outlast the duration of the sensory stimuli, reverberatory mechanisms are required which can sustain the appropriate level of arousal as well as the internal representations of the external events concerned. This reverberation calls for positive feedback loops in addition to the local cortical feedback loops which the cortical representations themselves demand (Section 10.3). Most observers agree that these loops must include the reticular formation and non-specific thalamus (Figure 10.4). Transection of the brain at the intercollicular level produce conditions in which emotional reactions to a stimulus do not outlast the stimulation.

In our analysis three categories of reverberatory loops are of paramount importance from the general organizational point of view. One category concerns the sustained arousal which may be triggered by novel stimuli. Insofar as the novelty is detected in the representational areas of the cortex and the resulting global arousal mediated by the reticular formation, these loops must be closely related to both these structures.

The second and third categories comprise the reverberatory loops required for sustained focused attention and sustained arousal respectively when the evaluation centres judge a stimulus object to be significant in the context in which it is perceived. On our reading of the evidence, these loops embrace the evaluation centres of the cortex or limbic system and are completed by the intralaminar nuclei of the thalamus in the one case and via the reticular formation and reticular nucleus of the thalamus in the other (cf. Section 10.3).

The hippocampus appears to enter the attentional loops in an activating capacity while at the same time maintaining an inhibitory relation to the reticular formation and hence to the arousal loops. By contrast the amygdala appears to enter these loops only in an activating capacity. Possibly the hippocampus may exert part of its inhibitory influence on the arousal loops already in the amygdala. If the hippocampus is ablated, electrical discharges recorded in the amygdala whenever the animal is exposed to novel events fail to subside when the animal becomes familiar with the event.

Although slow stimulation of the intralaminar nuclei may produce sleep, fast stimulation evokes cortical arousal. But the quality of this arousal differs essentially from reticular arousal. Reticular arousal has a general cortical distribution and is long lasting. The EEG arousal response produced by stimulation of the reticular formation may last several minutes. The EEG arousal produced by thalamic stimulation, on the other hand, is very short-lived (a few seconds only). Also there appears to be a region to region correspondence between the place of stimulation and the responding cortical areas, i.e. the EEG effects appear to have a loose topographical organization.

Sharpless and Jasper have pointed out that whereas the reticular system is capable only of crude differentiation between stimuli and produces long-lasting persistent changes in the level of reactivity, the activating systems of the higher centres must be able to produce rapid but brief shifts in the reactivity of the central nervous system if the animal is to adjust to rapid and often slight changes in the significance of environmental events. The properties of the reticular formation are ill-adapted to the sudden and brief changes in reactivity which a changing environment demands. The non-specific thalamic nuclei, on the other hand, appear to be better equipped for this purpose.

Both the hippocampus and the fornix have connections to the midline thalamus. There are also pathways from the hippocampus to the hypothalamus and from the associated mamillary bodies to the midline thalamus. Either set of pathways could serve to complete the loops to the relevant representational systems in the posterior cortex.

The reverberatory circuit proposed by Papez was mentioned in Section 8.3. Various alternatives to this circuit have since been proposed by a number of investigators. For example, the fact that hippocampal seizures readily spread to the limbic cortex and frequently remain confined to these areas has been held against the Papez circuit and has led to the suggestion of an even smaller loop based on reciprocal links between the hippocampus and cingulate gyrus. Other investigators have suggested more comprehensive loops including the reticular formation, the intralaminar nuclei, amygdala, subthalamus and septum.

As has been mentioned, Parmeggiani and others have recorded the 'echo' obtained round the Papez circuit following stimulation of the hippocampus. The impulses covered the circuit in about 50–60 milliseconds. The records also show that this feedback response is inadequate to maintain the circulation of volleys round the circuit without concomitant hippocampal activation by septal inputs. Thus there may well be a hierarchy of loops. However, the whole situation is a complex one in which no simple answer has so far been able to do justice to all the evidence.

3. *Memory functions.* In so far as it is true to say that the consolidation of the memories in the temporal lobe and elsewhere requires that the respective internal representations of experienced events are maintained in an active state over a certain period of time, we must expect that the limbic system also plays an important part in the stamping in of memories. I shall return to this question in Section 10.6.

4. *Reward and punishment.* We saw in Section 6.7 that positive and negative outcomes of responses exert their learning effects partly through two general organization systems which are subject to close reciprocal relationships. According to the interpretations given at the time, punishment zones are zones which during ontogeny have become assimilated amongst the foci mediating the generalized components of aversive reactions and incremental arousal, whereas reward zones are zones which have become assimilated among the foci mediating the reciprocal effects. From what has gone before it follows that we must expect to find such foci primarily in the drive system and evaluation system of the brain. The abundance of such foci in the limbic system is not therefore surprising when seen in this context. Since these are in part acquired associations, we must expect that the exact sites at which self-stimulation can be obtained are neither stereotyped nor constant. Several investigations have indeed shown that stimulation of a given region may be either reinforcing or inhibiting, depending on the training procedures used and the environment in which the tests are conducted.

10.6 SHORT-TERM AND LONG-TERM MEMORY

When the eye scans a novel scene, as when I enter a room for the first time, there will be many shapes which are familiar and which I recognize at once as a chair, table, book, window etc. Although I may never before have seen chairs, tables, books or windows quite like the ones I see now, the figural elements of which the shapes are composed and the manner in which they transform in response to self-induced movements are familiar enough to activate an ensemble of preformed internal representations which, in the context in which they are elicited, evoke the appropriate categorizing reactions.

There is also much that is new, both in points of detail and, particularly, in the spatial arrangement of the objects concerned. But the novel elements essentially consist of novel combinations of familiar elements (lines, angles, squares, triangles, rectangles) and relations (distances, directions). In the mature brain the experience of a novel scene essentially consists of the activation of established representations in novel combinations at many different levels.

We have a great deal of experimental evidence to show that the brain registers these novel combinations initially only in a very labile form. Traumatic events like concussion or electroconvulsive shocks extinguish this registration irretrievably. This suggests that the memory of the scene initially consists of no more than a sustained activation (through self-excitation) of the combinations of representations called up by the scene. The question of the necessary feedback loops was discussed in Sections 10.3 and 10.5.

Hilgard and Marquis[110] suggested in 1940 that recent memory was a reverberatory process which would later be followed by permanent changes in the excitability of one neuron by another. This two-stage model of memory functions has since found widespread acceptance. Penfield and Milner[193] first suggested in 1957 that bilateral lesions in the hippocampus interfere with retention of memory before consolidation takes place. It is clear from our previous analysis that this does not mean that storage necessarily occurs *in* the hippocampus. The hippocampus may merely act as a link (though presumably an adaptive and selective one) in the reverberatory circuits which sustain the patterns of excitations that form the neural representations of the significant external events until permanent structural or chemical storage has been accomplished. The actual sites of the permanent storage must be the many sites on whose adaptive plasticity the formation, evaluation and effective use of these neural representations depend.

Lesions in the hippocampus tend to interfere with any learning task in which the meaning of a stimulus has to be compared with the meaning of a preceding stimulus. Typical examples are tasks involving alternation behaviour or successive discrimination. The deficits are particularly noticeable when the successive stimuli are separated by an interval in which distraction may occur. In human subjects Milner[168] found that after right temporal lesions impairment in stylus maze learning (and in remembering the correct sequence of turns in the maze) occurs if and only if the bulk of the hippocampus had been removed. Memory deficits were particularly pronounced if both the hippocampus and hippocampal gyrus were removed.

Utilizing a simple but effective technique for measuring changes in short-term retention Stepien and Sierpinski[237] found that the impact of distracting stimuli was particularly marked with bilateral damage to the hippocampus. They interpreted this as suggesting that the hippocampus plays an important role in preserving the recent memory traces when the person turns his attention to something else.

A number of other investigators have stressed the importance of the hippocampus and allied limbic structures in recent memory[48]. Patients with large bilateral lesions in this area may show a general inability to remember recent events even though their memory for earlier events remains unimpaired. Such loss of recent memory has also been reported from lesions near the orbital surface of the frontal lobe in the course of fibres from the uncinate bundle. Recent memory may also be disrupted by stimulation of the reticular formation or of the intralaminar nuclei of the thalamus. But the hippocampus appears to be the kingpin in the reverberatory feedback system. It is frequently suggested in the literature that the memory storage of discrete events presupposes the existence of two or three parallel but structurally distinct systems: one system in which the recognition of the external events takes place at the time of their occurrence, and a second system to which the respective representational patterns of excitation are transferred for memory storage after they have been found to be significant. Possibly this second system would in turn consist of two parallel systems: one for temporary storage and one for permanent storage. The suggestion appears to be based on the assumption that the representations set up by the topical perception of an event must be moved out of the way so as not to interfere with the representations which will be set up by the perception of subsequent events. The networks occupied by what is being perceived now must be cleared to make room for what will be perceived next.

However, our analysis has shown that whereas this must obviously apply to the primary afferent pathways, it need not apply to the networks in which object recognition takes place, that is to say, the networks in which these primary afferent inputs trigger organized ensembles of cells which represent the particular features, properties or relations that characterize the perceived events. These representations consist of aggregates of patterns of excitations which, as we have seen, reflect aggregates of expectations relating to the way the sensory inputs transform as a function of time and, more especially, as a function of our own activities. These are representations of abstract qualities of the stimulus objects which are activated by the primary sensory inputs but which are not to be identified with them. It follows from our analysis of the nature of these representations (Chapters 7 and 9) that there is no reason to assume that the sustained activation of a neural representation signifying that there is an A which is expected to change into a P, a B expected to change into a Q etc., will interfere with a representation signifying that there is an A expected to transform into an X, a C expected to transform into a Y etc., despite the fact that these two sets have a common member. As we have seen in our simple network paradigms the representations of *an A expected to transform into a P* and *an A expected to transform into an X* engage no common neurons. Hence we need not assume that the neural representations which are activated by the primary sensory inputs and which signify the abstract qualities of what we perceive must interfere with subsequent perceptions if they are prolonged by reverberation beyond the duration of the original sensory inputs. Even in the extreme case of eidetic memory only abstractions are retained (Section 11.2). Nor need we necessarily assume that the 'transfer' of an event from short-term memory to permanent memory implies a physical transfer of the information to a different network. It may mean no more than the transition from initially unstable forms of registration to more stable ones within the same network.

Naturally, after the passage of a significant and attended event, the reverberating brain must be able to tell that the event is now a thing of the past. But it has plenty of information available to make the discrimination. The primary sensory stimuli relating to the event are now absent. Moreover, expectations regarding the sensory consequences of particular movements that were triggered by the stimuli and which (we assume) are still reverberating in the brain, now remain unfulfilled.

Another point to be considered concerns the information content of the stream of excitations which, we imagine, sweeps from the representational and frontal evaluating cortices into the limbic system and then, to complete the loop, back through the midline thalamus to the representational cortices. The postulated function of this stream is to potentiate the neural representations of external events which the evaluation system judged to be significant in the motivational context in which they occur and to sustain the reverberation of these representations. This selective potentiation gives us the state of focused attention; the reverberation in turn would give us the initial stage of memory storage.

In the discussion of focused attention it is frequently assumed that the attentional mechanisms must augment the relevant modality while blocking irrelevant modalities. Thus if a visual stimulus is significant the visual afferents (or the reactivity of the cortex to visual afferents) must be augmented and the auditory afferents or reactivity diminished. Various mechanisms have been proposed for this function. However, this conception simplifies the matter too much. In most realistic cases the choice is not between modalities but between complex stimuli in the same modality. The central problem to be explained is how attention comes to focus on an apple when I am hungry and on a glass of water when I am thirsty. If we ignore this we arrive at false predictions. According to the above assumptions, if a cat is given a repeated click and then suddenly shown a mouse, click-evoked response should go down and visual responses evoked by a light flash should go up. When Horn tested these predictions with electrical recordings of cortical activity he found that the flash-evoked response amplitude in the visual cortex went down rather than up when the animal looked at the mouse. In other words, selective attention operates more powerfully on categories of representations within the same modality than on entire modalities.

Now it may be felt that if the limbic feedback stream is to potentiate the reverberation of individual representations selectively in the posterior representational areas of the cortex, it must carry a very high information content all round the feedback loop. This is not necessarily so. We need not assume that the signals travelling round the loop must be as complex as the representations they are to potentiate. If the signal flow from this loop enters the representational cell organizations in the posterior and inferotemporal cortex in the manner of 'contextual' inputs (Section 7.4) on which their synapses can align, the variety of signals required in the loop need not exceed the *number* of combinations of individual representations from which selection has to be made, regardless of the neural complexity of the individual representations concerned. A loose topographical organization of the feedback loop (as indeed it is found in the intralaminar nuclei) would also assist in this respect.

An elegant series of investigations carried out by Albert[7, 8] show that the processes which intervene between the initial perception of an event and its final storage in the memory are not as simple as a naive two-stage model might suggest.

Albert's technique was to use spreading depression (SD) in conjunction with the application of electrical polarization of the cortex and subcortical injections of local anaesthetics. His basic procedure was to depress one hemisphere of a rat by SD (induced by application of KCl) while the animal was given an avoidance task to learn. He then examined conditions affecting the transfer of learning from the trained hemisphere to the depressed one after this had regained its former reactivity. In normal circumstances one trial with both hemispheres intact suffices to transfer the conditioned response to the previously depressed hemisphere (cf. Section 6.5). Transfer is demonstrated by applying SD to the other hemisphere and observing behaviour at the next trial. Similar results had previously been obtained by Bureš[33].

Albert then studied the time course of the consolidation of this transmitted information in the receiving hemisphere and he examined the consequences of applying SD or polarization to this hemisphere at varying intervals after the transfer trial.

The results of his work suggest that between an initial (possibly reverberatory) phase, lasting about 3 minutes, and the final consolidation there exist two intermediate holding mechanisms. One of these holds the information for up to 3 hours and is capable of mediating memory recall. This mechanism is disrupted by SD but not by cathodal polarization. The second mechanism is inadequate for recall but sufficient for consolidation. This mechanism is disrupted both by SD and cathodal polarization. It has an apparent life of 11 hours. The consolidation itself appears to be completed in about 5 hours. Albert also found that it was possible to block the consolidation process with SD or *cathodal* polarization of the receiving cortex and then to restart it again by a subsequent application of *anodal* polarization to the same region.

These results no doubt lend themselves to more than one interpretation. However, it is worth noting that they are compatible with the hypothesis that the first mechanism comprises a phase of unstable synaptic potency changes together with the release of sensitizers or precursors which earmark these synaptic changes for subsequent consolidation. The second mechanism would then consist of the processes effecting the consolidation. These assumptions agree with Albert's last-mentioned result if we assume that the sensitizers or precursors themselves are not affected by SD or cathodal polarization.

Electroconvulsive shock (ECS) also interferes with recent memory and sometimes also with long-term memory. The nature of this interference is difficult to determine. Some writers have attributed the effect to interference with reverberation. On the strength of observations made on conditioned avoidance responses in rats, Misanin, Miller and Lewis[170] claim that the primary determinant of amnesia is that the 'memory-trace system must be in a state of change' at the time of the ECS. This would be compatible both with the suggestion that the ECS interferes with reverberation and the suggestion that it interferes with the initial unstable synaptic change or the precursors mentioned above. However, there are also other possibilities. ECS might interfere by inducing fear or by producing conditioned inhibition. Nielson and Fleming[177] have suggested a further alternative. They have pointed out that the 'amnesia' produced by ECS for recent events is temporary only and that the return of memory is hastened if the increased motor activity produced by ECS is prevented. ECS leaves a permanent change in brain excitability and Nielson observed that if the animal is conditioned after this excitability change has been produced (so that both learning and recall take place in identical conditions of excitability) the ECS does not lead to amnesia at all. This suggests that the amnesia following ECS is really a case of state-dependent learning. In other words, the amnesia occurs because the contextual patterns of internal neural excitations have been changed by the shock. (The classical paradigm for state-dependent learning is that a conditioned response established under the effect of a particular drug—strychnine, for example—can only be activated following the injections of the drug.)

Since the discovery in 1952 by Brattgard[25] that the RNA level in the retinal ganglion cells of the rabbit varies as a function of light stimulation, a number of investigations have confirmed the fact that neural activity stimulates ribonucleic acid and protein synthesis. This was soon followed by the suggestion that the final processes of memory consolidation may depend on protein synthesis. Flexner, Flexner and Stellar[67] have shown that in mice bilateral injections of puromycin into the hippocampus and temporal cortex interfere with memory consolidation, and puromycin is known to block protein synthesis. A number of other investigators have since obtained similar results. Some of these suggest that the protein synthesis is only required in the last phase of consolidation—after a period of about three hours, say. But there are also findings which suggest that the effects of puromycin on consolidation cannot simply be attributed to interference with protein synthesis. Cycloheximide also inhibits protein synthesis, but does not interfere with memory. Because of the different effects of puromycin and cycloheximide on memory Cohen, Ervin and Barondes[44] studied their effects on hippocampal activity, since hippocampal ablations are known to interfere with the consolidation of memory. It was found that puromycin produced marked abnormalities in hippocampal activity whereas cycloheximide did not. It is probable, therefore, that puromycin affects memory consolidation by interfering with the normal activities of the limbic system (see above). However, this whole area of research is still in a state of flux, which makes it hazardous to accept any verdict as final.

The discovery of the mechanisms for the storage of genetic information and of the role of RNA and DNA brought in its wake the suggestion that the storage of information in the memory may be based on similar principles. Already in 1948 von Foerster[68] had pointed out the large information capacity which base sequences in a macromolecule might afford. Many models have since been proposed on this basis. Hyden[122], for example, proposed a model in which the sequence of stimuli impinging upon a cell is presumed to alter the base sequence of RNA in some fashion. This new RNA then synthesizes proteins with particular configurations. It is postulated that this protein dissociates when the cell is subsequently stimulated with the same temporal pattern of nerve volleys. The resulting protein fragments then stimulate the release of transmitter substance.

The model illustrates one of the main difficulties that confront all models which attempt to expand the dimensions available for information storage beyond those afforded by the assumption of plastic changes in the synapses. Since the storage of the information must be channelled through the synapses and the retrieval through cell discharges, there are not enough information-bearing variables available at the level of neural transmission to exploit the extra storage capacity offered by macromolecules unless one falls back on such hypothetical variables as critical impulse frequencies or critical temporal micropatterns of impulses. However, the evidence for brain functions in which narrow frequency bands or temporal micropatterns assume critical significance is negligible in comparison with the wealth of data which testify to the paramount importance of line-labelling and levels of excitation (i.e. frequency *levels* as distinct from frequency *bands*). The fact that over a certain range the brain can learn to discriminate between different frequencies (flicker frequencies, for instance) does not prove the use of frequency coding as a standard routine in the brain. It is also very difficult to see how chains of networks tuned to particular frequencies, or chains of resonant cells, could yield the range of molar phenomena that can be explained by the view that plastic changes in synapses provide the most plausible neurological basis for learning.

In the experiments cited above Albert showed that ablation of the medial cortex of one hemisphere blocks retention of an avoidance response by a rat which learnt that response while the other hemisphere was disturbed by spreading depression. When the removed tissue was then homogenized and injected into the other hemisphere after this had recovered normal function, significant savings were obtained on retraining. Moreover, the savings were specific to the task learnt previously. This is only one of a number of injection experiments which have been performed in different laboratories and in respect of different forms of learning. The first of these to attract publicity were those of Zelman, Kabat and Jacobson[279] on planaria in 1963.

The results obtained by a number of investigators in this field are frequently cited in support of specific molecular coding of information in the brain. If the principal implications of these results can be substantiated (and at present there are many contradictory findings) they would indicate a considerable degree of chemospecificity of neurons or their synapses. But they would not disprove the thesis that from the organizational point of view synaptic changes are the crucial changes in learning.

10.7   MOTOR INTEGRATION

The transactions of the brain take place at a variety of anatomical levels and the subcortical levels make their own contribution to the evaluation of stimuli and the setting up of responses. However, at these lower levels the power of discrimination and the scope of the information taken into account are rudimentary by comparison with the cortical systems, and the motor reactions are poorly differentiated or mainly tonic in character. The reticular formation may be the core of the subcortical systems, but it is doubtful whether it can appreciate more than what may loosely be called the 'feeling tone' of a stimulus. Again the decorticate animal has no emotional reactions except rage and sexual reactions. It can adjust posture to gravity, right itself and walk. But it walks blindly; it cannot distinguish between different locations. Tactile placing is also absent. Nevertheless, even when the cortex is fully operational, each subcortical level contributes to the final outflow of motor information.

This parallel processing at different levels is a formidable obstacle in any attempt to visualize the functional organization of the brain. How can an orderly and informed response result when so many ill-informed systems contribute to the making of it? As we are mainly concerned with the higher brain functions which we believe to be concentrated in the cortex, we need not pursue this question at great length. All the same it will help if we can form a general idea of how this integration appears to be effected in practice.

Some of the main descending systems of the brain were illustrated in Figure 6.6. There are three somatotopic representations of the musculature in the cortex. The best defined representation is in the primary motor area (area 4) which lies rostral to the central fissure (Figure 6.5). A second representation lies in a small area in the lateral prolongation of the precentral gyrus. The third (area 8), extensive but less clearly defined, extends from area 6 forwards and comprises also the frontal eye-fields. Motor efferent fibres, however, do not originate only in these areas. Some have their origins in the somatosensory cortex, the parietal areas and the temporal lobe. Crosby introduced the term 'supplementary motor areas' for all regions of the cortex, outside the primary motor area, where stimulation elicits movement.

The motor efferent outflow from the cortex descends along two parallel systems:

1. *The pyramidal tract.* This descends via the pons to the appropriate levels of the spinal cord where the fibres terminate either on intercalated neurons or directly on motoneurons. According to Russell and De Myer 29% of the pyramidal fibres arise in area 6, 31% in the precentral motor cortex (area 4) and 40% in the somatosensory cortex (areas 3, 1, 2) and parietal cortex (areas 5, 7).

2. *The extra-pyramidal system.* These fibres also originate both in the primary and supplementary motor areas. But they relay at various intermediate subcortical stations where their impulses are integrated with efferents from other structures.

The highest integrating stations along this extra-pyramidal path are formed by the basal ganglia (caudate nucleus, putamen and globus pallidus—Figure 6.6). The caudate nucleus receives many cortical inputs and also acts as an important efferent outlet for the limbic system and, together with the putamen, for the centromedian nucleus of the thalamus. Both caudate and putamen project to the globus pallidus. This in turn projects to the subthalamus, red nucleus (Figure 6.8) and various lower structures. From the basal ganglia some fibres proceed to the substantia nigra where they integrate with direct efferents from frontal, parietal and temporal areas before descending to the spinal cord. Other pathways from the basal ganglia project on the subthalamic nucleus and there join a cascade of efferent pathways which takes in the red nucleus, midbrain tegmentum, inferior olive and other centres.

Final integration takes place in the spinal cord itself. It would be wrong to form the impression that skilled movements are organized in the motor cortices. A more fitting picture is to think of skilled movements as organized in the first instance subcortically from a confluence of efferents originating in a wide range of cortical and subcortical areas. The primary motor cortex is a complementary device to which stimuli taken from various stations of the efferent pathway are fed back and which generates from these stimuli and from the information sources at its disposal various corrective, differentiative and otherwise improving contributions to motor performance. Without area 4, for example, there is a permanent loss of fine movements, particularly of hand and foot. But man can still walk quite well without the leg area of the precentral motor cortex. Circumcision of the primary motor cortex does not impair skilled movements, thus showing that such movements are primarily organized subcortically.

The main upward stream of stimuli to the primary motor cortex (including area 6) is channelled through (and modulated in) the nucleus ventralis lateralis and nucleus ventralis anterior of the thalamus. It is drawn mainly from the cerebellum, globus pallidus and red nucleus. The projections from the cerebellum form part of the cerebellar loops mentioned in Section 8.1 (cf. Figure 8.3).

To achieve the appropriate degree of refinement the primary motor cortex also draws upon inputs from several cortical areas and a wealth of proprioceptive information. Conceivably, too, it owes much of its special powers to the ability of cortical networks to register the temporal order in which events occur (Chapter 7) and to take this into account in shaping their own outputs. Although the primary motor cortex is organized somatotopically, stimulation shows that partly organized movements rather than specific muscles are represented in the various regions. And the responses are always context-sensitive, depending on the initial position of the limb and the stimulation that went before. The size of the area given over to particular functions depends on the variety of movements which they are generally called upon to perform.

In general, the higher the level at which integration occurs the more detailed and comprehensive is the information which is brought to bear on the stream of efferent impulses produced. As we pass from the spinal level to the cortical each contribution grows in precision and in the degree to which it brings the response into an appropriate relation to the organism as a whole and, finally, to the environment. This integration, therefore, cannot be a question of the lower levels simply modulating the stream of efferent impulses descending from above, for the higher levels are the better informed levels and must therefore be given overall control. This is achieved in practice by the higher levels exploiting or suppressing (as the case demands) reflex mechanism existing at the lower levels—adding their own refining impulses when necessary. In a sense one can say that the higher levels play on a keyboard of lower reflex arcs. Areas are found in the diencephalic region, for example, whose stimulation facilitates one conditioned reflex but inhibits another and other areas where the reverse occurs. Even the efferents from the reticular formation play on lower reflex arcs. Throughout this system suppression takes a particular form: generally it is achieved, not through axons from inhibitory neurons situated at the upper level, but through excitatory axons which suppress the system concerned by activating an antagonistic one. The final inhibition, therefore, frequently happens further downstream than one might otherwise expect. Hence the control of movement is largely a process of acting on the balance between rival or antagonistic systems right down to the final balance between flexors and extensors.

Thus, even when there is no overt behaviour, a constant stream of impulses descends from the higher to the lower centres. The net effect is inhibitory, all unwanted reflex elements being cancelled against antagonistic elements. Disequilibrium results through the loss of one member of a balanced pair. Acts improve during learning as the upper levels add selective restriction to selective restriction. Hence removal of a competing stimulus from an upper level may at once facilitate some coarse stimulus at a lower level.

The final excitation achieved is partly tonic (enduring) and partly phasic (transient). The tonic component may act on the gamma neurons in the spinal cord, thus resetting the 'zero point' of the gamma-efferent mechanism mentioned in Section 5.4. The phasic component may act directly on the alpha neurons (although some alpha neurons have also a tonic action).

The stretch reflex produced by the gamma-efferent mechanism is not the only spinal reflex which can act as a substrate in the control of movement. Another example of such a reflex is limb withdrawal to noxious stimuli. This forms the lowest element in avoidance reactions. But the part it plays in highly organized withdrawal responses is decided by the higher centres. The studies of Denny-Brown[53], in particular, have shown that at the level of the midbrain avoidance is still a coarse and tonic response. The same applies to the main antagonistic system, the grasping response. This is also tonic and coarse at the midbrain level. But under cortical control it comes to act as substrate reaction in delicately adjusted visual and tactile grasping behaviour. These two antagonistic systems are balanced at the level of the basal ganglia. The fine movements which may occur in tactile exploration and palpation show the delicacy with which this balance may be controlled. The basal ganglia also appear to be concerned in the elaboration of specialized motor reactions to the environment by modifying labyrinthine reactions.

Obviously we must assume that some of the brain's learning systems have a higher controlling status than others. This affects the required flow of information. In general when the outputs of a learning system X depend for their final effects on contributions from a learning system Y, integration being effected in an integrating unit IU, either of two theoretical conditions must be satisfied if X is to have overall control:

1. Outputs from X enter Y as 'demand' inputs (cf. Section 5.2) which remain constant until a particular goal is reached in consequence of the outputs of Y. The function of Y then is to effect some or all of the detailed correlations demanded by the goal. Its role is purely submissive.
2. X receives feedback from Y or IU which informs about the outputs and learning changes of Y and thus enables X to adjust its own outputs accordingly. In this case, therefore, the role of Y is not wholly submissive

although X retains overall control. Some of the ascending connections to nuclei which give off descending fibres (Figure 6.6) may possibly discharge this particular feedback function.

10.8   THE GROUND PLAN

Throughout this chapter we have been concerned with the organization of behaviour based on the internal representations or 'models' the brain forms of the outer world and of the relation of the agent to that world. To reduce the magnitude of the problem we have concentrated mainly on visual representations. We have covered somatic representations only to the extent to which they are relevant in relation to the visual representations and we have ignored completely the olfactory and auditory sensibilities.

Although the higher brain functions are mainly the province of the cerebral cortex it is evident that their mechanisms cannot be fully understood except in conjunction with the action of particular subcortical structures such as the cerebellum, the limbic system, the thalamus, the hypothalamus and the reticular formation. Each of these structures has of necessity been brought into the picture at one stage or another. But we still have to see these various structures as parts of a single coherent organization. In the present section I shall attempt to complete a schematic outline of this organization in so far as it relates to the particular mechanisms we have been interested in.

Each of the cortical areas we have dealt with depends for its main subcortical afferents on a correlated region of the *thalamus*. The specific sensory afferents to the primary sensory areas of the cortex, for example, are transmitted by the specific thalamic relay nuclei (e.g. lateral geniculate nucleus for the primary visual cortex, ventroposterior nucleus for the primary somatic cortex). The association areas of the cortex also have their correlated thalamic nuclei (e.g. lateral posterior nucleus and pulvinar for the parietal and temporal association areas). Sensory inputs of a given modality may therefore reach a cortical association area both from the cortical primary area and from a specific thalamic relay nucleus via a thalamic association nucleus. Phylogenetically the latter are the older connections. It is widely held that the various cortical areas also project reciprocally to their correlated thalamic nuclei, but these projections are less well established. Their precise functions are unknown. From a general informational point of view we may possibly interpret them as completing the reciprocal connections we have postulated for any pair of units engaged in parallel functions.

The third set of thalamic nuclei are the 'intrinsic' or 'diffuse' thalamic nuclei which lie in the most medial and midline location in the thalamus. These comprise the intralaminar nuclei and the reticular nucleus of the thalamus (which forms the diencephalic head of the ascending system of the reticular formation). Whereas the association nuclei receive most of their inputs from other thalamic regions and project rather discretely to association areas of the cortex, in accordance with their 'attentional' and 'arousal' functions the diffuse thalamic nuclei draw on rather more comprehensive input sources. Although their ascending projections are structured, they are not discretely confined to specific cortical regions.

An attempt has been made in Figure 10.6 to extend the schema of Figure 10.4 so as to display these and a number of other relevant structures of the brain according to the particular functional significance we have come to attach to them. Although this presentation of a functional ground plan of the brain called for some drastic distortions and extravagances (such as presenting the thalamic nuclei as a linear array) it helps us to see at a glance the functional significance we have come to attribute to the units and projections shown.

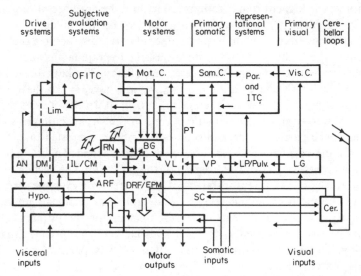

Figure 10.6. The suggested organizational ground plan of the brain arranged according to vertical columns designating specific functions. See also Figure 10.4 and text and Appendix C. Key: AN, anterior nucleus of thalamus; ARF, ascending reticular formation; BG, basal ganglia; Cer., cerebellum; CM, centromedian nucleus; DM, dorsomedial nucleus; DRF, descending reticular formation; EPM, extra-pyramidal motor system; Hypo., hypothalamus; IL, intralaminar nuclei; ITC, inferotemporal cortex; LG, lateral geniculate body; Lim., limbic system; Mot. C., motor cortex; OFITC, orbitofrontal–insulotemporal cortex; Par., parietal cortex; Pulv., pulvinar; PT, pyramidal tract; RN, reticular nucleus of thalamus; SC, superior colliculus; Som. C., somatic cortex; Vis. C. visual cortex; VL, ventrolateral nucleus; VP, ventroposterior nucleus

The diagram is divided into vertical columns, the heading of each column denoting the main functional contribution of the structures appearing in the column. The main cortical regions that have engaged our attention are shown in the upper set of blocks. Their associated thalamic nuclei are entered on the horizontal bar below. Only two specific afferent systems are shown: the visual, which relays in the lateral geniculate nucleus (LG), and the somatic, which relays in the nucleus ventralis posterior (VP). The two main vertical columns represent respectively the ascending reticular formation (ARF) and the descending reticular formation (DRF). For simplicity this has been combined with the mesencephalic nuclei of extra-pyramidal motor system (EPM). The separation between the ascending and descending reticular formation must be understood in a purely symbolic sense only. Anatomically they are not separable since many reticular neurons have both ascending and descending axon collaterals. The limbic system (Lim.) has been entered as a single unit to which we assign both 'drive' and 'evaluating' functions. (This dual role does not apply to all limbic structures, but it does seem to apply to the amygdala, for example.) The hypothalamic complex has reciprocal connections with the dorsomedial nucleus of the thalamus (DM) and with the anterior nucleus (AN) and intralaminar nuclei (IL). DM projects to the orbitofrontal-insulotemporal cortex (OFITC), AN to the cingulate gyrus. These are among the main projections through which the limbic and cortical evaluation centres may be informed about the current drive state of the organism. However, the reader will recall that there are also extra-thalamic projections from the hypothalamus to the limbic system.

Descending projections from the evaluation cortex pass to the limbic system (e.g. amygdala and hippocampus) and from there to the hypothalamus, intralaminar nuclei and reticular formation. According to our tentative hypotheses the main functional significance of this descending information flow lies in the part it plays in the 'attentional' feedback loops which eventually ascend again to the representational areas of the cortex via the diffuse (but organized) projections of the intralaminar nuclei (for phasic components and specific attention) and the reticular nucleus of the thalamus (for tonic components and general arousal).

Our analysis has led to the suggestion that visual and somatic information is integrated in the posterior association areas of the cortex in a manner which yields internal representations of the outside world and the body schema. These processes of feature extraction and integration are continued into the frontotemporal areas at increasing levels of abstraction and integration. In close association with the limbic system (Lim.) this complex (OFITC) evaluates the representations in the light of the current drive state of the organism. Efferents from this subjective evaluating system control action programmes via the motor cortex, the basal ganglia (BG) and other extra-pyramidal structures. We have also seen that a particular segment of these outputs must return to the representational cortex. The subcortical arcs of this reflux form the 'attentional' pathways mentioned above. The probable role of the hippocampus and amygdala in these loops was discussed in Section 10.6.

Since we assume that the thalamic nuclei associated with particular cortical regions perform functions similar to those regions (though in a more rudimentary form) we must expect to find projections from the thalamic evaluating systems to the motor cortex and extra-pyramidal motor systems. The projections from the centromedian nucleus (one of the intralaminar nuclei) to the nucleus ventralis lateralis (VL) and basal ganglia (BG) may be interpreted in this light. The reader will recall that VL also acts as a gate for the ascending outputs to the motor cortex from the cerebellum (Cer.). Similarly, the projections from the intralaminar nuclei to the nucleus lateralis posterior (LP) and pulvinar (Pulv.) may be interpreted as the thalamic equivalent of the obligatory projections from the evaluation systems to the representational systems.

The *basal ganglia* (BG) form the subcortical head of the extra-pyramidal motor system (Section 10.7). One of their main functions is to interrelate cortical and subcortical mechanisms of movement with diencephalic motivational mechanisms and to give priority to specific stimulus–response sequences. However, the internal globus pallidus is not primarily an effector centre. Via VL and the nucleus ventralis anterior (not shown) it exerts a restraining influence on the motor cortices. The partial function of the basal ganglia as an efferent outlet for the evaluation systems may be illustrated by unit recordings made by Travis, Sparks and Hooten[254] from the globus pallidus in monkeys during food-motivated behaviour. Many units were found to be inhibited during particular sequences of food-motivated behaviour, such as carrying a food pellet to the mouth. No such inhibition was found when the same movements were executed with inedible objects.

Skilled movements, as we have seen, are essentially organized subcortically. The diagram shows the main pathways along which the resulting patterns of excitation reach the precentral motor area for refinement and added precision.

The prominence given to the *primary cortical motor area* sometimes leads to the impression that this is where movements are initiated. As we have seen, this strays far from the truth. Our analysis of how goals are formed and how they come to be executed also underlines the fallacy of the idea. It is known that destruction of this area in no way impairs our general ability to execute fully goal-directed movements within the practical limits imposed by the lesion. Conversely, stimulation of the motor cortex does not create a feeling of 'I want to' in relation to the elicited responses. On the other hand, if the association areas are destroyed, the patient can perform fine movements but in a meaningless fashion only. The primary motor cortex also projects to the extra-pyramidal motor system. After section of the pyramidal tract stimulation of area 4 can still cause synergic movements, but they are poorly localized and slow in starting and stopping. Conversely the extra-pyramidal system on its own cannot function without the priming and 'set' established by the pyramidal system.

Of the intralaminar nuclei, the *centromedian nucleus* (CM) is probably the most powerful correlator at the thalamic level. It distributes widely to the thalamic association nuclei and also receives afferents from them. It is affected by visceral factors via the limbic system. It is also a convergent centre for impulses from the bulbar reticular formation and from the cerebellum. Some investigators believe the centromedian receives additional information from the inferotemporal and parietal cortices (possibly also from the primary cortices) and that it integrates some of this information for final dispatch to the motor system. This would be in line with the general evaluating functions we assign to this and the other intralaminar nuclei. Its main influence over the motor systems appears to be inhibitory: if the nucleus is destroyed every intention of moving causes involuntary contractions or spasms. Its outputs probably affect the motor system in two ways: partly through modulating the stream of cerebellar (and other) impulses which are gated through VL on the way to the motor cortex and partly through its efferents to the basal ganglia.

The evaluating functions of the centromedian nucleus are illustrated by the fact that stimulation of this nucleus activates a response conditioned to the stimulation only if the relevant drive is present. Stimulation has also been observed to increase fear and restlessness in a situation in which the animal expects a shock. The nucleus also appears to play a part in the evaluation of painful stimuli. I have mentioned already that the intralaminar nuclei receive projections from the pathways for pain. Noxious stimuli are known to be most effective in the centromedian and other intralaminar nuclei.

The *reticular formation* is a region of extreme convergence which runs from the spinal cord right up to the thalamus. Most of the neurons recorded in this network are seen to be polysensory. In a typical sample half the neurons may respond to stimulation from more than one limb, for example. It receives convergent collaterals from many sensory pathways, also from the spinothalamic tract and the superior colliculus. Its descending outputs have only diffuse motor effects but nonetheless form an essential substrate in the voluntary activities initiated in the higher centres.

The reactions of the reticular formation can habituate. Hence they come to depend on the significance of the stimuli rather than on their intensity. But although the reticular formation may receive instructions about the significance of stimuli from the higher evaluating centres, it is widely held to play its own primitive role in the evaluation of the general character of a stimulus and in programme selection. The ascending reticular formation has therefore been entered in the 'evaluation' column of the diagram.

The existence of chemoreceptors in the reticular formation has been mentioned. To symbolize their part in the hedonic drive system a branch of the reticular formation has been entered in the 'drive' column. Within the limits of its mainly tonic and relatively non-specific reactions the reticular formation thus really constitutes a kind of 'minibrain' within the total brain.

As already mentioned, reticular arousal of the cortex appears to be mediated mainly by the reticular nucleus of the thalamus (RN). This nucleus envelops large areas of the thalamus and also has projections to all cortical areas. Its activities contrast with the phasic and rather more discretely organized attentional activation which the intralaminar mediate mainly in the association areas of the cortex and the somatic sensory-motor field. High frequency stimulation of the reticular formation causes immediate and often long-lasting activation all over the cortex. Stimulation of the intralaminar nuclei, on the other hand, produces 'recruiting' responses in the cortex which do not outlast the duration of the stimulus. Maximal recruiting occurs in the association areas and the sensory-motor field. These recruiting responses are of the nature of surface negative potentials which follow the stimulus and grow in amplitude during the first few stimuli. They are blocked (both at the thalamic and cortical level) by reticular arousal. This effect expresses the inherent antagonism between general arousal and specific attention.

As Jasper and others have pointed out, reticular activation is not a simple volume control. It yields a structured flow of ascending excitations which reorganizes the excitatory and inhibitory patterns held in the dendritic networks of the cortex.

Reticular stimulation and states of attention generally increase the responses evoked by peripheral stimuli in the primary receiving areas of the cortex, but depress EEG responses in the association areas. At the same time they tend to diminish spontaneous activity and also multisensory effects in the primary areas. Conversely, states of inattention diminish primary responses and increase evoked responses in the association areas. On our tentative interpretation the decrease in evoked association responses following reticular stimulation is due to the mobilization of recurrent inhibition and to the decorrelation of unit activity this effects as part of the type of information processing we considered in Chapter 7 (see also Section 8.6).

The ascending reticular activating system also plays a crucial role in the control of *sleep and wakefulness*. Lesions in this area may produce permanently sleepy animals. Total destruction causes permanent coma. During sleep the specific sensory pathways remain open, but presumably the internal representations of the outside world and of our relations to it are largely suspended. Although sleep itself, and the different phases of sleep, are controlled by a separate system of nuclei in the brainstem, arousal from sleep and the concomitant reconstitution of these internal representations requires reticular activation, and so does the maintenance of the state of wakefulness once it has been reconstituted. The possibility has been mentioned that this general activating effect may be mediated or assisted through the liberation of activating agents of a chemical nature.

The subject of sleep raises the question of *consciousness*. In the present context the only pertinent sense of 'consciousness' is the sense in which we would say, for example, that at a particular stage the patient 'lost (or regained) consciousness'. Although this use of the term is familiar enough experience has shown that even this dichotomy is difficult to define adequately either in behavioural or clinical terms. The criterion I have suggested in Chapter 3 is simply whether the brain of the patient at the time was or was not sustaining coherent internal representations or 'models' of the outer world and of his relations to that world. Since we have already interpreted 'voluntary' activity as activity based on such coherent internal representations, 'consciousness' understood in the above sense appears as a necessary condition for voluntary activities—although, of course, involuntary activities may also occur in a state of consciousness. I shall return to these questions in the next chapter.

The key function of the reticular formation in maintaining wakefulness suggests that the sustained activation of internal models of the outside world requires the support of some measure of reticular activation even after habituation to insignificant stimuli has taken place and general arousal has been replaced by the higher mechanisms of focused attention acting through the intralaminar nuclei. The intracortical associative feedback loops on which the representational functions of the cortex depend may not be able to sustain these representations unless some of this activating support from the ascending reticular formation is forthcoming.

By this account the dreaming phase of sleep would be an intermediate state in which some of the cell organizations involved in these cortical representations spring to life erratically and in haphazard succession, without ever reaching the level of the coherent and comprehensive models which full wakefulness demands. It is known that special switching machinery in the brainstem prevents the dreamer acting out his dreams. This in turn prevents the motor activities that could test and correct the aggregate of expectations which, as we have seen, are embodied in the cortical models of the outer world and the body scheme. (If this switching machinery is damaged in the cat the animal will be seen catching imaginary mice.)

During sleep the cortex is not inactive. As we know, it may even respond to complex sensory stimuli, as when the sleeper's name is called. Arousal from sleep would then depend on whether the frontal evaluation of such complex stimuli can raise the attentional loop activity to a pitch at which comprehensive and coherent models of the external realities come to be fully reconstituted and maintained.

CHAPTER 11

Thought and Language

11.1 PERCEPTION AND CONSCIOUSNESS

It would require a lengthy treatise to cover all the shades of meaning in which the concept of consciousness has appeared in the literature and the interpretations that have been attached to it. But, as we know, meanings are volatile and elusive things unless they can be firmly anchored in publicly observable events or operations, or unless they can be defined in terms of concepts which in the final analysis satisfy this condition. The strength of the natural sciences lies in the extent to which they have accepted this discipline in the choice and development of their own concepts. At the same time, of course, the scientist must acknowledge that concepts defined on these presuppositions may cover no more than a fraction of the many aspects of experience that have troubled Man's reflections on the nature of self-awareness.

The task of the neurologist, therefore, is to search for concepts of consciousness which satisfy the primary canons of science while at the same time capturing as much as possible of the sense (or senses) in which the term is commonly used. In this endeavour it is important to maintain a consistent point of view. The scientist approaches the human subject as an outside observer. This does not imply that 'consciousness' can only be defined scientifically in behavioural terms, if by behaviour we mean the overt activities of the observed individuals. If it is profitable to do so, it is equally legitimate to define 'consciousness' in terms of internal reactions of the brain, provided these internal reactions can be defined in scientifically acceptable terms—for instance, in terms of patterns of neural excitations which satisfy certain clearly specifiable conditions. Nor does it matter in the present semantic context if these reactions are purely hypothetical and not *in practice* observable or measurable. From the standpoint of science it is perfectly meaningful to talk about atomic events at the centre of the sun even if *in practice* there exists no known way of observing the occurrence of such events. To say this is not to commit oneself to the philosophy of logical positivism, but merely to affirm some of the proven canons of scientific endeavour.

A tentative definition of consciousness was given in Section 3.4. According to this interpretation, the most significant step we have taken is to have given precision to the idea of the brain forming internal representations of the surrounding world, of the physical self (body schema) and of the relations of the self to that world. We have also seen in what sense it is possible to think of neural networks which can form such representations as the result of experience and learning (Chapters 2, 7 and 9).

It will help at this stage to recapitulate briefly the basic structural principles of the networks we have envisaged. We have seen that the internal representations of the characteristic properties and relations of objects, events or situations in the outer world may be thought of as representations of particular aggregates of expectations concerning the way in which sensory inputs transform in consequence of our own movements and shifts of attention. 'Expectation' is here used in the objective sense in which it denotes a state of adaptedness which is directively correlated to the fact that in a given situation an event A tends to be followed by an event B. The power to form internal representations of external objects, events, properties or relations therefore calls for sets of cells or cell-groups which are each capable of representing a particular expectation of this type and which during learning form associative linkages, thus forming organized aggregates which can be triggered *en bloc* in appropriate circumstances. This collective activity thus produces a pattern of outputs which is characteristic of the aggregate of expectations concerned, hence of the respective environmental object, event, property or relation.

In the common case in which the formation of these internal representations is based on the reafference principle the outputs of these organized cell aggregates have to characterize a particular functional relationship (in the mathematical sense) between two sets of variables—one set representing movements executed by the organism and the other the resulting sensory input transformations. For simplicity we symbolized this functional relationship as $s = f(m)$ (Chapter 7).

We noted at the time that any function (in this mathematical sense) denotes a set of ordered pairs of elements. In this case the ordered pairs are pairs of signal configurations (s and m). The first requirement, therefore, is the existence of cells or cell-groups which are selectively responsive to particular combinations of s and m. There must be enough of these (and each endowed with sufficient powers of discrimination) to yield an adequate sample of the combinations that are possible within the relevant range and domain of s and m. The sample is adequate if it prevents confusion with other functional relationships the subject may have to distinguish in respect of the variables concerned.

To account for the required associative linkages between the appropriate members of the sets of representative cells or cell-groups, we assumed that the aggregates of cells representing the appropriate set of combinations of s and m, i.e. the appropriate set of transformation expectations, become jointly conditioned to 'contextual' inputs representing the empirical conditions or situations in which the combinations were consistently experienced during the learning phase.

A more sophisticated mechanism results if the outputs of the representative cells are fed back to their shared input systems by way of associative feedback circuits of the kind illustrated in Sections 7.5 and 7.6. In this case the relevant representative cells would gradually become responsive to each other and function as a closed system which is capable of reverberation and can maintain the activity of the respective cell aggregates beyond the duration of the activating stimuli.

If this second mechanism is combined with the first we can arrive at a system in which the required cell aggregates are triggered by perceptive inputs but through self-reexcitation maintain their activity beyond the duration of the original triggering stimuli.

The above cell organizations were called the 'latent' representations of the external world, whereas the pattern of outputs resulting from a triggering of the cell organizations by a given sensory input was called the 'activated' representation.

Since the latent representations are based on past experience they form the basic 'memory store' on which perception depends. In conjunction with the categorizing reactions it elicits, the activation of a representation by a sensory input configuration constitutes the act of 'recognition' and this sense implies a 'read out' from the memory store. Errors in perception result when a sensory input triggers the wrong cell organization, i.e. 'calls up' the wrong 'model'. Unlike a number of other theories, the present theory requires no scanning of the memory store, nor separate 'comparators' or 'coincidence detectors'. Given the state of the organism, including its state of attention, the current sensory inputs either do or do not activate a given latent representation. The factors which decide this depend on the particular networks concerned and the synaptic alignments they have formed as the result of previous experience (see Chapters 7 and 9). The neural organizations which constitute the latent representations are their own 'coincidence detectors', for, as we have seen, once a 'model' (i.e. organized aggregate of expectations) has been activated the networks we have envisaged can detect if the current sensory input transformations fail to match the expectations.

The general principles reviewed above are particularly important in respect of the spatial relations that characterize the three-dimensional manifold of the body and its surroundings. Although the brain may use various auxiliary clues (accommodation, texture, size) for determining relations such as distance, for example, the internal criteria for the correct interpretation of those clues remains the same, viz. whether the interpretations result in expectations which correctly map the manner in which sensory inputs transform in response to self-induced movements. Thus, in Chapter 9 it was suggested that the stable image of a shape or a scene is represented in neural terms by patterns of excitation representing a totality of expectations regarding the set of projections that will strike the retina in all possible positions of the eye. Though the projections are unstable, the set of expectations is not.

Similarly the neural organization which maps expectations of how the stable image changes in response to head- and body-movements serves to represent the three-dimensional relationships of the objects contained in the given scene. Finally, the manner in which the objects transform in response to interfering activities on the part of the perceiving subject serves as a basis for his perception of particular properties of the objects.

It may seem that this account places undue emphasis on motor activity and the consequences to be expected from motor activity. But, as Sperry[233] has pointed out: 'all brain excitation has ultimately one end, to aid in the regulation of motor coordination. Its patterning throughout is determined on this principle. It follows that efforts to discover the neural correlates of consciousness will be more successful when directed on this basis than when guided by arbitrary correlations with psychic experience, stimulus patterns, or outside reality, or by analogies with various types of thinking machines'. In other words we must expect the prognostic machinery of the brain to be largely preoccupied with the expected consequences of motor activity.

The perception of dynamic events, as distinct from static objects or situations, depends on similar neural principles—except that in this case the brain must also be able to register changes in sensory inputs as functions of time independently of the organism's own movements. Primarily this means registering the serial order of sequences of sensory inputs. Examples of possible neural networks which can perform this task were given in Section 7.5, 7.6 and 9.2. These networks, too, depend on associative feedback systems.

As the result of repeated and consistent experiences of many situations and of their significance in relation to its current drive states, the organism comes to react in particular ways to the models which are activated by its current sensory inputs. Some of these reactions may be purely internal, others may result in overt behaviour. In so far as these reactions come to generalize over particular sets of situations they impose a categorization on them. The same applies to the objects and events which form part of the situations the organism encounters. In this manner objects and events, as well as entire situations, come to be divided into classes distinguished by particular features or properties. Shapes come to be recognized as circles, squares or triangles; solid objects as cubes, spheres, rods and as hard, soft, hot or fragile. These categorizing reactions complete the analysing functions of the brain. They are reactions to the called-up models. Hence they are reactions not only to the current sensory inputs but also to the transformation expectations these inputs elicit. In this sense the categorizations transcend the immediate evidence of the senses.

Medical textbooks tend to define consciousness as a state of awareness of and attention to surroundings. This pragmatic view is a useful starting point, provided we realize what it implies. It is clear that 'awareness' of surroundings here means more than mere sensory contact, because even in sleep all specific sensory pathways are kept open. It means in addition the activation of organized perceptions in which objects are identified and seen in their proper spatial relation to other objects and to the perceiving subject. In other words 'awareness' here implies a state of the brain in which it forms internal models of the self, of its surroundings and of the relation of the one to the other. Only in this sense can we say that the conscious individual perceives objects in their context (Section 3.4). The reader will recall in this connection that to the extent to which these internal models are based on positive feedback loops they are capable of self-reexcitation and hence of being sustained even if some sensory pathways are temporarily shut off (as when we close our eyes) or if the senses are temporarily engaged in a manner which causes part of the modelled situation to lie outside the field of perception. Thus my brain can sustain a model of the room in which I move even if parts of that room lie outside my current field of vision. The same capabilities enable me to move in a familiar room with a fair degree of confidence even in the dark or with the eyes shut. As I move through the room the model is reinforced or corrected by tactile and proprioceptive sensations.

It is perfectly compatible with this interpretation that the awareness of which I am speaking may at times prove to be a graded form of awareness. As we pass from sleep to wakefulness more and more of the objects which at first are only dimly perceived gain in clarity and begin to fall into place. We are not fully conscious until they have fallen completely into place—in other words, until the internal models of the physical self and its surroundings have become fully reconstituted and integrated. Although I have suggested that the cell organizations which form these models are mainly cortical organizations dependent on associative feedback of an intracortical nature, we had to assume that the sustained activation of these models in bulk depends also on excitatory support from the ascending reticular formation. The suggestion lies close at hand that once wakefulness has returned this activation in turn is maintained by feedback from the activated models via the evaluation centres and limbic structures (Chapter 10).

As the internal models of the physical self and of the external world come to be fully activated, external objects begin to be seen in their proper spatial context. The same applies also to discrete peripheral stimuli. When a discrete stimulus is applied to the body, a pinprick for instance, this also now comes to be incorporated in the models and thus perceived in its proper spatial context. A painful stimulus applied to my left arm, let us say, now elicits not only excitations which (through line-labelling) are implicitly representative of its location, but also excitations which are explicitly representative of the relation of that location to the rest of my body. The pain has become a fully *projected* sensation. These excitations take the form of patterns of neural discharges which represent a variety of expectations regarding the sensory consequences, for instance, of bringing the other arm into contact with the injured arm, of scratching the afflicted area etc. The aggregate of these expectations amounts to an explicit neural representation of the fact that the pain is a pain *in my left arm*. They are part of a wider set of expectations concerning the general sensory effects of bringing limbs into contact with each other or with body surfaces. These sensory effects include not only the transformations of tactile and proprioceptive sensations but also of the visual inputs. The arm is experienced as *my* arm only to the extent to which its afferent signals are integrated with the body schema. It appears to become a foreign body when, for instance, the proprioceptive apparatus on which the body schema depends is destroyed.

The use of 'my' in the above context implies a unity, in the first instance the unity of the physical self. The unity of the body finds expression in the movements which the body permits in conjunction with the character of the transformations of sensory inputs that result from these movements. The duality of my arms or legs finds expression in the same manner. In terms of internal representations the unity of the physical self finds expression in a family of characteristic transformation expectations the brain assimilates during ontogenesis.

Since we have been able to define both the difference between voluntary and involuntary activities and the unity of the self mentioned above in terms of neural functions, it is conceivable that the brain can abstract these qualities from its internal representations and the associated networks. This could then account for my ability to distinguish voluntary from involuntary movements and to recognize an act as an act *willed by me*. Penfield has reported that if a patient is made to move a limb by electrical stimulation of the pyramidal tract there is no awareness of stimulation except awareness of the movement and the patient will often say in the end 'you made me do it'. On the other hand, stimulation in the second sensory area sometimes causes a patient to say 'I want to' make certain movements. These facts support the suggestion that the neurological distinction between voluntary and involuntary movements is essentially that between movements which occur as a reaction to the internal representations of the physical self or its surroundings and movements which do not. Movements resulting from pyramidal tract stimulation clearly do not.

Given a neural basis for my awareness that a given movement is a movement *willed by me* we can also conceive of a neural basis for my awareness that a picture I see is a picture *seen by me*. The picture is experienced as a picture seen by me because it changes or vanishes in consequence of movements of which I am aware that they are movements *willed by me*. In other words the neural basis for my *self-conscious* experience of *seeing* the picture (as distinct from mere perception) may be conceived of as a set of expectations which have formed on internal representations of eye- or body-movements coupled with representations of the fact that the movements are *self-induced* movements, i.e. movements *willed by me*.

Our tentative interpretation of consciousness as the state of a person in which the brain forms and sustains coherent internal representations of the physical self, of its surroundings and of the relation of the one to the other goes a long way towards meeting the sense in which 'consciousness' is commonly used. It gives us a neurophysiological interpretation of the 'awareness of self' as a complement of 'awareness of surroundings'. If medical textbooks concentrate on the latter aspect to the exclusion of the former it is probably only for the pragmatic reason that awareness of surroundings is more readily detectable in overt behaviour than awareness of self.

In one respect this interpretation of self-awareness does not go far enough. Awareness of self includes an awareness of our *inner experiences*. The question is what we mean by 'inner experiences'. William James said that his own search for the 'I' revealed only feelings of tension chiefly in the mouth and the throat. This means an awareness of sensations which are related to the physical self in much the same way as the pinprick I mentioned above. Such sensations would be fully covered by our interpretation of consciousness. But, as we have seen above, we can go further than this. We can identify my 'inner experience' of seeing an object with the awareness that the object is *seen by me*. The neural correlates of that awareness were outlined above.

The internal representations which come to be called up when I examine the chair in front of me elicit certain categorizing reactions, such as those that I would express verbally by calling the chair 'large', 'comfortable', 'broken' etc. I may or may not express such categorizations verbally. I may merely act upon them without naming them. There may also be categorizations for which there exists no name in my vocabulary. To express these verbally I may have to circumscribe them in terms of categorizations for which I can find a name, as explained in Section 2.3.

Similarly, the internal representations of the self, and the states through which these pass, may elicit categorizing reactions which I may or may not express verbally. If I express them verbally the question arises whether the criteria that distinguish one such category from another are accessible to outside observers. They may be, as when they relate to my body posture. They may not be, as when they relate to a pain in my left elbow. In the latter case they are 'introspective'. By *mental states* we mean states of the individual which are categorized on this basis (Section 3.3).

From the methodological point of view the crucial fact about 'mental states' is that there exists no procedure for attaching verbal labels to these categories which could ensure a completely consistent and uniform use of these labels by different individuals. Nor, indeed, is it meaningful to ask whether two individuals apply the same categorization. We can only say that two individuals apply the same categorizations if in applying these categorizations they would divide the same set of objects into identical subsets. This is plainly precluded in the case of introspective judgements. From a scientific point of view, therefore, verbal evidence based on introspection is admissible only within strictly circumscribed limits.

If we add the internal representations of these self-categorizing reactions to the internal representations of the physical self (body schema) we arrive at internal representations of the self which comprise also the 'inner experience' that many regard as an essential ingredient of awareness of self. In Section 3.4 'consciousness' was accordingly defined as awareness of self (in this comprehensive sense), of the surrounding world and of the relation of the one to the other. 'Awareness' in turn was defined in terms of internal representations and the generalized reactions to them through which we impose a categorization upon them, the latter being essentially a descriptional function, an edited commentary on the 'content' of the internal representations. Finally, the 'stream of consciousness' was interpreted as the succession of mental states through which the subject passes.

11.2 MEMORY AND IMAGINATION

At the beginning of this chapter we reviewed the manner in which the brain may come to form cell organizations amounting to *latent* representations of familiar objects or events and their distinctive features, elements or properties. In each case the cell organization maps not only sensory inputs but also aggregates of expectations of how these inputs will transform in consequence of particular actions or acts of attention. Perception consists of the triggering of such organizations by the current sensory inputs. The resulting pattern of excitation constitutes the *activated* mode of the representations.

Whenever the networks concerned contain positive feedback elements (as suggested for a number of networks in Chapters 7 and 9) there exists the theoretical possibility of such representations being sustained beyond the duration of the stimuli which triggered them. We may assume that in suitable conditions such organizations may also spring into action 'spontaneously' and sustain a free running mode of activity. In these cases, therefore, we would have network conditions suitable for neural processes of the kind involved in reproductive memory and the free play of the imagination.

In a broad sense all enduring changes produced in the nervous system by particular experiences may be called memory changes. But the memory functions concerned in the recollection of past events are of a more sophisticated type, for they imply the reactivation of complex representations (and categorizing reactions) relating to the original events. In other words, they imply a 'spontaneous' activation of latent representations which have formed as the result of particular experiences. They are 'spontaneous' only in the sense that the activation now occurs in the absence of sensory stimuli similar to those which took part in the original experiences and in the formation of the neural organizations concerned. The same applies to the representations which are activated in the free play of the imagination. But there are important differences. The internal representations which are activated in the recollection of past events occur in combinations and in a serial order which are true to the original events. In the free play of the imagination, on the other hand, they occur in combinations and temporal sequences which may be unrelated to any concrete experiences of the organism. Their basic constituents are based on experience, but the combinations or the temporal sequence in which they come to be activated are not. In imagining a unicorn I draw on my experience of horses and horns, but the combination has no experienced prototype (disregarding pictures or descriptions expressing someone else's imaginings).

However, the faculty of imagination obviously involves more than the mere activation of previously experienced elements in new combinations. In imagining a unicorn we do not just form two internal representations, one of a horse and one of a horn. We form an integral representation of a very particular kind, viz. one in which the horn sprouts from the horse's head in a plausible position. That is to say the reactivated elements are actively combined into a new representation and one that is subject to strict tests for consistency or plausibility and other forms of censorship. There is an element here of critical (and in that sense genuine) creativity. Although there is a random element, the element is subject to comprehensive restraints which we must think of as learnt inhibitions of the highest order of sophistication.

In addition the activation of representations in the imagination and in memory recall is obviously subject to processes of facilitation, selection or restraint which arise from the general context in which our mental processes run their course. In the processes of rational thought the restraints may be very specific (Section 2.3). Even in the sensory activation of internal representations which occurs in the normal processes of perception a variety of contextural influences may be operative. For instance, the ease with which a model comes to be called up in sensory perception sometimes depends to a significant extent on the kind of thing I am expecting at the time.

The question arises how the brain can distinguish in neural terms between representations which are activated in the perception of actual events and representations which are activated by way of memory recall or in the free play of the imagination. According to our analysis there are two sets of criteria immediately available to the brain. One concerns the level of abstraction at which the representations are activated. I shall return to this point presently. The other arises from the very nature of internal representations. Since the neural representations of external objects, events or situations are really representations of aggregates of expectations relating to the way in which sensory inputs transform in consequence of our activities, the representations activated in memory recall or the imagination stand out by virtue of the fact that the respective expectations remain totally unmatched by our current sensory inputs and input-transformations. And this is something the networks we have envisaged can easily detect.

The further question of how the brain may distinguish between remembered and imagined events is much more difficult to answer. I shall not attempt to tackle it in this volume—except for pointing out that one distinction, which I tried to formulate in neurophysiological terms in Section 11.1, may be relevant. This is the distinction between neural representations of objects or events that I perceive and neural representations of the fact that the objects or event are *perceived by me.*

The feeling that the internal representation of some event relates to past experience is probably based on a variety of factors relating to the internal consistency and coherence of the representations concerned, to the context in which the events were experienced etc. But if at the time of the original occurrence of the events my brain also registered the events as *events experienced by me* (in the sense discussed in Section 11.1) this could later furnish an effective criterion for distinguishing between remembered and imagined events since this element will be absent in the latter. The very sophistication of these processes and the abstract level of the categorizing reactions which they presuppose, may account for the genuine difficulties younger children have in making the distinction.

In the 'spontaneous' activities of the imagination or memory recall, only those classes of representational cells can become activated which function at (or beyond) a level of organization at which there exist the necessary positive feedback circuits. We have seen that we must assume that there are 'cascades' of successive network organizations in the representational cortex which function according to similar principles but deal with successively higher levels of analysis and abstraction.

How detailed or relatively 'concrete' our imaginings or recollections can be, therefore depends in theory on the lowest level in these cascaded networks at which the positive feedback conditions are satisfied. However, although the higher levels receive inputs from the lower levels, they can function independently of these inputs if they themselves contain positive feedback circuits. Thus the low-level details may be entirely absent from the content of our imaginings or recollections. As we know, neither the memory nor the imagination generally function at a precisely detailed pictorial level. In this sense Shorter[222] is right in describing imagining as more like depicting in words than like painting a picture. The details that are left out are not represented in a vague or ambiguous way. They are simply not referred to in the activated representations at all. As Dennett[50] has pointed out, my not going into details about hair colour in imagining a man, does not mean that his hair is coloured 'vague' in my imagining. His hair is simply not 'mentioned' in my imagining at all. This accords with the general descriptional view of awareness we arrived at in the last section.

Although in theory representations may be revived in the memory or injected into the imagination from the lowest level upwards at which positive feedback occurs, in practice it appears that the very lowest levels (such as the mechanism for stable image creation) do not exhibit spontaneous activation despite their positive feedback connections. They may prolong an activated representation beyond the duration of the stimulus for brief periods (e.g. during saccadic movements of the eye), but they do not as a rule become activated in the absence of the proper sensory stimulation. A rare exception to this rule occurs in the phenomenon of eidetic memory. Children capable of eidetic memory images can read off the details of the remembered scene with almost photographic precision. The fact that these eidetic images appear to be superimposed on the subject's normal field suggests that the images consist of representations recovered at very low levels of abstraction, indeed even within the mechanism for stable image creation. As the representations activated in eidetic memory are independent of the current visual inputs they remain fixed in relation to the visual field when the eyes move. Hence they appear to move with the eyes, rather in the manner of after-images.

This raises an interesting point: at what level of feature analysis would 'spontaneous' activations of latent representations (as in memory recall or the imagination) cease to interfere with (or appear to be superimposed upon) representations activated by current sensory inputs in the normal processes of perception?

This is not so much a question whether the brain has criteria available for distinguishing between the two, as a question whether the one set of representations occupies units required for the other. In the images of eidetic memory the brain has such criteria available in the fact that these images do not transform in response to movements of the eyes, head or body. But the images still interfere with perception. If models called up in the memory or imagination are not to interfere with the normal processes of perception surely the main condition must be that the former representations are called up at a level of abstraction at which all expectations have been eliminated which relate to a specific position either in the visual field or in the stable image of the given scene (cf. Section 10.6). Probably the lowest of these levels are the levels at which the brain abstracts explicit representations of individual spatial relations between discrete pairs of objects. At these levels representations of objects and their *relative* spatial relations can be activated without 'mention' of the position of the objects within the visual field or stable image of the scene. Hence they would not now interfere with (or appear superimposed upon) the contents of the visual field or stable image of the scene.

The reader will recall that the lowest of these levels is the one at which the brain registers the eye movements that accompany shifts of attention from one given object to another. This forms the basis of explicit representations of the relative position of the objects seen. These processes (and the adequate stimulus substitution which enables the representations subsequently to be elicited without prior execution of shifts of attention) function at a higher level than the processes involved in the creation of the stable image itself.

In the above account we have interpreted the phenomena of reproductive memory and imagination in terms of the 'spontaneous' activation of neural organizations (or fragments thereof) which are of the nature of latent representations of objects, events or situations which have grown from a wealth of experience of sensory inputs and of the manner in which they transform in response to self-induced movements and attentional behaviours.

Obviously the factors that control such 'spontaneous' activation of latent representations must involve complex questions of contextual inputs to the cortical regions concerned and of tonic activations which may involve the whole machinery of goal-directed activity. Many of the processes involved in memory recall and the imagination are of the nature of a search terminated only by the activation of latent representations (or combinations thereof) which satisfy specific criteria of relevance to the situation in which the subject happens to be engaged at the time. However it would take us too far to attempt an analysis of these particular factors even if I were competent to do so.

11.3   LANGUAGE FUNCTIONS

One of the aims of this volume is to arrive at some idea of the type of neural mechanisms that could account for the special competences of the human brain. The subject of language is complex enough at the logical and semantic level. When it comes to trying to visualize the neural correlates of speech production and speech comprehension the difficulties assume astronomical proportions. For the time being we can only hope to arrive at some idea of these neural processes by concentrating on essentials and simplifying the variables concerned as much as possible. In Section 2.3, for example, we confined ourselves to the cognitive principles involved in the production of simple descriptive sentences. In the present section I shall continue to consider only the most characteristic elements in the phenomena we are interested in. And I shall confine myself to the narrative, hence descriptive, use of language. My aim is a speculative one: given the problems the brain has to solve in the descriptive use of language, what kind of neural organization should we expect to find in the light of our previous results?

Descriptive sentences typically serve to convey that some (real or imagined) object or event is of a certain kind, i.e. is a member of a certain class of objects or events. At an elementary level they have a straightforward subject–predicate form such as 'The strong man threw a blue ball'.

We noted in Section 2.3 that if we had command over a vocabulary of such proportions that it could furnish a single word (name) for every object or class about which we might wish to communicate, all descriptive utterances could be cast into the form of simple two-word sentences. Failing this, each 'unnamable' object or class of objects must first be specified in terms of the intersection of an adequate set of 'namable' classes. The unnamable object or class must therefore first be 'seen' as an intersection of namable classes. We have called this the 'cognitive resolution' of the unnamable object or class.

Thus 'the strong man' in the sentence quoted above denotes an unnamable object which is here specified in terms of two namable classes (the class of all men and the class of all strong objects) and finally pinpointed by the use of the definite article (see below). The predicate of the sentence assigns this particular man to a further class. This class, too, is unnamable and is here specified in terms of three classes: the class of ordered pairs of objects standing in the relation of a thrower and the object thrown, the class of balls and the class of all blue objects. Finally, as indicated by the past tense, the class membership which forms the essential content of the message is asserted only conditionally, viz. only for some (unspecified) point of time which precedes the time of utterance of the sentence.

The type of cognitive resolution concerned in these processes was illustrated diagrammatically in Figure 2.6. The set of namable classes appearing in such resolutions must be sufficient to prevent confusion with alternative objects or classes to which the message might relate. This depends on the circumstances in which the communication is made. 'The table is clean' is unequivocal only in circumstances in which no other tables present themselves as possible objects of reference or in which alternative tables have been removed from the field of attention by previous utterances. The use of the definite article here indicates that this is assumed to be the case.

Given the conceptual resolution of the unnamable objects or classes in terms of namable classes, a further cognitive process is required before a proper sentence structure can be produced in the established code of our language, because this code relies on the use of a special 'lexical' categorization of the namable classes occurring in the resolution. This additional categorization is based on a closed set of criteria. These concern questions such as whether the namable classes are classes of objects, of properties or of actions, whether the objects are singular or plural, male or female etc. This is the universe of grammatical distinctions, such as those between nouns and adjectives. They are required by the code used to express the cognitive resolution. They may also distinguish between contingent and constant properties. Compare, for example 'John is brutal' with 'John is a brute'.

We must now take a closer look at these basic cognitive processes and see if we can visualize types of neural organization which could learn to accomplish the required processes within the framework of the general network types and overall connectivities we have envisaged so far.

Let us start with the *conceptual content* of the messages conveyed in simple descriptive sentences.

Regardless of whether the message relates to the present, the past or the future, the neural correlate of this conceptual content presupposes a set of internal representations in the sense in which this phrase has been used throughout this volume, and of appropriate categorizing reactions to these representations (Sections 2.3 and 11.1). To distinguish between message contents relating to the past, present or future the internal representations concerned must also include either explicit representations of the time factor or representations of contexts which determine the time factor implicitly.

The neural correlates of internal representations of objects, events or situations and of their properties, features or relations have been discussed at various stages in this volume. They were reviewed again in Section 11.1.

Depending on the significance different aspects of objects (events, situations) assume in our practical transactions with the environment, the brain develops generalized, and hence categorizing, reactions to the aggregates of relevant internal representations.

Thus we arrive at the neural correlates of *concepts* of trees, horses, solids, liquids etc. Since these categorizations are generalized reactions to internal representations and since these representations may encompass a multitude of expectations concerning the consequences of possible actions, it is evident that concepts go beyond the immediate data of perception. Nor are concepts just collections of physical properties. The concept of a particular class of objects, for instance, may relate to the uses to which the object can be put (houses, knives, lamps). This illustrates that some concepts may be based on aggregates of internal representations which are the product of elaborate exercises of the imagination. Since by definition categorizing reactions are reactions which generalize over a particular set of internal representations, concept formation is a process of *abstraction*: it abstracts from the difference between the members of the set. Categorization, generalization and abstraction are all aspects of the same process.

One can see from this account that concepts of even comparatively simple objects may be based on expectancies covering sensory transformations resulting from a great variety of attentional, exploratory or interfering behaviours. They depend, therefore, on neural excitations derived from a great variety of cross-modal products of sensory information and movement information. It follows that the neural correlate of any concept of objects or their properties must have a fairly diffuse distribution in the brain.

Typically the purpose of a descriptive message is to convey that some object or event is of a certain kind, i.e. belongs to a certain class. Typically, too, the purpose of the message is to cause the listener to picture certain objects or events. It goes without saying that the speaker must first be conscious of the fact that the object or event is of this kind. However, in neural terms this presupposes more than just having an internal representation of the object and having the appropriate categorizing reaction. It presupposes in addition an internal representation of the fact that the relevant categorizing reaction was elicited by the object in question. I shall return to this point presently.

To get a broad idea of what is involved in the production and comprehension of descriptive statements, let us start with a hypothetical world in which all the main problems have been drastically simplified and assume that our vocabulary is so comprehensive that it contains a name for every object and class of objects about which we may wish to communicate. Our language would then require no more than simple two-word sentences like 'John tall', 'Teddy brown', 'Peter angry' etc. It would be not unlike the simple two-word combinations that are typically found in two-year-old children. To introduce a grammar, assume that the correct word sequence is subject–predicate. For the time being we shall also ignore the motor skills required to utter the selected words and the perceptual skills required to identify apprehended words. We shall look only at the problems arising in connection with word selection, lexical classification and the serial order in which the words are produced.

Consider the case in which I want to express the fact that a teddy bear known as Teddy is brown, i.e. that this particular object belongs to a particular class, viz. the class of all brown objects. It is easy to see that in neural terms this presupposes more than just an explicit internal representation of the teddy bear and an explicit categorizing reaction specific to the colour brown. It requires in addition an explicit internal representation of the fact that the brownness is part of the teddy bear, i.e. that the reaction 'brown' is elicited by this particular object. I must be aware of the fact of association of object and property. In other words, the fact of association must appear explicitly in my internal representation.

At the simplest level this explicit internal representation may be conceived in terms of two complementary patterns of neural excitations:

(A) excitations representing the expectation that when I look at this object I get the impression of brownness, and

(B) excitations representing the expectation that when I cease to look at this object the impression of brownness ceases too.

Similarly, the fact that the teddy bear is fragile may typically be represented internally by

(A) expectations to the effect that the object breaks if I drop it, in conjunction with

(B) expectations to the effect that if I do not drop it, the object remains intact.

We saw in Chapter 7 how expectations may be represented in terms of
patterns of neural excitations and what kind of networks could make the
required cell organizations possible.

To produce simple descriptive two-word sentences of the type we are en-
visaging here the brain has to learn

  (i) to select the appropriate word for the object to which the attentional,
       exploratory or interfering behaviours mentioned in the expectations
       (A) and (B) are applied;
 (ii) to select the appropriate word for the categorizing reactions to which
       these expectations relate;
(iii) to distinguish the lexical category of these names (one being an object
       name, the other a property name);
(iv) to utter the two names in the conventional order, as dictated by their
       lexical category.

All this is a question of learning a correct set of responses to a particular
situation. This raises no special problems except in one respect. How can the
brain learn the necessary skills to the point at which, without further learning,
it can produce the correct utterances in respect of *novel* combinations of known
objects and known properties? In other words, how can it learn the grammar
of this particular language as distinct from merely learning particular applications of this grammar? The importance of this point was stressed in Section
2.3.

In the present case it means that the mechanisms for speech production
must have explicit information available as regards the lexical categories of
the words (e.g. in the form of excitations in specific fibre groups) and must
learn to let the serial order of the utterances be governed by this information.
This is not difficult to visualize in neural terms.

Speech comprehension, on the other hand, makes more complex demands
on the networks of the brain. Broadly speaking, to learn to comprehend our
simple two-word sentences the brain must learn

  (i) to recognize the words occurring in a perceived sentence and their
       individual significance;
 (ii) to recognize their lexical category;
(iii) to recognize the serial order in terms of the lexical categories;
(iv) to generate from these outputs the appropriate internal representations
       and (if the listener is to become explicitly aware of the message content)
       also expectations of the type mentioned under (A) and (B) above.

The class of these expectations as regards the attentional, exploratory or interfering behaviours to whose consequences they relate is determined by the class name occurring in the sentence, while their class as regards the object to which these behaviours are applied is determined by the object name. It is clear that these delimitations could be learnt for individual object words and class words independently of the particular combinations in which they occur in particular sentences. (Just as having learnt to paint a chair red I know how to paint a table red.)

Task (iv) is obviously the critical part of the whole process of speech comprehension. Moreover, the neural events we want the message to elicit in the brain of the listener are under-determined. If the listener has no previous experience of a *brown* teddy bear, neither the required internal representations of the object nor the expectations mentioned above can be produced by way of triggering a cell organization which is already in existence. At this stage, therefore, there must be a creative jump. If no brown teddy bear has been experienced before there must at this stage occur a process of creative synthesis similar to the creative processes I mentioned in connection with the faculty of the imagination (Section 11.2). I mentioned at the time that the imagination does not generally function at a very detailed pictorial level. A lot of details may go unmentioned. And, indeed, it may not be the intention of the speaker to evoke a detailed image in the listener's mind. But in the most common forms of human communication it is the speaker's intention to evoke some kind of imagery in the listener's mind and to the extent to which this is imagery of something not previously experienced by the listener, the communication presupposes active participation of the listener's imagination, including the processes of critical censorship that assure the coherence and plausibility of the results.

To fulfil their proper function in these creative processes the perceived object name and class name must enter this process of creative synthesis in a dual role, viz. as general activating stimuli and as specific restraints. Whatever details are omitted or randomly added in the imagination (such as posture and location of the teddy bear), the imagined object must be identifiable with Teddy and it must be brown.

The suggestion lies close at hand that in this particular case the censorship mentioned above includes tests to check whether the end products of the creative process are consistent with the perceived sentence, i.e. whether they would have found expression in an identical sentence if they had to be communicated verbally. If this suggestion is correct it would support the belief, frequently voiced by psycholinguists, that the machinery for speech comprehension leans heavily on the machinery involved in preparing a sentence for production.

According to this account of speech comprehension the process of learning the grammar of the language (as distinct from learning particular applications

of the grammar) would consist mainly of learning the control functions specified under this heading in our discussion of speech production (above), as
well as learning to use the object name and class name occurring in the message as appropriate constraints in the creative synthesis which the message
evokes in the brain of the recipient.

So much for the simple hypothetical case in which all objects and classes
we wish to communicate about are namable. We must now return to the
world of reality in which this is the exception rather than the rule.

In the circumstances in which the natural languages function few of the
objects or classes about which we may wish to communicate are namable.
Hence we now need additional mechanisms which enable these unnamable
objects or classes to be adequately specified in terms of namable objects or
classes.

At a naive level of thought one could imagine a mechanism which simply
lists all namable classes to which a given unnamable object is known to belong.
The perception of an object elicits a number of categorizing reactions in the
brain. For some of these we have a name in our vocabulary, names like
'brown', 'fragile', 'tall', 'strong' etc. We could therefore imagine a neural
mechanism which would simply facilitate all words in our vocabulary that
correspond to any of the categorizing reactions elicited by the perceived
object. However, this would obviously be a highly redundant process. It
would generate absurdly redundant lists of ceaselessly growing proportions
as we continue to examine the object. Hence there must be some form of
selection from among the set of class names which are facilitated by our
categorizing reactions to the perceived object. In practice it is only necessary
to specify the object to the extent required to avoid equivocation in the circumstances in which the utterances occur. Hence the appropriate selective
processes must obviously depend on highly skilled faculties. It is not surprising that these skills appear to develop only slowly as the result of experience
and learning (witness the typical beginning of any story told by a child:
'There was that man, you see, and he . . .').

This process of selective potentiation of the appropriate object names or
class names may perhaps best be compared with the process of learning that
a given goal can best be reached through a particular combination of acquired
motor skills. In this comparison the categorizing reaction corresponding to
the unnamable class would take the place of the 'demand signals' and the
potentiation of an appropriate set of class names would take the place of the
selected motor skills.

However, to think at this stage already of the potentiation of strings of
speech movements would obviously be jumping several stages too far ahead.
The organizational aggregates which come to be potentiated at this stage are
not as yet representative of actual words, let alone of speech movements.
They are precursors which may perhaps best be described as '*word-equiva-*

lents' or '*word-roots*'. At this stage it is still an open question, for example, what word endings will be employed or in which serial order the words will be uttered.

Detailed investigations by Goodglass[89] and his coworkers of lesions in the frontal areas held responsible for the production of word structures indeed suggest that in the process of producing a word we have to distinguish a stage of having words in some sort of abstract pattern from a stage in which the abstract pattern is converted into its phonic form. The frontal areas concerned in this conversion extend over area 44 and the adjacent part of area 45 (Figure 6.5). They are generally known as Broca's areas, after Paul Broca who with Bouilland was one of the first to point out that damage in these areas results in disturbance of language output. It is assumed that these areas exercise their phonic programming influence partly via the areas of the motor cortex related to the movements necessary for speech and partly via the subcortical structures involved in these movements (basal ganglia, cerebellum etc.).

Thus the collection of existing neural organizations on which the mechanisms concerned with word availability and word selection depend, would be a vocabulary of word-equivalents or word-roots rather than a vocabulary of preprogrammed utterances. Word selection may then be conceived as a process in which some of these organizations come to be potentiated in consequence of the categorizing reactions elicited by the perceived object, the potentiation being subject to the selective (i.e. inhibitory) mechanisms adumbrated above.

A further complication is that the learning of words clearly appears to be a separate process from the learning of syntax, as indeed we would expect it to be. When we have learnt a new class name and its lexical category we do not in addition have to learn how to use it in different sentence structures. This functional separation is also suggested by the pathology of speech and language disorders, as we shall see presently.

The classification of the different types of aphasia resulting from brain lesions is a difficult and controversial subject. There is hardly ever a pure loss of easily categorized language functions. But as Jakobson[125] has pointed out, a notable dichotomy runs through the various disorders. Whereas some mainly disturb word selection, others mainly affect word combination and serial order. In Luria's 'efferent aphasias', for example, the selection of content words is unimpaired, but the combination of words and their serial order may be severely disturbed[152]. Speech may degenerate to a succession of telegraph-style utterances. Grammatical words such as conjunctions, prepositions, pronouns and articles disappear. Roots of words are better preserved than grammatical endings, tense or gender. The nominative may be the only case that survives. These aphasias appear to essentially link with lesions in Broca's areas. In Luria's 'sensory aphasias' on the other hand, syntactic wholes are generally preserved (including grammatical words) but content words are lost. The main disruption appears to be in the word–object relation.

It is generally held that the posterior association cortex of the dominant hemisphere is critically implicated in mediating this relation, in particular the supramarginal gyrus (area 40, Figure 6.5) and the angular gyrus (area 39). The latter appears to be implicated in naming visual objects and in the recognition of written words. Lesions in this area impair naming and reading. Word identity ceases to exist outside the context in which the word occurs. The patient cannot find the required word if it is context free. But comprehension and repetition of perceived speech remain generally unimpaired.

Another important area concerned in these functions is Wernicke's area (area 22, Figure 6.5). According to a widely accepted view the auditory pattern of perceived words is set up in this area, so that, for example, comprehension of a written word would involve evocation of the auditory form in this area by the visual inputs via the angular gyrus. Conversely it is assumed that if a word has to be spelt, the auditory pattern is passed to the angular gyrus where it elicits the visual pattern. For patients with lesions in area 22 the meaningfulness of words is lost (auditory receptive aphasia).

The posterior areas are linked with Broca's areas by the arcuate fasciculus. If lesions in this fasciculus sever the connection between Wernicke's area and Broca's area, then, according to the same model, comprehension should remain unimpaired and speech should remain fluent (though abnormal), but repetition of perceived speech should be severely impaired. This syndrome, first predicted by Wernicke, is known as 'conduction aphasia' and has in fact been observed.

We left our speculative outline of the process of speech production at the point at which the appropriate word-equivalents had been selected. The outputs of the neural organization which determines this selection must be paired with information specifying the lexical category of the words before the next phase of the operations can begin. This information is required for the modification of the words at the point of insertion into the sentence and the serial order in which they are inserted (as well as the 'grammatical' words that must be added). In effect this means that the operations of the next phase are formed as a function both of the pattern of these selective outputs and of the 'lexical' class of the activated output channels. By this I mean a classification of the relevant channels according to whether they derive from neural representations of objects, actions, properties etc. According to our analysis, it is clear from the manner in which these neural representations are formed that this information would lie available in the identity of the fibre groups which are activated in the perception and recognition of the objects, actions, properties etc.

We may pause at this point and summarize the initial processes I have listed so far. They are shown diagrammatically in Figure 11.1 in which I have

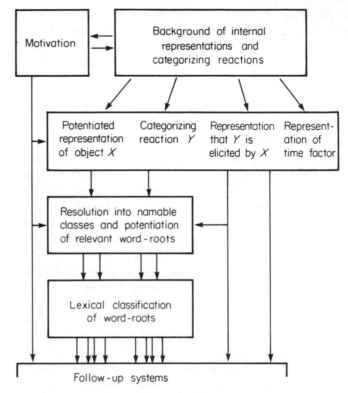

Figure 11.1. Synopsis of the suggested processes in the preparatory stages of sentence production

assumed a primary message content to the effect that an unnamable object X is a member of an unnamable class Y. The diagram speaks for itself. Apart from the factoring out of the time reference (i.e. representations which relate to the conditional validity of the intended message and which will find expression in the tense of the sentence) the main processes shown have been reviewed at various points of this chapter. I have inserted the time reference for the sake of completeness only. It would take us too far to analyse this factor even at the cursory level at which we have only been able to analyse the other processes. The mechanisms indicated in the diagram, of course, cover only the main preparatory processes that must go into planning a sentence for production. There is much more to follow. On the evidence the functions symbolized in the diagram appear to be mainly performed in the posterior association areas (parietal and temporal). This includes the formation of the equivalents of the content words, but not of the grammatical words.

The most important point to make about the outputs of these preparatory mechanisms is that to all intents and purposes we must regard them as concurrent and static. They are simultaneous outputs which remain essentially constant throughout the production phase of the sentence. They reflect the outcome of a preparatory structuring and elaboration of the message content which must precede the production of the verbal utterances that give physical expression to the message. Although the outputs of these preparatory mechanisms contain the lexical information required for the sentence structure no question of the serial order of utterances or the insertion of grammatical words has arisen so far. The outputs we are concerned with at the moment form the neural substrate of the plan that must be set up before speech production starts. They control the sentence *as a whole*. Their general role in the follow-up mechanisms that produce the appropriate string of verbal utterances is therefore similar to that of 'demand signals' in the common mechanisms of behavioural control (Chapter 5).

Next, the language mechanisms need a neural organization which receives these static outputs as demand inputs and uses the information they contain to generate a temporal sequence of neural events which will eventually result in the appropriate string of verbal utterances. Some of the main conditions this organization must satisfy may be gathered from our analysis of the simple 'lambda' models introduced in Chapter 7. To remind us of the kind of connectivities that can produce serialization Figure 11.2 illustrates a simple lambda network which can learn to convert a constant input pattern into any required temporal sequence of outputs. The constant inputs enter the system by way of 'demand inputs' (Section 5.2). A second input system is provided by

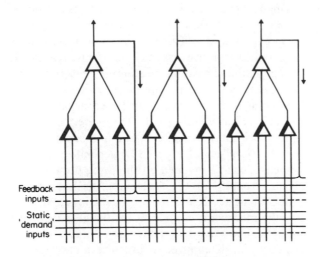

Figure 11.2. Simple model of lambda network capable of translating static input pattern into dynamic output pattern. The system can learn to respond to a static 'demand' input with a programmed succession of outputs

associative feedback channels from subsets of lambda neurons joined by OR gates. In consequence of this arrangement, the identity of the lambda neuron firing at any one time is determined both by the demand inputs and by the feedback inputs, the latter being determined by the identity (subset) of the last lambda neuron to fire. As each feedback input gives way to the next a temporal sequence of outputs results which the system can learn to fashion as an appropriate function of the current pattern of demand inputs. In other words, given appropriate reinforcement control, the system can thus learn to produce any desired dynamic output sequence in response to any given pattern of static demand inputs. Owing to the grouping of the lambda neurons the system also permits the same output to occur in more than one of the response sequences it learns to assimilate.

The most important feature of this very elementary paradigm is the system of positive feedback loops (recurrent axon collaterals). This is important because, as we saw in Chapter 7, such a system is also inherently capable of triggered chain reactions which mimic acquired response sequences. It will be suggested presently that triggered chain reactions of this type may play an essential part in the mechanisms of both speech perception and speech comprehension.

Granted then that the system of Figure 11.1 is followed by systems which can generate a temporal sequence of neural events from the static demand inputs they receive from the former system, the next question concerns the nature of the first *serial* neural events that are now produced. In theory it would be possible for these follow-up systems to generate straight away the appropriate command signals for the speech muscles. But if this were the case all speech movements would have to be learnt from scratch for any new sentence the brain has to master. This is clearly not the case in practice. The position changes radically if we assume that sentences can not only be *formally analysed* into atomic meaning-bearing elements but that they are also *physically produced* in terms of such atomic units, each in turn being expressed in a chain of muscle activations which can be learnt once and for all time. Such an atomic unit is the *morpheme*. In the interest of maximal learning economy, therefore, we must expect that the first serializing system which follows the preparatory system of Figure 11.1 generates a temporal sequence of neural events which can be mapped on the string of morphemes that constitute the surface structure of the sentence. This implies converting the equivalents of the content words into appropriate strings of morpheme equivalents and adding the morpheme equivalents of the grammatical words.

The next question then must be whether the outputs of this morphemic serializing system are translated directly into speech movements, or whether there exists yet another intermediate apparatus, viz. one which receives these outputs as demand inputs and generates from each input pattern the neural equivalent of a string of *phonemes*. In other words, is there a second, semi-autonomous, serializing system which converts each of the morphemic input patterns into a string of output patterns each of which triggers a phoneme, in the sense of a particular preprogrammed set of speech movements?

The 'duality of patterning' (i.e. patterning at both morphemic and phonemic levels) is generally accepted as a feature of the natural languages. However, the degree of autonomy of these processes is still in dispute. It appears to be true to say that the rate at which individual muscular events occur throughout the speech apparatus is of an order of magnitude (several hundreds per second) which calls for a certain degree of automation. Thus there must be combinations of muscular events which are 'preprogrammed' and merely require to be triggered at the right moment. However, it also appears to be true that the time required for the activation of all muscles that enter into the production of a single speech sound may be as much as twice as long as the duration of the sound itself. Hence there must be a certain degree of anticipation and overlap. Motor outputs required for one phoneme may have to be initiated during the preceding one. It has also been found that the muscular activity associated with one phoneme is frequently influenced by phonemes that precede or follow it. Even more significant is the observation that the segmentation of morphemes into phonemes which we appear to register in the acoustic *perception* of speech and which we take for granted in the functional analysis of language, is not in fact matched by a segmentation in the acoustic *production* of speech (Figure 11.3). Phonemes certainly appear to be very real in speech perception but their discreteness in speech production is less certain.

Perceptually, speech sounds indeed seem to follow one another like a train of independent speech segments. No matter how carefully or how often we listen to a sequence of tape-recorded words played back at the original speed, we always hear a clear cut succession of phonemes.

This strongly suggests that phonemes have physiological reality in the mechanisms of speech *perception*, in the sense that the auditory inputs appear to trigger a string of discrete neural events which can be mapped on the phonemes and in which each event begins at the termination of the previous one. We can picture these discrete events as the triggering of neural organizations which have formed during learning in the same manner as the neural organizations we discussed in connection with other forms of perception. The question is: do these organizations form during reinforced practice of speech *perception* or reinforced practice of speech *production*?

There are those who feel that if traditional learning theory invoking external reinforcement is to apply at all production must come first. Liberman[148], for example, holds that the acquired distinctiveness of phonemic contrasts follows from cues supplied by articulation. This belief in the physiological reality of phonemes in speech production is supported by certain speech disorders in which individual phonemes are preserved but their serial order is

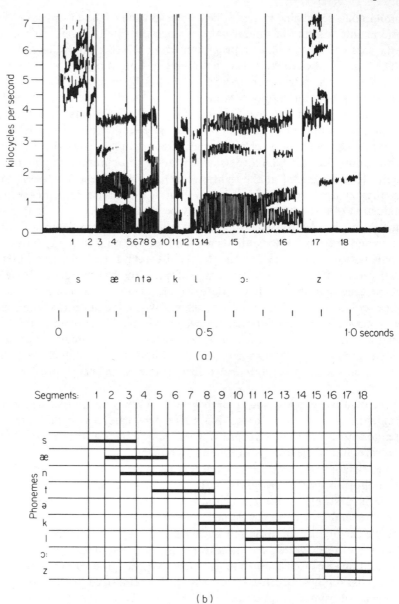

Figure 11.3. Perceptually, speech sounds seem to follow one another like a train of independent speech segments. Acoustically, however, there is considerable overlap. (a) Spectrogram of the words *Santa Claus*. Vertical lines mark acoustically differentiated segments. (b) Assignment of phonemes to acoustic segments (From Lenneberg[147], after Fant and Lindblom, *Studies of minimal speech and sound units*[63]. Reproduced by permission of Gunnar Fant)

disturbed: individual phonemes may advance in the string in which they are due, or there may be a propensity for spoonerisms.

On the other hand the overlap shown by spectrographic analysis (Figure 11.3) compels the conclusion that if strings of discrete neural phoneme-equivalents enter into speech production at all they cannot be the sole controllers of organized speech movements.

Another significant observation which argues against the above motor theory of speech perception concerns the known cases of children with congenital defects in speech production who learnt to understand speech even though they were literally speechless. The perceptual skill here evidently developed unaided by speech production. Furthermore, it is known that during infancy language comprehension generally develops *ahead* of language expression.

A possible way out of these difficulties and apparent contradictions is suggested by the known importance of auditory feedback in speech production. Auditory feedback appears to play an important part both in shaping the neural organizations that govern speech production and in the actual production of speech.

It is well known that the congenitally deaf never learn to produce speech that sounds like that of a normal hearing person, however carefully they may be trained. Correction by matching to auditory criteria thus seems indispensable for learning correct speech. We also know that interference with auditory feedback produces notable speech disturbances. Normally we hear our own voice the very instant speech is produced. If a delay is artificially introduced between the time we actually speak and the time the sounds we produce reach our ear, speech may be severely disrupted. The most characteristic effect is a drawing out of vowels. This shows that the mechanisms of speech perception participate in speech production by way of one or more feedback loops.

Given the importance of auditory feedback loops we may find a possible solution in the schema of Figure 11.4 (solid lines only). System I here symbolizes the system of internal representations and categorizations which was detailed in Figure 11.1 and which we have placed in the posterior association areas (parietal and temporal). System II is the serializing system (postulated above) for generating temporal sequences of morpheme-equivalents from the static outputs of System I. This includes the formation and insertion of grammatical words. On the evidence cited above one would be inclined to place this system in Broca's area. System IV represents the motor apparatus directly implicated in speech production. This would include the relevant areas of the motor cortex and the subcortical structures implicated in the execution of speech movements. Direct links from II to IV are suggested by the phenomena of inter-phonemic interference and by the fact that motor commands relating to one phoneme may have to be triggered already during the preceding phoneme (see above). System III is the phonemic perception system. By this we

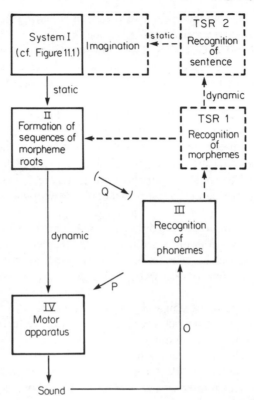

Figure 11.4. Schematic outline of suggested organization for speech production (solid lines) and speech perception (broken lines), with System III participating in both in an essential capacity

mean a system in which the distinctive features of individual phonemes (see below) come to be represented by assemblies of neurons which during learning come to be linked through synaptic alignment on recurrent collaterals directly or indirectly derived from other members of the assembly. We assume that, once formed, these assemblies will be triggered by auditory inputs containing the respective phonemes. The auditory feedback is formed by pathways O and P. On the evidence one would be tempted to assume that this system lies in area 22.

Although we have described system III as a perception system, its feedback functions obviously also make it part of the production system. It is plausible to assume that to the extent to which System III participates in speech production by way of the feedback loop it participates also in the reinforcing effects of successful production. In other words, it may undergo learning changes both during speech production and speech perception. Seen in this light the question whether the neural organizations that mediate speech perception do or do not first form in the course of speech production, becomes merely a question of whether the egg came first or the hen.

It is conceivable that System III enters speech production also in a more direct capacity: there may exist links Q (bracketed arrow) which enable the phonemic organizations in III to be triggered also by inputs from System II. System III would then participate in a direct production chain (I–II–III–IV) and might undergo plastic changes also in consequence of these relationships. This would lessen the dependence of the production apparatus on the auditory feedback loop.

Clearly the actual networks must be very much more complicated than the simple paradigms I have used to illustrate particular aspects of the matter. System III, for example, must be able to factor out phoneme identity from a great variety of sounds produced by speakers of different voice qualities. This appears to be a question of factoring out a finite set of feature contrasts in the auditory inputs. The well known analysis of Jakobson and coworkers has shown that individual phonemes can be thought of as aggregates of feature contrasts of the type nasal/oral, strident/mellow, vocalic/non-vocalic etc. It is claimed that each phoneme can be specified by listing the appropriate binary value in a specific set of such contrasting pairs of features. Jakobson believes that a total range of twelve such contrasts suffices to cover all phonemes. It is conceivable that this skill of phoneme perception develops according to the 'analysis-by-synthesis' principle first proposed by Stevens and Halle. According to this hypothesis the primary function in phoneme perception would be to match the 'foreign-made' phonemes of received speech with the 'home-made' phonemes of produced speech.

The perception of phonemes is only the first stage in speech perception and comprehension. To complete these processes the brain needs systems which can register strings of phonemes, interpret them as strings of morphemes and finally convert these temporal sequences of neural events into spatial distributions of neural excitations which can trigger stable representations of the meaning of the sentence. The rudimentary principles of neural networks that can convert a temporal sequence of neural input patterns into a characteristic spatial distribution of outputs, were illustrated in Chapter 7.

The systems concerned are indicated by broken lines in Figure 11.4, proceeding on the assumption that we are here dealing with a two-stage process in which the first stage (TSR 1) extracts the morphemes from the temporal sequence of phonemes and the second stage (TSR 2) converts the temporal sequence of morphemes into a static pattern of output excitations which are characteristic of the message content. Presumably these systems, too, would be located in area 22.

We have now reached a stage which parallels the processes involved in learning to comprehend the simple hypothetical language we discussed at the beginning of this section, a language composed of only two-word sentences.

The reader will recall that we began that analysis with the assumption that individual words and their serial order could be successfully identified. The processes which must occur in the natural languages to achieve comprehension of the string of identified morphemes have to solve the same basic problems as the processes we discussed at the time—except that the syntactical elements are now very much more complex. In the earlier case there were only two such elements: the lexical category and serial order of the perceived words. Now we have something very much more complex.

To isolate these syntactical elements it is expedient to introduce the notion of a *sentence frame*. Broadly speaking a 'sentence frame' means the structure that results if we remove the 'content-morphemes' but leave the closed class of morphemes that make up the word-modifiers and grammatical words. Thus 'The ——s who ——ed ——ly' is the sentence frame of 'The boys who talked quietly'. Essentially therefore, the sentence frame contains the components whose use and serial order we learn when we learn the grammar of a language. Having mastered this closed class of morphemes and their correct application (given the deep structure of the sentence) our linguistic competences subsequently expand mainly by adding to the open class of content words which may be dropped into the spaces left open in the sentence frame. Broadly speaking, therefore, the sentence frame maps common features of the cognitive resolutions that precede sentence production.

It follows that in the present case the sentence frame in conjunction with the lexical categories of the content words really plays the same part in the process of speech comprehension as did the mere conjunction of lexical categories and serial order in the hypothetical two-word language considered earlier. In that simplified model the mechanisms of speech comprehension learnt the grammar of the language by learning to use the content words both as general stimuli to the imagination and as specific constraints, while using the lexical categories and serial order for determining the application of these constraints. In the present rather more complex case the brain has to learn to use the sentence frame in the same imagination-restraining way. And again it seems plausible to assume that these imaginational processes are subject to an additional censorship which tests whether their end products tally with the perceived sentence. Conceivably the tests, too, involve checking whether these end products would lead to the synthesis of similar sentences if they had to be expressed verbally.

As has been said, these creative processes need not necessarily function at very detailed or pictorial levels of representation. When I am told that it rains outside we need not suppose that the brain interprets this statement by imagining a detailed scene in which rain falls. We have seen that imaginative processes can function at various levels of abstraction. Though the neural events here are concrete enough, what they map may be highly abstract. Even so, introspection shows that in response to the statement that it rains outside we often do respond by vaguely imagining the garden or the street as they would look when it rains.

It follows from the above that at this stage, too, the mechanism of speech comprehension must be expected to lean on the mechanisms concerned in preparing sentences for production (our System I) in the manner adumbrated. To symbolize this I have taken the outputs from System TSR 2 (Figure 11.4) to a block labelled 'imagination' affiliated to System I. The feedback loop R is suggested by the internalization of communicative behaviour that appears to occur in verbal thinking, as well as by the need for 'productive' checks on comprehension.

In view of the diffuse nature of many of the processes that have been mentioned, it is not surprising that the evidence for their localization in the brain is relatively indecisive. With the exception of functions closely bound to the source of auditory inputs (for instance the auditory association areas 22) or to the final motor output (for instance the bulbar RF), or the naming of discrete visual objects (area 39 in conjunction with 22) the effect of brain lesions often points to no more than broad topographical divisions[77]. The uppermost of the systems shown in Figure 11.4 (System I and TSR 2) appear to implicate mainly the temporoparietal regions of the dominant hemisphere. Sensory aphasias are typically produced by lesions affecting these regions. Word-deafness is most frequently found to be correlated with lesions in the superior middle temporal lobe (area 22). At the other end of the hierarchy (System IV) there is a definite involvement of the excitable motor cortex and of the subcortical, diencephalic and mesencephalic regions which we must expect to participate in the execution of motor skills. Lesions in these regions produce disruption of articulation or phonation depending on the level of the affected site. Thus lesions in the basal ganglia may result in speech monotony and lesions in the cerebellum may cause changes in speech rhythms. According to our model this motor apparatus is programmed by System II, which we have placed in Broca's area.

Severance of the links between I and II produces the syndrome of conduction aphasia (see above). I have mentioned that the final processes of speech comprehension must be expected to lean heavily on the mechanisms concerned in preparing a sentence for production. In the final phase of comprehension the listener identifies with the speaker, as it were. In our model the relevant preparatory phase occurs in System I. This would explain why in conduction aphasia comprehension remains generally intact despite the probable dependence of speech comprehension on speech production.

In broad outline our model agrees with the results of Luria, Barton and others who have found that patients with more posteriorly located lesions tend to show more disturbances within the sphere of meaning whereas aphasics with anteriorly located lesions make more errors characterized by breakdown in word structure. More especially we have seen that aspects of language chiefly dependent on visuospatial orientation are largely sustained by the posterior parietal cortex. Lesions in these areas may occasionally produce 'disconnection' or 'isolation' syndromes which are modality specific. Geschwind[76], for example, has reported the case of a patient who could name objects he saw. But though he could manipulate and match objects by touch and had no tactile perceptual difficulties, he could not name the objects when blindfolded. The relevant sensory information, it seemed, could not reach the speech areas.

The less the information required for a specific linguistic task depends on our internal representations of the outside world and the more it depends on information lying available within the linguistic system itself, the less severe will be the impairment resulting from lesions in the association cortex. Thus Goodglass *et al.*[89] report that posterior patients may show much greater defects in object naming than in letter naming.

Following his extensive studies of word-frequency distributions in aphasics, Howes[117] came to draw a dividing line between two comprehensive systems which he calls the 'alpha' and 'beta' systems respectively. The alpha system receives inputs representing the information content of the message to be communicated. It emits outputs that through the function of the speech musculature give us the phonic form of words. This system may in some cases also create its own inputs, viz. inputs specially related to grammatical elements like conjunctions, prepositions, and pronouns. The beta system, on the other hand, has the task of integrating, coordinating and codifying the wealth of potential information that can be expressed verbally and of making a selection of words for a particular topic. Receiving inputs from the various sensory mechanisms, the limbic system, memory systems and others, the beta system normally inhibits the inputs from all such channels bar the relevant ones. Thus Howes' alpha and beta systems are broadly identifiable with our System II and I respectively, it being understood that the latter includes the 'drive' and 'motivational' elements indicated in Figure 11.1.

It follows from the analysis given in Chapter 10 that to the extent to which System I includes these drive and contextual elements, it cannot entirely be confined to the posterior cortex and, at the cortical level, also embraces evaluation areas in the frontal or limbic cortex.

It is important to stress in this connection that normal speech production is a goal-directed process. Hence the same general considerations concerning the required information flow apply here as those that were set out in Chapter 10. Thus the neural excitations corresponding to an *intended* message arise from the impact of signals reflecting the drive state of the speaker with signals derived from internal representations of the circumstances in which the verbal communication is made and of the scene to be described. According to the analysis given in Chapter 10, the frontal and limbic areas of the cortex are the primary cortical sites of this impact. The excitations resulting from this impact then potentiate particular organizations in the posterior representational systems. Thus frontal lobe lesions must also be expected to interfere with linguistic functions. The reported effects of frontal surgery are broadly as we would expect. Milner[168] has reported that the most noticeable linguistic defect after frontal lobectomy is lack of spontaneous speech and poverty of word fluency. Luria[153] has stressed the impairment of spontaneous monologue, or narrative speech, in patients with tumours of the dominant frontal lobe, and a disturbance in the 'regulatory function of speech' (i.e. in the control of voluntary and autonomic processes). Among earlier workers Kleist[133] noted the poverty of spontaneous verbal expression in patients with lesions of the left anterior frontal area, although they have no aphasias in the usual sense. Hamlin[99] found that after superior frontal surgery a significant loss remained even after a number of years, which was reflected in verbal and numerical tasks more clearly than in perceptual and construction tasks. Not surprisingly there was also a notable loss in attention, problem solving and other intellectual functions.

Mere repetition of perceived speech obviously makes lesser demands on

Table 1. Classification of Typical Aphasias by Syndromes (From E. Green, Aphasia and Psycholinguistics, *Cortex*, **6**, 1970. Reproduced by permission of *Cortex*).

Type of aphasia	Site of lesion	Spontaneous speech	Comprehension	Repetition	Naming
Broca's aphasia	posterior inferior frontal (System II)	non-fluent	intact	limited	limited
Wernicke's aphasia	posterior superior temporal (Systems III, TSR 1, TSR 2)	fluent	impaired	impaired	impaired
Conduction aphasia	arcuate fasciculus (link between Systems I and II)	fluent	intact	impaired	impaired
Isolation syndrome	association cortex (parts of System I)	fluent echolalic (reiterative)	impaired	intact	inpaired
Anomic aphasia	angular gyrus (part of System I)	fluent	intact	intact	impaired

the brain mechanisms than tasks in which comprehension is required. This is confirmed by the observation that in adult aphasiacs you can get repetition from almost every patient as soon as the motor mechanisms are working. These considerations suggest feedback loops immediately below System I, e.g. the feedback connection shown between TSR 1 and System II (Figure 11.4). The observation that children do not begin to imitate words or phrases until their language development is fairly advanced, and then tend to impose their own primitive grammar on the repeated sentences, suggests, according to our analysis, that the feedback loop concerned functions at this level rather than the next lower level.

In Table 1 I have reproduced an aphasia classification published by Green which roughly summarizes the five main forms of aphasia that are typically seen in his research unit[93]. Below the sites of the lesions cited by Green I have added the interpretations suggested by the theoretical model of Figure 11.4. Although Green warns that his table is not all-inclusive and although our own analysis has only dealt with broad principles and a selective range of phenomena, the table gives some indication of the extent to which our model does justice to the evidence furnished by typical language disorders.

System I, of course, is so comprehensive that the syndromes listed in Table 1 can be no more than a small sample of possible disturbances. Lesions which disturb more complex levels of activity, for example, may result in impairment of the proper relation of speech to the general stimulus situation and motivational context. R. Brain[23] mentions aphasias in which patients succeed in naming objects in their normal environment which they cannot name if the objects are presented artificially as part of a test. In other cases ('pragmatic' aphasias) there may be a ready flow of words but no apparent self-criticism. Again, in some aphasias the patient may be able to cope with simple sentences but not with combinations of sentences (Luria's 'dynamic aphasia'). Or he may be able to comprehend the simple instructions 'show me your ear' and 'show me your nose' but not the instruction 'show me your ear and nose' (Luria's 'amnesic' aphasia).

Although language functions are mainly located in the dominant hemisphere (and the lesions mentioned in this section generally refer to this hemisphere only) the minor hemisphere is not entirely excluded from language functions. Observations on split-brain patients show that the minor hemisphere can comprehend spoken or written words. Patients can learn to rearrange letters with the left hand to spell words denoting objects presented to the left halves of the visual fields. But in general the minor hemisphere proves to be better organized for non-verbal tasks, such as visual construction tasks. In the dominant hemisphere, on the other hand, the influence of the language system appears to be pervasive. The performance of this hemisphere suggests that language may here influence the categorizations imposed on the sensory data as well as the integration of these data. The asymmetrical distribution of linguistic functions over the two hemispheres is evident even when similar faculties appear to be involved. Thus damage to the left temporal lobe which leads to disturbance of phonemic hearing, may leave musical hearing untouched. Conversely there are data which indicate that damage to the right temporal lobe may lead to amusia without evoking any defects of phonemic hearing.

The Basic Concepts of Information Theory

A message is informative to the extent to which it tells us something we did not already know and so reduces or removes a prior uncertainty. Information theory accordingly defines the content of a message in terms of the prior uncertainty it removes. If we can find a precise measure for the uncertainty we can measure information in similar precise terms.

Consider an event x for which there are r alternative possibilities $x_1, \ldots, x_r$ and let p_i be the probability of the ith alternative. For instance, if I toss a coin there are two possible alternatives, if I cast a dice there are six and if I write down a letter of the alphabet there are twenty-six.

We first take the case when the alternatives are equally likely. Thus there are six equally likely outcomes for the dice, each with a probability of 1/6, and two possibilities for the coin, each with a probability of 1/2. If a dice and a coin are thrown out of my sight the message telling me the number on the dice removes a greater uncertainty than the message telling me the outcome of the tossing of the coin. Taking this as its cue, information theory defines the uncertainty removed in the first case as

$$H \text{ (dice)} = \log_2 6 \text{ bits}$$

and that removed in the second case as

$$H \text{ (coin)} = \log_2 2 \text{ bits}$$

The unit chosen is the 'bit', formed as a contraction of 'binary digit'.

In general the information content of a message is taken to be equal to the uncertainty removed and is accordingly defined for equally likely possibilities by

$$H(x) = \log_2 r = \log_2 \frac{1}{P}$$

The choice of a logarithmic function in these definitions conforms to the ordinary sense in which we think of information. For if *two* dice are thrown and I am told *both* outcomes I intuitively accept this as a message with twice the information content as in the single case. There are now 36 alternative

378

possibilities; so according to the definition the information content is $\log_2 36$ bits, which equals twice $\log_2 6$ bits.

According to the definition, a device with two stable positions, e.g. a relay, can store one unit of information, because there are here two possibilities and $\log_2 2 = 1$. N such devices can store N units of information because there are now 2^N possibilities and $\log_2 2^N = N$. This also agrees with what we would intuitively feel to be the information storage capacity of a bank of relays.

If the events are not equally likely, as in the case of a bent coin, the uncertainty is defined as the weighted average

$$H(x) = \sum_{i=1}^{r} p_i \log \frac{1}{p_i}$$

If, by way of estimate, in a series of n trials the probability of each event is equated with the relative frequency with which it occurs in the series so that

$$p_i = \frac{n_i}{n}$$

the formula for the average uncertainty (hence information) per event becomes

$$H(x) = \log_2 n - \frac{1}{n} \sum n_i \log_2 n_i$$

It is easy to show that $H(x)$ is maximal if all the probabilities are equal.

The quantity

$$R = 1 - \frac{H(x)}{H_{max}(x)}$$

is defined as the *redundancy*. This quantity is important because it can serve as an indication of the degree to which the information contained in a message could have been conveyed more economically (i.e. in terms of fewer signs or signals) if a better system had been used for coding it. Thus in a series of 100 throws of a bent coin one could specify the complete set of outcomes by means of 100 binary digits, taking '0' for 'heads' and '1' for 'tails', or vice versa. But as the probabilities are unequal in the case of a bent coin the redundancy formula shows that it must be possible to use a code requiring fewer digits. (It does not, however, tell us how to find that code!)

The redundancy concept is also important because it gives us an informational measure of the extent of patterning or organization in any set of discrete elements. Written English, for instance, has a considerable redundancy because the different letters of the alphabet occur with quite different relative frequencies and so do different combinations of letters and words. Thus owing to the frequency of words like 'the', 'that', 'there' etc. an 'h' occurring after a 't' in written English removes very much less uncertainty than it would if occurring in a random letter sequence. Taking observed frequencies into account Shannon, for example, has calculated that the redundancy of written English is of the order of 75%.

Redundancy is not necessarily a bad thing. It is precisely because of the high redundancy in our language that a transmitted verbal message may suffer errors in transmission without loss of information, thus spelling mistakes and printers' errors may remain innocuous.

Another important concept in information theory is that of *information transfer*, or *information sharing*. Take the case of a laboratory experiment in which a subject is presented with a series of alternative stimuli *S* and a record is compiled of his response *R* and of the relative frequencies of *S* and *R*. When there is *no* correlation between the responses and the stimuli (as when a blind person is asked to identify the colours of light spots projected on a screen) the average uncertainty of any stimulus–response combination, i.e. $H(S, R)$, must equal the sum of average uncertainty $H(S)$ of the stimuli and the average uncertainty $H(R)$ of the responses. But when there *is* a correlation between the stimuli and the responses, then $H(S, R)$ will be less than this sum. We may therefore define the *information transfer* between the stimuli and the responses by the formula

$$T(S; R) = H(S) + H(R) - H(S, R)$$

For the case of the blind subject this formula gives us $T(S; R) = 0$. At the other extreme, the case of a seeing person who invariably identifies the colours of the spots correctly, all the terms on the right-hand side of the formula are of equal magnitude and we get

$$T(S; R) = H(S) = H(R) = H(S, R)$$

A number of interesting results have been obtained about the information transfer characteristics of the nervous system. It has been found, for instance, that the amount of information a human subject can transmit in an experiment in which the subject is required to judge the absolute pitch of a note according to five categories, is of the order of 2–3 bits. This quantity turns out to be much the same for any other one-dimensional stimulus variable (loudness of tone, absolute size of shapes projected on a screen etc.). As the number of dimensions in which the stimuli may vary is increased, the transmitted information rises as a logarithmic function of the number of dimensions.

In certain cases we can also calculate the information transfer capacity per second of individual subjects. In conscious and deliberate human behaviour this is of the order of 10–100 bits per second. This may seem small in comparison with the information handling potential of a system composed of 10^{10} neurons. But it must be remembered that this system is not only capable of transmitting information about the stream of stimuli impinging on it at any particular moment, but also about a vast range of past experiences which have left their traces in the brain and affect its current behaviour patterns. Any simple and meaningful estimate of the redundancy built into the information processing machinery of the brain seems out of the question.

The concept of information transfer is not, of course, restricted to stimulus–response associations. $T(x; y)$ may be defined on any two variables for which we can make probability estimates.

When three variables, x, y, z, are involved we may consider the information transfer from any two (e.g. x, y) onto the third (z). This is defined by the formula $T(x, y; z) = H(x, y) + H(z) - H(x, y, z)$. We may also consider the information transfer from y to z if x is known or held constant, say $x = x'$. This quantity may be symbolized by $T_{x=x'}(y, z)$. It is determined by the formula $T_{x=x'}(y; z) = T(x, y; z) - T(x; z)$.

APPENDIX B

The Lambda System as a Maximum Intensity Filter

We investigate the parameters of a lambda module (Figure A.1) in which only the one lambda neuron discharges which experiences the maximum excitation from a given input pattern.

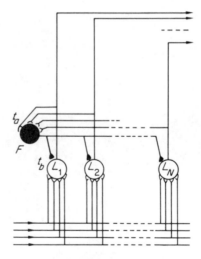

Figure A.1

In a different context and in respect of single-input neurons only, the problem was first investigated by W. K. Taylor.* Transposing his line of argument we assume that in the system of Figure A.1 the output frequency (f) of any neuron (including neuron F) is proportional to the amount by which EPSP − IPSP exceeds a constant threshold (a), and zero if EPSP − IPSP is less than this threshold. We also assume that the synapses on F have an equal and constant potency (t_a) and the synapses of the axon collaterals of F on the lambda neurons have an equal and constant potency (t_b).

*W. K. Taylor: A model of learning mechanisms in the brain. In N. Wiener and J. P. Schadé (eds.), *Cybernetics of the Nervous System*, Elsevier, Amsterdam, 1965.

Let 'synaptic potency' be defined as the ratio between the absolute value of the potential changes effected in the cell by an afferent fibre and the frequency of the afferent impulses effecting it. Thus for any lambda neuron we have

$$IPSP = f_F.t_b$$

where f_F is the discharge frequency of F.

Also, for any p,

$$f_p = \begin{cases} c[(EPSP)_p - IPSP - a] & \text{if this is positive,} \\ 0 & \text{otherwise,} \end{cases} \tag{i}$$

where a is the threshold and c is a constant.

For the inhibitory neuron F,

$$(EPSP)_F = t_a \sum_{p=1}^{N} f_p$$

$$(IPSP)_F = 0$$

where N is the number of lambda neurons in the module. Hence, for any p,

$$(IPSP)_p = t_b f_F \begin{cases} t_b c(t_a \sum_{p=1}^{N} f_p - a) & \text{if this is positive} \\ 0 & \text{otherwise.} \end{cases} \tag{ii}$$

We demand that

(a) only one lambda neuron, say L_j, discharges within the module, hence

$$f_j > 0$$
$$f_i = 0 \qquad \text{for all } i \neq j. \tag{iii}$$

and

(b) the frequency f_j of this discharge is to be proportional to $(EPSP)_j$:

$$f_j = K(EPSP)_j \tag{iv}$$

We have to find the conditions on the constants a, b, t_a, t_b, K and on the inputs such that (i), (ii), (iii) and (iv) are consistent.

To satisfy (iii), (ii) becomes

$$(IPSP)_p = \begin{cases} t_b c(t_a f_j - a) & \text{if this is positive,} \\ 0 & \text{otherwise.} \end{cases} \tag{v}$$

Assuming f_j has become large enough to make $t_a f_j > a$, so that F fires, and substituting (v) into (i) for L_j, we get

$$f_j = c[(EPSP)_j - t_b c(t_a f_j - a) - a]$$

Hence, from (iv),

$$t_a c a - a = 0,$$

hence

$$t_b c = 1 \tag{vi}$$

and $$K = b - t_b c^2 t_a K = c - ct_a K,$$

hence $$K = \frac{c}{1 + ct_a} \tag{vii}$$

Equations (vi) and (vii), therefore, state the conditions the parameters of the system must satisfy if the inhibitory mechanism is to perform as required.

It can also be shown from (v) and (vi) that to function in this manner the EPSP of the neuron which receives the greatest excitation from a given input pattern (neuron L_j) must exceed that of the neuron receiving the next highest EPSP, say neuron L_g, by an amount which is given by

$$(\text{EPSP})_g \leqslant Kt_a(\text{EPSP})_j$$

It follows that we need Kt_a as close as possible to 1, or we need ct_a as large as possible (cf. equation (vii)). As an example, suppose $c = 20$, $t_a = 1$, $t_b = \frac{1}{20}$, $a = 20$ mV. This gives $K = Kt_a = \frac{20}{21}$. Then the system works correctly if the largest EPSP exceeds 21 mV and if the next largest EPSP does not exceed $\frac{20}{21} \times$ the largest. If this condition is *not* fulfilled *two* lambda neurons fire.

These conditions are not particularly stringent. They do imply, however, that considerable variations in the individual synaptic potencies are possible on the input side. It must also be emphasized that we are dealing here only with a simple model composed of 'formal neurons' which represent only a selection of simple properties.

The Distribution of Learning Changes

The ground plan given in Figure 10.6 is an attempt to visualize in simple schematic form the main connectivities in the brain whose function may be interpreted in terms of the organizational relationships that have occupied us in this volume. Many of the learning changes that must occur in this system were dealt with in connection with the specific mechanisms discussed. A brief exposition may be added of how I believe that the elementary phenomena of classical conditioning relate to the various levels of organized activity that have been our main preoccupation.

On the whole these levels have been such that we had to think primarily in terms of cortical activities. Classical conditioning, on the other hand, is confined to responses which can be consistently elicited by known stimuli (Section 5.3), and this tends to favour the use of gross stimuli (electric shocks, buzzers, flashes of light) which are likely to exert their primary influence at subcortical levels. Except in the case of the cerebellum and hippocampus, the question of the plasticity of subcortical structures has not so far been one of our major concerns.

In contrast with instrumental conditioning classical conditioning does not appear to be highly dependent on cortical function. This has frequently been demonstrated in animals rendered decorticate by surgery and in animals in which cortical action was suppressed by the drug curare. Thus decorticate dogs can give conditional responses to auditory stimuli by loud barking or growling when electric shock is used as the US. Bilateral ablation of the cortical projection areas of either the CS or US produces impairment of complex and delicate discriminating powers but may not otherwise hinder conditioning. Sometimes the impairment is only temporary. Thus simple pitch discrimination may be lost postoperatively by bilateral ablation of the auditory cortex, but may be recovered with retraining.

In split-brain animals instrumental conditioning may be effected in the two hemispheres separately. Indeed Trevarthen[255] has shown that the split-brain monkey can learn simultaneously two different and opposite problems, one in each functionally independent hemisphere. But attempts to achieve a similar separation in classical conditioning have failed.

The cortex appears to enter into the associations formed in classical conditioning mainly in a refining and elaborating capacity. Thus Girden *et al.*[82] have found that when a dog is conditioned to lift a paw from a grid, the US being an electric shock applied through the grid, there is an early phase in which the CR resembles the gross vigorous escape movements produced by the shock itself. This is followed by a later, precise phase in which the gross bodily reactions are inhibited and merely a neatly adaptive raising of the paw remains. This second phase fails to occur in decorticate preparations.

That classical conditioning engages primarily the subcortical brain is also supported by the observation that in these particular routines the organism does not adjust to situations in which reinforcement (occurrence of the US) happens only intermittently, whereas in instrumental conditioning it does. Adjustment to such partial reinforcement implies an adjustment to temporal factors and probabilities which we are bound to see as a primarily cortical function (cf. Section 10.3).

In a broad sense, classical conditioning may be viewed as a process resulting in some measure of stimulus equivalence or 'adequate stimulus substitution'. Appropriate pairings of a previously neutralized stimulus (CS) with a second stimulus (US) to which there is an established response (UR) result in a capacity of the first stimulus to elicit a grossly similar response (CR). Although from a behavioural point of view we appear to be dealing here with a class of uniform phenomena, our theoretical discussions have made it clear that in physiological terms such stimulus equivalences may result from a variety of mechanisms.

The stimulus equivalences established in conditioning mean in effect that a new afferent signal is grafted on the unconditioned stimulus–response arcs. The nature of the mechanism effecting this grafting, therefore, must depend on the particular arc (or segment of arc) concerned. Following the researches of Loucks and others it is now generally accepted that this grafting cannot occur in the subcortical descending pathways of the existing arcs. As regards ascending pathways the fast afferent pathways to the cortex are also excluded, since the relay stations along these pathways do not provide for the degree of convergence needed to account for the full range of stimuli to which a given response may be conditioned.

At the subcortical level this points mainly at the polysynaptic non-specific ascending pathways through the reticular formation and the non-specific nuclei of the thalamus as possible sites for the grafting or 'closures'. For the coarse stimuli used in many conditioning experiments (loud clicks, bright flashes etc.) the mesencephalic reticular formation and midline thalamus or reticular nucleus are widely accepted as the most probable sites. The centromedian nucleus appears to be particularly important in this respect.

It is known that during conditioning the afferent excitation arising from the CS is deviated to the cortical areas specifically related to the US. Thus when a response normally elicited by a flash of light is conditioned to a loud click, the evoked potentials come to show increased activity in the visual cortex when the click is heard.

In the light of our analysis these observations take on a new significance. The afferents to the cortex which come to be activated by this deviation appear in our analysis as the rising output segments of the diencephalic and mesencephalic evaluation systems. In fact, all structures generally mentioned as possible sites for the 'grafting' processes appear as 'evaluating units' in our ground plan. This conclusion is supported by a number of observations. For example, conditioning is generally known to be difficult unless the US is one which in man would be called pleasant or unpleasant (receiving food, electric shocks etc.). In other words, the US must occur in a suitable motivational context—an observation which clearly points to the involvement of evaluation centres. Other examples will appear below.

To account for the overall plasticity of the nervous system we may have to assume that convergent 'contextual' input systems reach key neurons in all evaluation centres, where they may then become assimilated as adequate releasers for particular ascending and/or descending discharges. The dual character of the discharges of the evaluation centres was analysed in Section 10.1.

The following observation also points to the involvement of subcortical evaluation centres in classical conditioning while at the same time illustrating the importance of the cortical influences on these centres. When decorticate dogs are presented with an auditory CS paired with shock they no longer demonstrate coordinated leg withdrawal (see above); but as Sager et al.[213] have pointed out, there is no loss of affective reactions to the CS (bristling of hair, dilation of pupils etc.). The conditioned significance of the CS is not diminished. In fact the reactions are often exaggerated, presumably due to the absence of cortical inhibitory control over affective responses. Thus, although the cortex is not the site of the main linkages established in classical conditioning, it does appear to influence the nature of the final response.

Removal of this background of cortical influence may abolish a previously established CR. If after conditioning these influences are removed by suppressing cortical activity with curare, the CR may be lost (though it can be restored through retraining). The converse also applies. Girden and Culler[81] found that conditioning effected under curare is lost upon recovery from the effects of the drug (but may again be restored through retraining).

I have mentioned before that the rising activations of the evaluation systems are manifest in the cortex in certain 'late components' of the evoked potentials (Section 10.3, and see also Section 8.6). These only appear when the stimulus concerned has significance as a cue to performance. It follows that during conditioning only the late components should transfer from the potentials evoked by the US to those evoked by the CS. This indeed appears to be the case.

When a response is conditioned to a rhythmical stimulus of a given frequency so that this frequency can be used as a 'tracer' in electrical recordings taken from different subcortical structures, John[126] and Killam found that on occasions when the CR occurs spontaneously the tracer frequency appears in the hippocampus, mesencephalic reticular formation and intralaminar nuclei. This again supports the suggestion that the crucial response decisions are taken in the evaluation centres.

When two distinct responses are conditioned to two distinct frequencies and both frequencies are presented together, the frequency in whose favour the conflict is resolved appears in the same structures. If a habituated tracer stimulus is paired with shock the tracer frequency appears in all structures involved in the general alarm reaction. These are all parts of the evaluation systems or parts receiving projections from them.

Conditioning in which electrical stimulation to the cortex is used as CS is abolished if the amygdala are ablated. This reminds us that the diencephalic and mesencephalic evaluation centres receive afferents also from above, not just from below.

The actual degree of adaptive plasticity of the reticular formation is uncertain. Changes in the responses of units in the reticular formation during conditioning have been demonstrated in the rat by Bureš and Burešova[34]. At first in these experiments auditory stimuli caused no change in the activity of the monitored units whereas sciatic stimulation caused inhibition of unit activity. After pairing of sound with sciatic stimulation a number of times, sound alone caused inhibition. However, as the authors have stressed, these results show only that the reticular formation participates in the affected networks, not that it is the site of the plastic changes. (The same remarks apply to transient changes which have sometimes been recorded in other subcortical structures—even in the receptive fields of retinal ganglion cells, as observed by Weingarten and Spinelli[271].)

If plasticity does exist in the reticular formation, the structure of the network concerned is obscure. The reticular formation contains no short-axoned neurons and there is no recurrent inhibition or gridlike distribution of afferents which might suggest a system functioning along the lines of our hypothetical lambda systems. Something rather more along those lines, on the other hand, is to be found in the thalamus. In the ventrobasal nucleus of the thalamus, for example, the main relay cells are subject to recurrent inhibition and each specific afferent fibre makes contact with about 25 relay cells. The recurrent inhibition, therefore, acts on sets of neurons sharing specific afferent fibres. But they are small sets and if this arrangement (which is fairly typical for thalamic nuclei) is of the lambda type it could at best be a rudimentary form of lambda system.

It follows from the concept of grafting onto existing arcs that if a stimulus S_A is grafted as conditioned stimulus onto an arc determined by an unconditioned stimulus S_B, the exact site of grafting is unlikely to be the same as when in a different context S_B is grafted onto an arc determined by S_A as unconditioned stimulus.

Recent physiological evidence also suggests that the CS and US enter the grafting neurons on unequal terms, as did the 'contextual' inputs and 'forcing' or 'biasing' inputs in the theoretical models we explored in Section 7.4. This may be illustrated with reference to recordings taken by F. Morrell[172] in a visual association area of the cat which broadly corresponds to area 19 in man. Although we are not here dealing with phenomena which satisfy all the criteria of classical conditioning, the results are nevertheless illuminating. In this area Morrell recorded a large number of individual cells each of which was selectively responsive to a particular category of visual inputs. The preferred stimulus configuration was usually complex. A typical cell, for example, might be maximally responsive to a dark bar on a light background oriented along a particular line stopped at one end. Another might be responsive to a vertical bar moving from right to left. Owing to the statistical nature of the responses their characteristics are best seen in a post-stimulus histogram in which discharge frequencies are summated over a number of trials. Figure A.2 (top line) illustrates the responses of one such cell to the presentation of a black bar on light background.

The majority of these cells also responded to tactile and other stimuli, for example to an electric shock administered to the contralateral limb (second line). The responses in this case were very different from those elicited by the preferred visual stimulus.

When the visual stimulus was combined with one of the others, electric shock of the hind limb, for example, a new complex histogram resulted rarely attributable to a simple linear summation of the firing pattern for the separate stimuli (third line).

Following a series of trials with paired stimulation the original test stimulus was again presented alone. In the great majority of the cells the response patterns to this visual stimulus were as before, but in about one sixth of the cells the subsequent test stimulations evoked stable response patterns with a marked resemblance to those elicited by the combined stimuli (bottom line). Somewhere in the brain the visual stimuli had become grafted onto an afferent pathway as adequate releasers for the non-specific excitations previously elicited only by the electric shock. And this was no symmetrical relationship: the shock alone would not elicit the response pattern of combined stimuli.

A different example of afferent signals entering convergent structures on unequal terms is furnished by records Morrell obtained from cells in which the

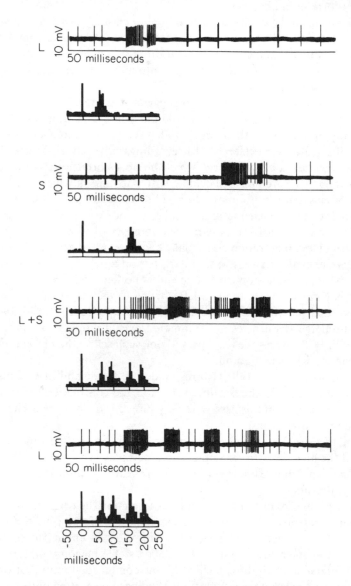

Figure A.2. Experientially-induced modification of response pattern. Cell responded to a dark horizontal bar and also to electric shock to the contralateral hindlimb (S). Combining these two stimuli (L + S) resulted in a histogram very different from that which might occur from simple linear addition of the two separate responses. Furthermore, after 40 trials of such paired stimuli, the original visual stimulus (L) was presented alone. It elicited a pattern much more like that elaborated by paired stimulation than like that which it produced prior to pairing. The histograms are sums of 20 trials. The single traces are the most representative of the overall pattern in each group of 20 (From Morrell[172])

non-preferred stimulus was ineffective. Thus there would be a cell which responded only to illumination of its receptive field in the contralateral (left) eye. Stimulation of the ipsilateral eye produced no alteration in the spontaneous firing rate or pattern. Yet when the two eyes were stimulated simultaneously over a number of trials a reorganization of firing patterns occurred and, when at the end of the paired trials the preferred stimulus (contralateral eye) was reintroduced in isolation, a complex response resulted which retained the two additional components contributed or elaborated during paired stimulation.

The hypothetical configurations we discussed in Section 7.4 suggest a very simple model for the type of differential input conditions and synaptic transfer that may account for these phenomena. The main assumption we make in this model is that the inputs from the foreign modalities enter the convergent neurons as 'contextual' inputs whereas inputs from the dominant or preferred modality as 'forcing' or 'biasing' inputs. It will be recalled that we coupled these distinctions with the assumption that only the synapses involved in the 'contextual' inputs undergo learning changes.

The model is symbolized in Figure A.3. Two modalities are envisaged (I, II). Cell P_I is a cell of the primary cortex for modality I, selectively responsive to a particular input pattern in this modality. Cell A_I belongs to an association area dominated by modality I. Cell C_{II} belongs to a convergent, possibly subcortical, system dominated by modality II and supplying contextual inputs to large areas of the cortex including cell A_I. Cell A_I also receives collaterals from primary cell P_I as forcing inputs. Other collaterals of the same axon act on C_{II} as contextual afferents. As has been said, we assume that synapses relating to contextual inputs undergo learning changes, but forcing or biasing synapses do not.

Let St_I and St_{II} represent particular stimuli in modalities I and II respectively. Assume also that initially C_{II} is insufficiently receptive to discharges of

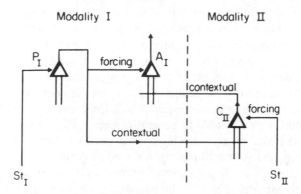

Figure A.3. Model of simple neural organization that could yield the kind of effects illustrated in Figure A.2. For explanation see text

P_I to fire in the absence of the additional stimulation St_{II}. It follows that if St_I is paired with St_{II} A_I receives a double input with different latencies and, we may assume, respond in a distinctive fashion. But if repeated pairing results in the assimilation by C_{II} of discharges from P_I as adequate stimuli, St_I alone will subsequently result in a double input to A_I and thus elicit a similar distinctive response in A_I even in the absence of St_{II}. The responses of A_I to St_{II} occurring without St_I, on the other hand, remain the same as before. This is a naive model of the kind of dominance relations which could account for phenomena of the type illustrated in Figure A.2.

A case similar to Morrell's second example I cited results if we take St_I and St_{II} to represent stimuli to the contralateral and ipsilateral eye respectively and assume that St_{II} enters C_{II} via biasing synapses. Initially, therefore, C_{II} responds only to the paired presentation of St_I and St_{II}. During repeated pairings C_{II} increases its responsiveness to discharges from P_I but not to St_{II} since we assume that biasing synapses undergo no learning changes. Hence after repeated pairings St_I will evoke the combined response in A_I, but St_{II} alone remains ineffective. Alternatively we could assume that the afferent fibres conveying St_{II} to the cell C_{II} are of the nature of forcing fibres but that the particular stimulus chosen for St_{II} did not excite these fibres with sufficient intensity to result in a forcing action.

In truth, of course, the matter is bound to be very much more complex than our simple model suggests. The contextual inputs to cortical neurons reflect on-going activities in a variety of complex systems, cortical as well as subcortical. Some of these inputs may relate not only to current spatial distributions of excitation in these systems but also to the serial order in which they occurred. Nor is it necessarily the case that an integrative or representational area related to one particular modality receives all its inputs in that modality from the respective cortical projection area. Finally, evaluation systems at more than one level may be involved in the activating and attentional signals which rise to the cortex (and which along their pathway absorb the central stimulus equivalences established during classical conditioning).

One is accustomed to think of learning as a process in which initially coarse and generalized responses become progressively more circumscribed and refined if the successful outcome of any particular form of action demands this. But, as has been pointed out before, it is also often important that any initially limited stimulus–response association which the organism may have formed should in due course be able to generalize over a wider range of input conditions. In the past chapters we have come across a number of examples in which the progressive substitution of wide 'contextual' inputs for rather more specific local inputs as adequate stimuli for particular responses was of obvious advantage to the organism. All the paradigms we introduced as suggestions for the way in which the brain may form internal models of the outside world, assumed substitutions of this kind.

Investigations into the receptive fields of cortical neurons suggest that something of this nature happens in an elementary form already in or near primary receiving areas. Phenomena of this type, for example, have been described by Brooks[31] for the primary somatic cortex in the cat. Many cells in this area are sensitive to touch or pressure when this is applied to a narrowly circumscribed and constant area of the body surface. These cells with 'fixed local fields' contrast with others which are responsive to stimuli over a much wider constant area and probably receive their inputs via extra-lemniscal pathways. But there is also a category of cells whose fields (either local or wide) are labile and expand upon repetition of the stimuli. Brooks believes that the fixed wide fields are labile fields which have reached conditional limits of expansion. Sometimes in the primary somatic area and frequently in adjacent areas the labile phase extends not only over somaesthetic and kinaesthetic signals for the whole body but also over visual and auditory signals. The natural time course of this variability is unpredictable in the unrestrained animal. Under laboratory conditions, however, the non-specific discharges initially follow the specific ones within a fraction of a second and with repetition tend to grow into frank responses from widened receptive fields. This second phase can last up to several hours, depending on the amount of stimulation given. This appears to be a clear example in which convergent 'contextual' inputs (possibly including attentional inputs) in due course come to substitute for more restricted 'forcing' inputs as adequate stimuli for the release of particular outputs.

Bibliography

1. Abercrombie, M. L. J., 'Eye movements and perceptual development', in *Aspects of Developmental and Paediatric Ophthalmology* (Eds. P. Gardiner, R. MacKeith and V. Smith), Heinemann, London, 1969.
2. Adey, W. R., N. C. R. Merrillees and S. Sunderland, 'Corticifugal influences on intrinsic brain stem conduction in cat and monkey', *J. Neurophysiol.*, **20**, 1–16.
3. Adler, A., 'A case of visual agnosia', *Trans. Amer. neurol. Ass.*, **70**, 168 (1944).
4. Adler, A., 'Course and outcome of visual agnosia', *J. nerv. ment. Dis.*, **3**, 41–51 (1950).
5. Adrian, E. D. and B. H. C. Matthews, 'The interpretation of potential waves in the cortex', *J. Physiol.*, **81**, 440–71 (1934).
6. Aiken, L. S. and D. Brown, 'Feature utilization of continuously varying attributes in visual pattern classification', *Perception and Psychophysics*, **9** (2A), 145–9 (1971).
7. Albert, D. J., 'The effect of spreading depression on the consolidation of learning', *Neuropsychologia*, **4**, 49–64 (1966).
8. Albert, D. J., 'The effects of polarizing currents on the consolidation of learning', *Neuropsychologia*, **4**, 65–77 (1966).
9. Anand, B. K. and J. R. Brobeck, 'Hypothalamic control of food intake', *Yale J. Biol. Med.*, **24**, 123–40 (1951).
10. Andersen, P. O., 'Structure and function of archicortex', in *Brain and Conscious Experience* (Ed. J. C. Eccles), Springer, New York, 1966.
11. Arbib, M. A., *The Metaphorical Brain*, Wiley–Interscience, New York, 1972.
12. Armstrong, D. M., *A Materialistic Theory of the Mind*, Routledge and Kegan Paul, London, 1968.
13. Ashby, W. Ross, 'The set theory of mechanism and homeostasis', *Artorga*, Communication **76** (1965).
14. Aquinas, St. Thomas, *Summa Theologica*, new translation and edition by various hands under Fr. Thomas Gilby (Gen. Ed.), McGraw-Hill, New York, 1963 onwards.
15. Basowitz, H., S. J. Korchin, D. Oken, M. G. Goldstein, and H. Gussak, 'Anxiety and performance changes with a minimal dose of epinephrime', *Arch. Neurol. Psychiat.*, **76**, 98–105 (1956).
16. Beloff, J., *The Existence of Mind*, MacGibbon and Kee, London, 1962.
17. Beritashvili (Beritoff), I. S., 'The characteristics and origin of voluntary movements in higher vertebrates', in *Progress in Brain Research*, Vol. I (Eds. G. Moruzzi, A. Fessard and H. H. Jasper), Elsevier, Amsterdam, 1963, pp. 340–48.
18. Berlyne, D. E., 'The development of the concept of attention in psychology',

in *Attention in Neurophysiology* (Eds. C. R. Evans and T. B. Mulholland), Butterworths, London, 1969.

19. Beurle, R. L., 'Functional organization in random networks', in *Principles of Self-organization* (Eds. H. von Foerster and G. W. Zopf), Pergamon Press, Oxford, 1962.
20. Birkmayer, W., *Hirnverletzungen*, Springer, Vienna, 1951.
21. Blakemore, C., E. T. Garner and J. A. Sweet, 'The site of size constancy', *Perception*, **1**, 111–19 (1972).
22. Blomfield, S. and D. Marr, 'How the cerebellum may be used', *Nature*, **227**, 1224–8 (1970).
23. Brain, R., 'The neurology of language', *Brain*, **84**, 145–66 (1961).
24. Braitenberg, V., 'Is the cerebellar cortex a biological clock in the millisecond range?' in *The Cerebellum* (Eds. C. A. Fox and R. S. Snider), Elsevier, Amsterdam, 1967.
25. Brattgård, S. O., 'RNA increase in ganglion cells of retina after stimulation by light', *Acta Radiol.*, Suppl. **96**, 80 (1952).
26. Brazier, M. A. B., *The Electrical Activity of the Nervous System*, Pitman Medical, London, 1968.
27. Brentano, F., 'The distinction between mental and physical phenomena' (translated by D. B. Terrell), in *Realism and the Background of Phenomenology* (Ed. R. M. Chisholm), Glencoe Free Press, London, 1960.
28. Brindley, G. S., 'The classification of modifiable synapses and their use in models for conditioning', *Proc. Roy. Soc. B*, **168**, 361–76 (1967).
29. Broadbent, D. E., *Perception and Communication*, Pergamon Press, New York, 1958.
30. Brodal, A., 'Some data and perspectives on the anatomy of the so-called extrapyramidal system', *Acta neurol. scand.*, **39**, Suppl. 4, 17–38 (1963).
31. Brooks, V. B., 'Variability and redundancy in the cerebral cortex', in *The Physiological Basis of Mental Activity* (Ed. R. Hernandez Peòn), pp. 13–32, Elsevier, Amsterdam, 1963.
32. Brooks, V. B., K. Kameda and R. Nagel, 'Recurrent inhibition in the cat's cerebral cortex', in *Structure and Function of Inhibitory Neuronal Mechanisms* (Eds. C. von Euler, S. Skoglund and U. Söderberg), Pergamon Press, London, 1968.
33. Bureš, J., 'Reversible decortication and behaviour', in *The Central Nervous System and Behaviour* (Ed. M. A. Brazier), J. Macy, New York, 1959.
34. Bureš, J. and O. Burešovà, 'Plasticity at the single neuron level', *Proc. 23rd Intern. Physiol. Congr., Tokyo*, **IV**, 359–64 (1965).
35. Burns, B. Delisle and B. Grafstein, 'The function and structure of some neurones in the cat's cerebral cortex', *J. Physiol.*, **118**, 412–33 (1952).
36. Burns, B. Delisle., *The Uncertain Nervous System*, Edward Arnold, London, 1968.
37. Buser, P., P. Ascher, J. Bruner, D. Jassik-Gerschenfeld and R. Sindberg, 'Aspects of sensorimotor reverberation to acoustic and visual stimuli', in *Brain Mechanisms* (Eds. G. Moruzzi, A. Fessard and H. H. Jasper), Elsevier, Amsterdam, 1963.
38. Campbell, H. J., *Correlative Physiology of the Nervous System*, Academic Press, London, 1965.
39. Carnap, R., 'The methodological character of theoretical concepts', in *Minnesota Studies in the Philosophy of Science*, Vol. II (Eds. H. Feigl and M. Scriven), Univ. of Minnesota Press, Minneapolis, 1956, pp. 36–76.

40. Chisholm, R. M., *Perceiving*, Cornell, New York, 1957.
41. Chomsky, N., *Syntactic Structures*, Mouton and Co., The Hague, 1957.
42. Chow, K. L. and H. W. Nissen, 'Interocular transfer of learning in visually naive and experienced infant chimpanzees', *J. comp. physiol. Psychol.*, **48**, 229 (1955).
43. Clare, M. H. and G. H. Bishop, 'Dendritic circuits: The properties of cortical paths involving dendrites', *Amer. J. Psychiat.*, **111**, 818–25 (1955).
44. Cohen, H. D., F. Ervin and S. H. Barondes, 'Puromycin and cycloheximide: Different effects on hippocampal electrical activity', *Science*, **154**, 1557–1558 (1966).
45. Colonnier, M. L., 'The fine structural arrangement of the cortex', *Arch. Neurol.*, **16**, 651 7 (1967).
46. Creutzfeldt, O. D., H. D. Lux and S. Watanabe, 'Electrophysiology of cortical nerve cells', in *The Thalamus* (Eds. D. P. Purpura and M. D. Yahr), Columbia University Press, New York, 1966.
47. Critchley, M., *The Parietal Lobes*, Hafner, New York, 1966.
48. Crosby, E., T. Humphrey and E. W. Lauer, *Correlative Anatomy of the Nervous System*, Macmillan, New York, 1962.
49. Delgado, J. M. R., W. W. Roberts and N. E. Miller, 'Learning motivated by electrical stimulation of the brain', *Amer. J. Physiol.*, **179**, 587–93 (1954).
50. Dennett, D. C., *Content and Consciousness*, Routledge and Kegan Paul, London, 1969.
51. Denny-Brown, D., *The Basal Ganglia*, Oxford University Press, London, 1962.
52. Denny-Brown, D., 'The midbrain and motor integration', *Proc. R. Soc. Med.*, **55**, 527 38 (1962).
53. Denny-Brown, D., *The Cerebral Control of Movement*, Liverpool University Press, Liverpool, 1966.
54. Douglas, R. J. and K. H. Pribram, 'Learning and limbic lesions', *Neuropsychologia*, **4**, 197–220 (1966).
55. Drewe, E. A., G. Ettlinger, A. D. Milner and R. E. Passingham, 'A comparative review of the results of neurophysiological research on man and monkey', *Cortex*, **6**, 129 63 (1970).
56. Eccles, J. C., *The Physiology of Synapses*, Springer, New York, 1964.
57. Eccles, J. C., 'Cerebral synaptic mechanisms', in *Brain and Conscious Experience* (Ed. J. C. Eccles), Springer, Berlin, 1966.
58. Eccles, J. C., 'Mode of operation of the cerebellum in the dynamic loop control of movement', *Brain Research*, **40**, 73–80 (1972).
59. Eccles, J. C., M. Ito and J. Szentàgothai, '*The Cerebellum as a Neuronal Machine*', Springer, New York, 1967.
60. Estes, W. K., 'Toward a statistical theory of learning', *Psychol. Rev.*, **57**, 94–107 (1950).
61. Evans, C. R. and T. B. Mulholland (Eds.), *Attention in Neurophysiology*, Butterworths, London, 1969.
62. Evarts, E. V., 'Effects of sleep and waking on spontaneous and evoked discharge of single units in visual cortex', *Fed. Proc.*, **19**, 808–37 (1960).
63. Fant, G. and B. Lindblom, 'Studies of minimal speech and sound units', *Speech Transmission Lab.*, *Quarterly Progress Report*, **2**, 1–11 (Royal Institute of Technology, Stockholm) (1961).
64. Feigl, H., *The 'Mental' and the 'Physical'*, Vol. 3, Minnesota Studies in the Philosophy of Science, Minneapolis, 1958, pp. 370–457.

65. Festinger, L., C. A. Burnham, H. Ono and D. Bamber, 'Efference and the conscious experience of perception', *J. Exp. Psychol. Monograph*, **74** (1967).
66. Findlay, J. N., *Values and Intentions*, Allen and Unwin, London, 1961.
67. Flexner, J. B., L. B. Flexner and E. Stellar, 'Memory in mice as affected by intracerebral puromycin', *Science*, **141**, 57–9 (1963).
68. Foerster, H. von., *Das Gedächtnis*, Deuticke, Vienna, 1948.
69. Fox, A. C., 'The structure of the cerebellar cortex', in *Correlative Anatomy of the Nervous System* (E. C. Crosby, T. Humphrey and E. W. Lauer), Macmillan, New York, 1962.
70. Fox, S., 'Evoked potential habituation and sensory pattern preference as determined by stimulus information', *J. Comp. Physiol.*, **58**, 257–72 (1964).
71. Fox, C. A. and R. S. Snider (Eds.), *The Cerebellum*, Elsevier, Amsterdam, 1967.
72. Freedman, N. L., B. M. Hafer and R. S. Daniel, 'EEG arousal decrement during paired-associate learning', *J. Comp. Physiol.*, **61**, 15–19 (1966).
73. Gaito, J., *Macromolecules and Behaviour*, North Holland Publishing Co., Amsterdam, 1966.
74. Gastaut, H., 'The role of the reticular formation in establishing conditioned reactions', in *Reticular Formation of the Brain* (Ed. W. H. Jasper), Little Brown, Boston, 1957.
75. Gergen, J. A. and P. D. MacLean, *Ann. N.Y. Acad. Sci.*, **117**, 69 (1964).
76. Geschwind, N., 'The varieties of naming errors', *Cortex*, **3**, 97–112 (1967).
77. Geschwind, N., 'Disconnexion syndromes in animal and man', *Brain*, **88**, 237 and 585–644 (1965).
78. Gesell, A., 'Infant vision', *Scientific American*, Feb. 1950.
79. Gibson, E. J., R. D. Walk and T. J. Tighe, 'Enhancement and deprivation of visual stimulation during rearing as factors in visual discrimination learning', *J. Comp. Physiol. Psychol.*, **52**, 74–81 (1959).
80. Gibson, J. J. and E. J. Gibson, 'Continuous perspective transformations and the perception of rigid motion', *J. Exp. Psychol.*, **54**, 129–38 (1957).
81. Girden, E. and E. Culler, 'Conditioned responses in curarized striate muscle in dogs', *J. Comp. Psychol.*, **23**, 261–74 (1937).
82. Girden, E., F. A. Mettler, G. Finch and E. Culler, 'Conditioned responses in a decorticate dog to acoustic, thermal and tactile stimulation', *J. Comp. Psychol.*, **21**, 367-85 (1936).
83. Glaser, E. M., *The Physiological Basis of Habituation*, The University Press, Oxford, 1966.
84. Globus, A. and A. B. Scheibel, 'Pattern and field in cortical structure: the rabbit', *J. Comp. Neur.*, **131**, 155–72 (1967).
85. Globus, A. and A. B. Scheibel, 'The effect of visual deprivation on cortical neurons. A Golgi study', *Exp. Neurol.*, **19**, 331–45 (1967).
86. Gloor, P., 'Amygdala', in *Handbook of Physiology* (Eds. J. Field, H. W. Magoun and V. E. Hall), Section 1, *Neurophysiology*, Vol. II, American Physiological Society, Washington, 1960, pp. 1395–1420.
87. Goldrich, S. G., F. J. Pond, P. Livesey and J. S. Schwartzbaum, 'Electrically induced after discharges in inferotemporal cortex of monkeys', *Neuropsychologia*, **8**, 417–29 (1970).
88. Goldstein, K. and M. Scheerer, 'Abstract and concrete behaviour; an experimental study with special tests', *Psychol. Monogr.*, **53**, No. 2 (667, 674–5, 677–8), 941.

89. Goodglass, H., B. Klein, P. Carey, and K. Jones, 'Specific semantic word categories in aphasia', *Cortex*, **2**, 74–89 (1966).
90. Grastyan, E., 'The hippocampus and higher nervous activity', in *The Central Nervous System and Behaviour* (Ed. M. A. Brazier), J. Macy, New York, 1959.
91. Grastyan, E., 'The significance of the earliest manifestations of conditioning in the mechanisms of learning', in *Brain Mechanisms and Learning* (Ed. J. F. Delafresnage), Blackwell, Oxford, 1961.
92. Gray, E. G., 'Ultrastructure of synapses of the cerebral cortex and of certain specializations of neuroglial membranes', in *Electron Microscopy in Anatomy* (Ed. Boyd *et al.*), Edward Arnold, London, 1961.
93. Green, E., 'Aphasia and psycholinguistics', *Cortex*, **6**, 216–35 (1970).
94. Gregory, R. L., 'On how little information controls so much behaviour', in *Contemporary Problems in Perception* (Eds. A. T. Welford and L. Houssiadas), Taylor & Francis, London, 1970.
95. Grice, G. R., 'An experimental study of the gradient of reinforcement in maze learning', *J. Exp. Psychol.*, **30**, 475–89 (1942).
96. Gross, C. G., D. B. Bender and C. E. Rocha-Miranda, 'Visual receptive fields of neurons in inferotemporal cortex of the monkey', *Science*, **166**, 1303–6 (1969).
97. Gross, C. G., C. E. Rocha-Miranda and D. B. Bender, 'Visual properties of neurons in inferotemporal cortex of the macaque', *J. Neurophys.*, **35**, 96–111 (1972).
98. Guthrie, E. R., *The Psychology of Learning*. Harper, New York, 1935 (revised 1952).
99. Hamlin, R. M., 'Intellectual functions 14 years after frontal lobe surgery', *Cortex*, **6**, 299–307 (1970).
100. Harmon, L. D. and E. R. Lewis, 'Neural modelling', *Physiol. Rev.*, **46**, 513–91 (1966).
101. Harmon, L. D., R. T. Kado and E. R. Lewis, 'Cerebellar modelling problems', in *To Understand Brains* (Ed. L. D. Harmon), New York: in press.
102. Head, H., *Studies in Neurology*, 2, Frowde, Hodder & Stoughton, London, 1920.
103. Head, H., *Aphasia*, Cambridge University Press, 1926.
104. Hebb, D. O., *Organization of Behaviour*, Wiley, New York, 1949.
105. Held, R., 'Plasticity in sensory-motor systems', *Scientific American*, **213**, No. 5, 84–94 (1965).
106. Held, R. and J. Bossom, 'Neonatal deprivation and adult rearrangement: complementary techniques for analyzing plastic sensory-motor coordination', *J. Comp. Phys. Psychol.*, **54**, 33–7 (1961).
107. Held, R. and A. Hein, 'Movement-produced stimulation in the development of visually guided behaviour', *J. Comp. and Phys. Psych.*, **56**, 872–6 (1963).
108. Helmholtz, H. von., *Handbuch der Physiologischen Optik*, Vol. III, Leopold Voss, Leipzig, 1867.
109. Hernandez-Peòn, R. and M. B. Sterman, 'Brain functions', *Ann. Rev. Psychol.*, **17**, 363–94 (1966).
110. Hilgard, E. R. and D. G. Marquis, *Conditioning and Learning*, Appleton, New York, 1940.
111. Hilgartner, C. A. and J. F. Randolph, 'Psycho-logics', *J. Theoret. Biol.*, **23**, 285–338 (1969).

112. Hoesen, G. W. van, D. N. Pandya and N. Butters, 'Cortical afferents to the entorhinal cortex of the rhesus monkey', *Science*, **175**, 1471–3 (1972).
113. Holmes, O. and J. Houchin, 'Units in the cerebral cortex of the anesthetized rat and the correlations between their charges', *J. Physiol.*, **187**, 651–71 (1966).
114. Holst, E. von, and H. Mittelstaedt, 'Das Reafferenzprinzip', *Naturwissenschaften*, **37**, 465–76 (1950).
115. Horridge, G. A., *Interneurons*, W. H. Freeman, London, 1968.
116. Houk, J. C., 'On the significance of various command signals during voluntary control', *Brain*, **40**, 49–53 (1972).
117. Howes, D., 'Hypotheses concerning the function of the language mechanism', in *Research in Verbal Behaviour and Some Neurological Implications* (Eds. K. Salzinger and S. Salzinger), Academic Press, New York, 1967.
118. Hubel, D. H. and T. N. Wiesel, 'Receptive fields and functional architecture in two non-striate visual areas (18 and 19) of the cat', *J. Neurophysiol.*, **28**, 229–89 (1965).
119. Hubel, D. H. and T. N. Wiesel, 'Receptive fields and functional architecture of monkey striate cortex', *J. Neurophysiol.*, **195**, 215–43 (1968).
120. Hull, D., *Philosophy of Biological Science* (Eds. E. and M. Beardsley), Prentice-Hall, Englewood Cliffs, N.J., 1972.
121. Hull, C. L., *Principles of Behaviour*, Appleton Century-Crofts, New York, 1943.
122. Hyden, H., 'The Neuron', in *The Cell* (Eds. J. Bracket and A. E. Mirsky), Vol. IV, Academic Press, New York, 1960.
123. Iversen, S. D. and L. Weiskrantz, 'Perceptions of redundant cues by monkeys with inferotemporal lesions', *Nature*, **214**, 241–3 (1965).
124. Jacobson, E., 'Electrophysiology of mental activities', *Am. J. Psychol.*, **44**, 677–94 (1932).
125. Jakobson, R., 'Linguistic types of aphasia', in *Brain Function* (Ed. E. C. Carterette), Vol. III, Univ. of California Press, Berkeley, 1966.
126. John, E. Roy, *Mechanisms of Memory*, Academic Press, New York, 1967.
127. Johnson, L. E., 'Dynamic analysis of visual tracking', SRC—28B—63—8, Systems Research Centre, Case Institute of Technology, Cleveland, Ohio, 1962.
128. Jones, E. G., 'Interrelationships of parieto-temporal and frontal cortex in the rhesus monkey', *Brain Research*, **13**, 412–15 (1969).
129. Jouvet, M., 'Recherches sur les mécanismes neurophysiologiques du sommeil et de l'apprentissage négatif', in *Brain Mechanisms and Learning* (Eds. A. Fessard *et al.*), Blackwell, Oxford, 1961.
130. Jung, R., H. H. Kornhuber and J. S. Da Fonseca, 'Multisensory convergence on cortical neurons', in *Progress in Brain Research* (Eds. G. Moruzzi, A. Fessard and H. H. Jasper), Vol. I, Elsevier, Amsterdam, 1963, pp. 207–240.
131. Jus, A. and C. Jus, 'Étude de l'extinction par répétition de l'expression EEG du réflexe d'orientation et de l'action du frein externe sur les réactions EEG aux différents stimuli chez l'homme', in *Moscow Collegium on Electroencephalography and Higher Nervous Activity* (Eds. H. H. Jasper and G. D. Smirnov), *EEG Clin. Neurophysiol.*, Suppl. 13 (1960).
132. Kennedy, D., A. I. Selverston and M. P. Remler, 'Analysis of restricted neural networks', *Science*, **164**, 1488–96 (1969).
133. Kleist, K. *Gehirnpathologie*, Barth, Leipzig, 1934.

134. Kilmer, W. L., W. S. McCulloch and J. Blum, 'Some mechanisms for a theory of the reticular formation', in *Systems Theory and Biology* (Ed. M. Mesatovic), Springer, New York, 1968.
135. Klee, M. R., 'Different effects on the membrane potential of motor cortex units after thalamic and reticular stimulation', in *The Thalamus* (Eds. D. P. Purpura and M. D. Yahr), Columbia Univ. Press, New York, 1966.
136. Kleene, S. C., *Introduction to Metamathematics*, van Nostrand, Princeton, 1952.
137. Kohler, I., 'Sitzber', *Oesterr, Akad. Wiss., phil.-hist. Kl.*, **227**, 1 (1951).
138. Kohler, I., *Die Pyramide* 3, Nos. 5–7 (1953).
139. Kohler, I., *The Formation and Transformation of the Perceptual World* (translated by H. Fiss), *Psychological Issues*, **3**, 1–173 (1964).
140. Köhler, W., *The Mentality of Apes*, Harcourt Brace, New York, 1925.
141. Kornhuber, H. H., 'Motor functions of cerebellum and basal ganglia', *Kybernetic*, **8**(4), 157–62 (1971).
142. Krechevsky, I., '"Hypotheses" in rats', *Psychol. Rev.*, **39**, 516–32 (1932).
143. Krnjević, K., M. Randić and D. W. Straughan, 'Cortical inhibition', *Nature*, **201**, 1294 (1964).
144. Krushinsky, L. V., 'Solution of elementary problems by animals on the basis of extrapolation', in *Cybernetics of the Nervous System* (Eds. N. Wiener and J. P. Schadé), Elsevier, Amsterdam, 1965.
145. Lashley, K. S., *Brain Mechanisms and Intelligence*, Univ. of Chicago Press, Chicago, 1929.
146. Lashley, K. S., 'Patterns of cerebral integration indicated by the scotomas of migraine', *Arch. Neurol. Psychiat.*, **46**, 331–9 (1941).
147. Lenneberg, E. H., *Biological Foundations of Language*, Wiley, New York, 1967.
148. Liberman, A. M., 'Some results of research on speech perception', *J. acoust. soc. Amer.*, **29**, 117–23 (1957).
149. Livingstone, R. B., 'Central control of receptors and sensory transmission systems', in *Handbook of Physiology* (Ed. J. Field), American Physiological Society, Washington, 1960.
150. Llewellyn Thomas, E., 'Movements of the eye', *Scientific American*, June 1966.
151. Lømo, T., 'Frequency potentiation of excitatory synaptic activity in the dentate area of the hippocampal formation', *Acta. Phys. Scand.*, **68**, Suppl. 227, 128, (1966).
152. Luria, A. R., 'Factors and forms of aphasia', in *Disorders of Language* (Eds. A. V. S. de Reuck and M. O'Connor), Churchill, London, 1964.
153. Luria, A. R., *Higher Cortical Functions in Man*, Basic Books, New York, 1964.
154. MacLeod, R. B., 'Teleology and theory of human behaviour', *Science*, **125**, 477 (1957).
155. MacKay, D. M., in *Mechanization of Thought Processes*, A National Physical Laboratory Symposium, Vol. II, Her Majesty's Stationery Office, London, 1959, p. 607.
156. MacKay, D. M., *Information, Mechanism and Meaning*. The M.I.T. Press, Cambridge, Massachusetts, 1969.
157. MacKay, D. M., 'Cerebral organization and the conscious control of action', in *Brain and Conscious Experience* (Ed. J. C. Eccles), Springer, New York, 1966.

158. Mackworth, J. F., *Vigilance and Habituation*, Penguin, London, 1969.
159. Melzack, R., 'The perception of pain', *Scientific American*, Feb. 1961.
160. Marr, D., 'A theory of cerebellar cortex', *J. Physiol.*, **202**, 437–70 (1969).
161. Marr, D., 'A theory for cerebral neocortex', *Proc. Roy. Soc. Lond. B*, **176**, 161–234 (1970).
162. McGeoch, J. A., *The Psychology of Human Learning*, Longmans, New York, 1942.
163. McGhie, A., *Pathology of Attention*, Penguin, London, 1969.
164. Miller, G. A. and N. Chomsky, 'Finitary models of language users', in *Handbook of Mathematical Psychology* (Eds. R. D. Luce, R. Bush and E. Galanter), Wiley, New York, 1963.
165. Miller, N. E., 'Some reflections on the law of effect produce a new alternative to drive reduction', in *Nebraska Symposium on Motivation* (Ed. R. J. Jones), Univ. of Nebraska Press, Lincoln, 1963.
166. Millikan, C. H. and F. L. Darley (Eds.), *Brain Mechanisms Underlying Speech and Language*, Grune and Stratton, New York, 1967, pp. 132–135.
167. Milner, B., 'Intellectual function of the temporal lobes', *Psychol. Bull.*, **51**, 42–62 (1954).
168. Milner, B., Brain mechanisms suggested by studies of temporal lobes', in *Brain Mechanisms Underlying Speech and Language* (Eds. C. H. Millikan and F. L. Darley), Grune and Stratton, New York, 1967.
169. Milner, P., 'The cell assembly: Mark II', *Psychol. Rev.*, **64**, 242–52 (1957).
170. Misanin, J. R., R. R. Miller and D. J. Lewis, 'Retrograde amnesia produced by electroconvulsive shock after reactivation of a consolidated memory trace', *Science*, **160**, 554–5 (1968).
171. Monod, J., *Chance and Necessity* (translated by A. Wainhouse), Collins, London, 1972.
172. Morrell, F., 'Electrical signs of sensory coding', in *The Neurosciences: A Study Program*, Rockefeller University Press, 1967, pp. 452–69.
173. Moruzzi, G., 'Synchronizing influences of the brain stem and the inhibitory mechanisms underlying the production of sleep by sensory stimulation', in *Moscow Colloquium on Electroencephalography of Higher Nervous Activity* (Eds. H. H. Jasper and G. D. Smirnov), *EEG Clin. Neurophysiol.*, Suppl. 13 (1960).
174. Mountcastle, V. B., 'Functional properties of the somatic afferent system', in *Sensory Communication* (Ed. W. A. Rosenblith), Wiley, New York, 1961.
175. Myers, R. E. and C. Swett, 'Social behaviour deficits of free-ranging monkeys after anterior temporal cortex removal', *Brain Research*, **18**, 551–6 (1970).
176. Neisser, U., *Cognitive Psychology*, Meredith, New York, 1967, p. 256.
177. Nielson, H. C. and R. M. Fleming, 'Effects of electroconvulsive shock and prior stress on brain amine levels', *Exp. Neurology*, **20**, 21–30 (1968).
178. Nissl, F., 'Experimentell-anatomische Untersuchungen über die Hirnrinde', *Versamml deutscher. Nat. Aerzte in Heidelberg*, 1911.
179. Noda, H. and Ross W. Adey, 'Firing of neuron pairs in cat association cortex during sleep and wakefulness', *J. Neurophysiol.*, **33**, 672–84 (1970).
180. Noda, H. and Ross W. Adey, 'Firing variability in cat association cortex during sleep and wakefulness', *Brain Research*, **18**, 513–16 (1970).
181. Noda, H., R. B. Freeman and O. Creutzfeldt, cited in 'Nerve cells that keep the world steady', *New Scientist*, 24 Feb. 1972.

182. Noda, H., S. Manohar and Ross W. Adey, 'Correlated firing of hippocampal neuron pairs in sleep and wakefulness', *Exp. Neurol.*, **24**, 232–47 (1969).

183. O'Brien, J. and S. S. Fox, 'Single cell activity in cat motor cortex', *J. Neurophysiol.*, **32**, 267–84 (1969).

184. O'Keefe, J. and J. Dostrovsky, 'The hippocampus as a spatial map. Preliminary evidence from unit activity in the freely-moving rat', *Brain Research*, **34**, 171–5 (1971).

185. Olds, J. A. and P. Milner, 'Positive reinforcement produced by electrical stimulation of septal area and other regions of rat brain', *J. Comp. Physiol.*, **47**, 419–27 (1954).

186. Orban, G., R. Wissaert and M. Callens, 'Influence of brain stem oculomotor area stimulation on single unit activity in the visual cortex', *Brain Research*, **17**, 351–4 (1970).

187. Oscarsson, O., in 'Satellite Symposium of the XXV International Physiological Congress', *Brain Research*, **40**, 100 (1972).

188. Paillard, J., 'The patterning of skilled movements', in *Handbook of Physiology* (Eds. J. Field, H. W. Magoun and V. E. Hall), Section 1, *Neurophysiology*, Vol. III, American Physiological Society, Washington, 1960, pp. 1679–1708.

189. Papez, J., 'A proposed mechanism of emotion', *Arch. Neurol. Psychiat.*, **38**, 725–43 (1937).

190. Parmeggiani, P. L., A. Azzaroni and P. Lenzi, 'On the fundamental significance of the circuit of Papez', *Brain Research*, **30**, 357–74 (1971).

191. Patton, H. D., 'Control of autonomic outflows: the hypothalamus', in *Neurophysiology* (T. C. Ruch, H. D. Patton, J. W. Woodbury and A. L. Towe), W. B. Saunders, Philadelphia, 1965.

192. Pavlov, I. P., *Conditioned Reflexes* (translated by G. V. Anrep), Oxford University Press, London, 1927.

193. Penfield, W. and B. Milner, 'The memory deficit produced by bilateral lesions in the hippocampal zone', *A.M.A. Arch. Neurol. and Psychiat.*, 1957.

194. Penfield, W. and L. Roberts, *Speech and Mechanism*, Princeton University Press, 1959.

195. Phillips, C. G., 'Changing concepts of the precentral motor area', in *Brain and Conscious Experience* (Ed. J. C. Eccles), Springer, New York, 1966.

196. Piaget, J., *The Origins of Intelligence in Children*, International Universities Press, New York, 1952.

197. Piaget, J., *The Child's Construction of Reality*, Routledge and Kegan Paul, London, 1955.

198. Porter, R. W. and D. McK. Rioch, 'Visual impairment induced by lesions of the midbrain in the chimpanzee', *Anatomical Records*, **142**, 321 (1962).

199. Pribram, K. H., 'The intrinsic systems of the forebrain', in *Handbook of Physiology* (Eds. J. Field, H. W. Magoun and V. E. Hall), Section 1, *Neurophysiology*, Vol. II, American Physiological Society, Washington, 1960, pp. 1323–44.

200. Pribram, K. H., 'Reinforcement revisited: a structural view', in *Nebraska Symposium on Motivation* (Ed. M. R. Jones), University of Nebraska Press, 1963, pp. 113–59.

201. Pribram, K. H., 'Memory and the organization of attention', in *Brain Function and Learning* (Eds. D. B. Lindsley and A. A. Lumsdale), Univ. of California Press, Berkeley, 1967.

202. Pribram, K. H., 'The limbic systems, efferent control in inhibition and behaviour', in *Progress in Brain Research* (Eds. G. Moruzzi, A. Fessard and H. H. Jasper), Vol. 27, Elsevier, Amsterdam, 1967, pp. 318–36.

203. Putman, H., 'Minds and Machines', in *Dimensions of Mind* (Ed. S. Hook), New York University Press, New York, 1960.

204. Raisman, G., W. M. Cowan and T. P. S. Powell, 'The extrinsic afferent, commissural and association fibres of the hippocampus', *Brain*, **88**, 963–96 (1965).

205. Ralston, H. J., 'Evidence for presynaptic dendrites and a proposal for their mechanism of action', *Nature*, **230**, 585–7, (1971).

206. Redding, F. K., 'Modification of sensory cortical evoked potentials by hippocampal stimulation', *EEG Clin. Neurophysiol.*, **22**, 74–83 (1967).

207. Riesen, A. H., M. I. Kurke and J. C. Mellinger, 'Interocular transfer of habits monocularly in visually naive and visually experienced cats', *J. Comp. Physiol.*, **46**, 166 (1953).

208. Rosenblatt, F., *Principles of Neurodynamics*. Spartan, Washington, 1962.

209. Rosenblatt, F., 'Recent work on theoretical models of biological memory', in *Computer and Information Sciences* II (Ed. J. T. Tou), Academic Press, London, 1967, pp. 35–56.

210. Rosenzweig, M. R., E. L. Bennett and M. C. Diamond, 'Brain changes in response to experience', *Scientific American*, Feb. 1972.

211. Ruch, T. C., H. D. Patton, J. W. Woodbury and A. L. Towe, *Neurophysiology*, W. B. Saunders, Philadelphia, 1965.

212. Ryle, G., *The Concept of Mind*, Hutchinson, London, 1949.

213. Sager, O., G. Wendt, M. Moisanu and V. Cirnu, cited in *Neurological Basis of Behaviour* (Eds. G. E. W. Wolstenholme and C. M. O'Connor), Little Brown, Boston, 1956.

214. Schilder, P., *The Image and Appearance of the Human Body*, Psyche Monogr. No. 4, Kegan, Trench & Trubner, London, 1935.

215. Scott, D. N., *An Annotated Bibliography of Research on Eye-movements published during the Period 1932–1962*. Defense Research Board, Toronto, 1962.

216. Sem-Jacobson, C. W. and A. Torkildsen, 'Depth recording and electrical stimulation in the human brain', in *Electrical Studies on the Unanesthetized Brain* (Eds. E. R. Ramsey and D. S. O'Doherty), Hoeber, New York, 1960.

217. Senden, M. von., *Raum- und Gestaltauffassung bei operierten Blindgeborenen vor und nach der Operation*, Barth, Leipzig, 1932.

218. Shannon, C. E. and W. Weaver, *The Mathematical Theory of Communication*, Univ. of Illinois Press, Urbana, 1949.

219. Sharpless, S. and H. Jasper, 'Habituation of the arousal reaction', *Brain*, **79**, 655–80 (1956).

220. Sherwood, S. L. (Ed.), *The Nature of Psychology* (a selection of papers, essays and other writings by the late Kenneth J. W. Craik), The University Press, Cambridge, 1966.

221. Sholl, D. A., *The Organization of the Cerebral Cortex*. Methuen, London, 1956.

222. Shorter, J. M., 'Imagination', *Mind*, LXI, 528, 1952.

223. Skinner, B. F., *The Behaviour of Organisms*. Appleton–Century, New York, 1938.

224. Skinner, B. F., 'Are theories of learning necessary?' *Psychol. Rev.*, **57**, 193–216 (1950).

225. Skinner, B. F., *Beyond Freedom and Dignity*, Jonathan Cape, London, 1972.
226. Smart, J. J. C., *Philosophy and Scientific Realism*, Routledge, London, 1963.
227. Smith, W. M., 'Visually-guided behaviour and behaviourally-guided vision', in *Contemporary Problems in Perception* (Eds. A. T. Welford and L. Houssiadas), Taylor & Francis, London, 1970.
228. Smythies, J. R., *Brain Mechanisms and Behaviour*, Blackwell, Oxford, 1970.
229. Sokolov, E. N., *Perception and the Conditioned Reflex*, Pergamon Press and Macmillan, London, 1963.
230. Sommerhoff, G., *Analytical Biology*, Oxford Univ. Press, London, 1950.
231. Sommerhoff, G., 'The abstract characteristics of living systems', in *Systems thinking* (Ed. F. E. Emery), Penguin, London, 1969.
232. Sperry, R. W., 'Cerebral regulation of motor coordination in monkeys following multiple transection of sensorimotor cortex', *J. Neurophys.*, **10**, 275–94 (1947).
233. Sperry, R. W., *American Scientist*, **40**, 291, (1952).
234. Sperry, R. W., 'Cerebral organization and behaviour', *Science*, **133**, 1749–1757 (1961).
235. Sperry, R. W., 'Brain bisection and mechanisms of consciousness', in *Brain and Conscious Experience* (Ed. J. C. Eccles), Springer, Berlin, 1966.
236. Sprague, J. M., W. W. Chambers and E. Stellar, 'Attentive, affective and adaptive behaviour in the cat', *Science*, **133**, 165–73 (1961).
237. Stepien, I. and S. Sierpinski, 'The effect of focal lesions of the brain upon auditory and visual recent memory in man', *J. Neurol. Neurosurg. Psychiat.*, **23**, 334–40 (1960).
238. Stratton, G. M., 'Eye movements and the aesthetics of visual form', *Philosophische Studien*, **20**, 336–59 (1902).
239. Strawson, P. F., *Individuals*. Methuen, London, 1959.
240. Sutherland, N. S., 'Visual discrimination of orientation and shape by octopus', *Nature*, **179**, 11–13 (1957).
241. Teuber, H. L., 'Alterations of perception after brain injury', in *Brain and Conscious Experience* (Ed. J. C. Eccles), Springer, New York, 1966.
242. Thach, W. T., 'Discharge of Purkinje and cerebellar nuclear neurons during rapidly alternating arm movements in the monkey', *J. Neurophysiol.*, **31**, 785–97 (1968).
243. Thach, W. T., 'Discharge of cerebellar neurons related to two maintained postures and two prompt movements', *J. Neurophysiol.*, **33**, 527–47 (1970).
244. Thierman, T., 'A signal detection approach to the study of set in tachistoscopic recognition', *Perceptual and Motor Skills*, **27**, 96–8 (1968).
245. Thompson, R. F., D. Denny and H. E. Smith, 'Cortical control of specific and nonspecific sensory projections to the cerebral cortex', *Psychon. Sci.*, **4**, 93–4 (1966).
246. Thompson, R. F., *Foundations of Physiological Psychology*, Harper and Row, New York, 1967.
247. Thorndike, E. L., 'Animal intelligence. An experimental study of the associative processes in animals', *Psychol. Monogr.*, **2**, No. 8 (1898).
248. Thorndike, E. L., *Animal Intelligence*, Macmillan, New York, 1911.
249. Tinbergen, N., *The Study of Instinct*, The Clarendon Press, Oxford, 1951.
250. Tinbergen, N., 'Specialists in nest-building', *Country Life*, 30 Jan. 1953, pp. 270–1.
251. Tolman, E. C., 'Cognitive maps in rats and men', *Psychol. Rev.*, **55**, 189–208 (1948).

252. Tolman, E. C., *Purposive Behaviour in Animals and Men*, Appleton–Century, New York, 1932.
253. Tolman, E. C., B. F. Ritchie and D. Kalish, 'Studies in spatial learning', *J. Exp. Psychol.*, **36**, 13 (1946), **36**, 221 (1946) and **37**, 39–47 (1947).
254. Travis, R. P., D. L. Sparks and T. F. Hooten, *Brain Research*, **7**, 455 (1968).
255. Trevarthen, C. B., 'Simultaneous learning of two conflicting problems by split-brain monkeys', *Amer. Psychologist*, **15**, 485 (1960).
256. Truex, C. R. and M. Carpenter, *Human Neuroanatomy*, Williams and Wilkins, Baltimore, 1969.
257. Turing, A. M., 'Computing machinery and intelligence', *Mind*, Vol. LIX, No. 236 (1950).
258. Unger, S. M., 'Habituation of the vasoconstrictive orienting reaction', *J. Exp. Psychol.*, **67**, 11–18 (1964).
259. Uttley, A. M., 'Conditional probability computing in a nervous system', in *Mechanization of Thought Processes* (National Physical Laboratory Symposium), Her Majesty's Stationery Office, London, 1959.
260. Vernon, M. D., *The Psychology of Perception*, Penguin, London, 1962.
261. Vernon, M. D., 'Development of visual perception', in *Aspects of Developmental and Paediatric Ophthalmology* (Eds. P. Gardiner, R. Mackieth and V. Smith), Heinemann, London, 1969.
262. Virsu, V., 'Tendencies to eye movement and misperception of curvature, direction and length', *Perception and Psychophysics*, **9**, 65–72 (1971).
263. Voeks, V. W., 'Formalization and clarification of a theory of learning', *J. Psychol.*, **30**, 341–62 (1950).
264. Wallach, H., K. J. Frey and K. A. Bode, 'The nature of adaptation in distance perception based on oculomotor cues', *Perception and Psychophysics*, **11**, 110–16 (1972).
265. Walter, W. Grey, *The Living Brain*, Duckworth, London, 1953.
266. Walter, W. Grey, 'Slow potential waves in the human brain associated with expectancy, attention and decision', *Arch. Psych. Zeitschrift f.d. ges. Neurologie*, **206**, 309–22 (1964).
267. Walter, W. Grey, 'Can "attention" be defined in physiological terms?' in *Attention in Neurophysiology* (Eds. C. R. Evans and T. B. Mulholland), Butterworths, London, 1969.
268. Walter, W. Grey, R. Cooper, V. J. Aldridge, W. C. McCullum and A. L. Winter, 'Contingent negative variation: an electric sign of motor association and expectancy in the human brain', *Nature*, **203**, 380–4 (1964).
269. Warrington, E. K., 'Neurological disorders of memory', *Brit. Med. Bull.*, **27**, 243–7 (1971).
270. Watson, J. B., *Behaviourism*, Norton, New York, 1925.
271. Weingarten, M and D. N. Spinelli, 'Retinal receptive field changes produced by auditory and somatic stimulation', *Exptl. Neurol.*, **15**, 363–76 (1966).
272. White, B. L., P. W. Castle and R. M. Held, 'Observations on the development of visually-directed reaching', *Child Development*, **35**, 349–64 (1964).
273. Woodger, J. H., *Biological Principles*, Kegan Paul, Trench, Trubner, London, 1929.
274. Woodger, J. H., *The Axiomatic Method in Biology*, Cambridge University Press, London, 1937.
275. Yarbus, A. L., *Eye movements and Vision*, Plenum Press, New York, 1967.
276. Yarrow, L. J., 'The etiology of mental retardation: the deprivation model', *Cognitive Studies* (Ed. J. Hellmuth), Vol. 1, Brunner/Mazel, New York, 1970.

277. Young, J. Z., *The Memory System of the Brain*, McGraw-Hill, New York, 1966.
278. Zaporozhets, A. V., 'The development of perception in the pre-school child', in *European Research in Cognitive Development* (Ed. P. H. Mussen), Vol. 30, No. 2, Chicago: University of Chicago Press, 1965.
279. Zelman, A., L. Kabat, R. Jacobson and J. V. McConnell, 'Transfer of training through injection of "conditioned" RNA into untrained planarians', *Worm Runner's Digest*, **5**, 14–19 (1963).

Index

For quick reference only the first-named author of any joint publication is cited in this index.

Abstraction, 227, 357; *see also* Categorization
Accommodation, 136
Action potentials, 137
Active representations, 219
Adaptation, asymmetry of, 83
concept of, 17, 21
conventional use of the term in neurophysiology, 136
general concept of, 93, 94
meaning of, 75ff.
ontogenetic, 88
phylogenetic, 81
Adequate stimulus substitution, 180, 201ff., 273, 386
in cerebellum, 238
Adey, W. R., 243
Adler, A., 270
Aesthetic sensibilities, 73
Afferent convergence, 155
Afferent divergence, 155
Albert, D. J., 330, 332
Alignment, of lambda neurons, 200
Allocortex, 240
Alpha/beta systems of Howes, 374
Alpha rhythm, 161
Amnesia, 331
Amygdala, 241, 323
Analog operations, 185
Anand, B. K., 322
AND gates, 186
Anthropomorphism, 57, 74, 90; *see also* Metaphors
Anticipatory reactions, 114
Aphasias, 362, 373
Green's classification of, 375
Appetitive behaviour, 105

Appropriateness, concept of, 39, 93
the brain's criteria for, 167ff.
Aquinas, St. Thomas, 24
Arbib, M. A., 11
Aristotle, 23, 24
Arousal, 116, 159ff.
cortical, 165, 255, 257
general, 314
Association areas, of cortex, 145
Associative feedback, 207
Ashby, W. Ross, 92
Attention, 159ff., 300ff.
mechanism of, 329
selective, 292
Attention system, 301, 307
Attentional loops, 307, 315, 339
Attentional responses, 265ff.
Auditory feedback, 369
Awareness, 348
nature of, 68, 69
Axons, 137

Back-reference period, 85
Basal ganglia, 146, 306, 340
Basket cells, cerebellar, 235
cortical, 251
Basowitz, H., 53
Behaviour lines, 76
Behaviour talk, 54
Behaviourism, 34, 63, 64
Beritoff, I. S., 29
Berlyne, D. E., 161, 163
Beurle, R. L., 4
Biasing inputs, 205
Birkmayer, W., 287
Blomfield, S., 239
Body schema, 243, 287, 294ff.

Boutons, 138
Brain, R., 376
Brain talk, 54
Brainstem nuclei, 146
Braitenberg, V., 238
Brattgard, S. O., 331
Brindley, G. S., 4
Broadbent, D. E., 115
Broca's areas, 362
Brooks, V. B., 189, 393
Bureš, J., 388
Burns, B. Delisle, 254

Carnap, R., 53
Categorization, 34, 40
Causal relations, 76
Central vision, 273
Centralization, 275
Cerebellar cortex, 234ff.
Cerebellar loops, 237, 335
Cerebellar nuclei, 236
Cerebellum, 151, 233ff.
  lambda systems in, 238ff.
Chomsky, N., 46
Cingulate gyrus, 146, 241
Clare, M. H., 255
Classes, namable and unnamable, 42
Climbing fibres, 140
  cerebellar, 235ff.
  cortical, 255
Closures, 386
CNS (central nervous system), organization of, 144ff.
Coenetic variable, 85
Cognitive maps, 29, 30, 33, 288
Cognitive resolutions, 42, 44, 356
Cohen, H. D., 332
Coincidence detectors, 346
Collaterals, 137
Colliculus, inferior, 146
  superior, 146
Command, concept of, 10
Command signals, 124ff.
Comparators, 10, 118, 346
Compass, of directive correlation, 90
Complementary afferent innervation, 154
Complementary coding, 187ff.
'Complex' cells in visual cortex, 158
Computers, comparison with brains, 11ff.
Concepts, 40, 357
Conditioned reflex, 109

Conditioning, classical, 109, 385ff.
  instrumental, 110, 111, 153
Consciousness, 67, 342, 344ff.
  the nature of, 69, 72
Consolidation of memory, 170ff., 245, 293, 326, 330
Constancies, 36
Content, of messages etc., 39, 67
  of neural representations, 69, 71
Content words, 44
Contextual inputs, 205
Contiguity theory of learning, 171ff.
Contingent inputs, 125, 193
Contingent negative variation, 317
Contour-following, 267
Contrast enhancement, 186ff.
Coordination, the concept of, 89, 93
Cortex, cerebral, excitability of, 142
  structure of, 144
Correlated firing patterns, 195
  in association areas of cortex, 257
  in hippocampus, 247
Craik, J. W., 285
Creutzfeldt, O. D., 257
Cybernetics, 91

Darwin, 20
Decision functions, 303
Decorticate preparations, 152, 385, 387
Definitions, operational, 56
Degrees of adaptiveness, 82
Degrees of directive correlation, 83
Demand inputs, 125, 193
Demand signals, 125
Dendrites, 138
Dendritic conduction, 255
Dennett, D. C., 68, 353
Denny-Brown, D., 230, 336
Descartes, 3, 24, 59
Descriptive use of language, 41ff., 355
Determinism, 23, 77
Deterministic systems, 76
Digital operations, 185
Directive correlation, concept of, 6, 14, 54, 73, 74ff., 300
  definition of, 79
  executive, 88
  ontogenetic, 88
  phylogenetic, 88
  types of, 88
Directiveness, types of, 21
Domain (of a directive correlation), 105
Douglas, R. J., 244

Dreaming, 343
Drive, concept of, 106
Drive centres, 127, 179
Drive reduction, 111, 113
Drive strength, 107
Drive system, 320ff.

Eccles, J. C., 237, 239, 256
EEG (electroencephalograph) recordings, 161, 258ff.
Einstein, 5
Electroconvulsive shock (ECS), effects on memory, 331
Electroencephalograph (EEG) recordings, 161, 258ff.
Emotional reactions, 243, 306
Entorhinal area, 241
Epiphenomenalism, 59
EPSP (excitatory postsynaptic potential), 138
Equilibrium-seeking, 19, 86
Erismann, K., 288
Error-signal generators (ESG), 118ff.
Error-signals, 116ff.
    Class I, 119ff.
    Class II, 119ff.
Estes, W. K., 172
Evaluation, *see* What-evaluation
Evarts, E. V., 258
Expectancy, 112; *see also* Expectation
Expectancy waves, 316
Expectation, 30, 33
    in the representation of properties, 220ff.
Expectation, nature of, 112ff., 114ff., 300
    role of, 262
Extinction of responses, 110, 173ff., 182
Extra-pyramidal motor system, 146
Eye, as prehensile organ, 274ff.
Eye movements, control of, 308

Feedback systems, 85, 118ff.
Feedforward, 118
Feeding centres, 322
Feigl, H., 20
Fissures, 145
Fixation system, 301, 307
Flexner, J. B., 331
Foerster, H. von, 332
Forced acquisition, 201ff.
    in cerebellum, 238
Forcing inputs, 205
Forward inhibition, 189

Fovea, 266
Fox, S., 165
Frontal eye fields, 308
Frontal lesions, 317ff., 375
Frontal lobe, 145, 313
Frontal pole, 145
Fronto-temporal system, 311ff.
Frustration, 169
Functions, biological, 93
    mathematical, 25

Gamma-efferent mechanism, 336
Gamma-efferent system, 119
Gastaut, H., 165
Generalized reaction systems, 160, 177ff.
Gergen, J. A., 246
Gerstmann's syndrome, 296
Geschwind, N., 374
Gibson, J. J., 224, 264
Girden, E., 386, 387
Globus, A., 198, 255
Goal, concept of, 300
Goal-directed activity, nature of, 16ff.
Goal-directedness, concept of, 6, 17
Goals, neural representation of, 310
Goal-seeking, 18, 74, 86; *see also* Goal-directed activity
Goal-signals, 124ff.
God, teleological argument for the existence of, 24
Goldstein, K., 317
Golgi cells, 235
Goodglass, H., 362, 374
Grammatical code of natural languages, 44
Grammatical words, 44
Grastyan, E., 166, 243
Gray, E. G., 140
Green, E., 375
Gregory, R. L., 261
Grice, G. R., 167
Gross, C. G., 230
Guthrie, E. R., 171

Habituation, 142, 163ff., 285
    of arousal, 315
Hamlin, R. M., 375
Harmon, L. D., 4, 239
Head, H., 161, 295
Hebb, D. O., 263
Hedonic drive system, 321ff.
Held, R., 264
Helmholtz, H. von, 228, 284

Hierarchies, of directive correlations, 100ff.
of goals and subgoals, 17, 98ff., 103
Hierarchy, concept of, 98
Hilgard, E. R., 327
Hippocampal gyrus, 146
Hippocampus, 241ff., 243ff., 315, 323, 327ff.
lambda systems in, 246ff.
Holst, E. von, 216
Homeostasis, 87
Homomorphism, 26
Horizontal cells, of cortex, 251
Houk, J. C., 10
Howes, D., 374
Hubel, D. H., 9, 158, 265, 290
Hull, C. L., 110, 168
Hull, D., 20
Hyden, H., 332
'Hypercomplex' cells, in visual cortex, 158
Hypothalamus, 150, 152, 242ff., 321
Hypotheses in perception, 288

Idealism, 59
Identity thesis, 59
Imagination, 351ff.
Imaginative processes, 213
Imprinting, 168
Infant vision, 268, 274
Inferotemporal cortex, 241, 289ff.
responses in, 230
Information content, quantitative measure of, 378
Information profile of sensory inflow, 73
Information theory, 58, 91, 378ff.
Information transfer, 380
Information, transmission of, 73
Innate releasing mechanism (IRM), 103, 105
Input sharing, 188ff.
Insight, 29
Instinct, concept of, 104
Insula, 146
Insulotemporal system, 318
Integration, biological concept of, 93
Interference, and extinction, 173ff.
as cause of habit extinction, 142
Intermediate coding network, 210
Internal models, *see* Internal representations
Internal representations, concept of, 31

nature of, 288
of goals, 129
of the outer world, 25
structure of, 262
summary, 345
Intralaminar nuclei, 324, 341
Introspection, 53, 60
Invariance in shape recognition, 267, 278
Inverting prisms, 288
IPSP (inhibitory postsynaptic potential), 140
Isomorphism, 26
Isthmus, 146

Jacobson, E., 36
Jakobson, R., 362, 371
James, William, 350
John, E. Roy, 113, 388
Johnson, L. E., 10
Jouvet, M., 166
Jung, R., 257
Jus, A., 165
Juxtallocortex, 241

K-complexes, 161
Kennedy, D., 4
Kilmer, W. L., 4
Klee, M. R., 255
Kleist, K., 375
Klüver–Bucy syndrome, 292
Kohler, I., 288
Köhler, W., 29
Kornhuber, H. H., 238
Krnjević, K., 255
Krushinsky, L. V., 112

Lambda module, definition of, 191
Lambda networks in speech production, 365
Lambda neuron, definition of, 191
Lambda system, definition of, 189
Language, argumentative use of, 47
different uses of, 41
nature of, 38, 40, 42
Language functions, 355ff.
Lashley, K. S., 249
Latent learning, 168
Latent representations, 219
Late components, 258, 315, 387
Law of Effect, 110, 168
Learning, nature of, 9, 57, 88, 89, 113, 166ff.

Learning changes in lambda systems, 197ff.
Lexical divisions, 44
Liberman, A. M., 367
Limbic system, 146, 166, 241ff., 323ff., 339
Line-labelling, 136, 185
Livingstone, R. B., 244
Local responses, in dendrites, 140
Logical product, 26
Logical sum, 26
Luria, A. R., 362, 373, 375

MacKay, D. M., 11
Macromolecules and memory, 332
Markoff systems, 87
Marr, D., 4, 231, 239, 240, 273
Martinotti cells, 252
Maximum intensity filter (MIF), 191, 382
McCulloch, W. S., 4
McLeod, R. B., 20
Meaning, of messages etc., 39
Memory, concept of, 12, 213
short-term and long-term, 326ff.
two-stage model of, 327
see also Reproductive memory
'Mental' states, 51, 53, 60, 61, 63, 67, 68, 72, 350
Mental states, events or processes, 58
Metaphors, 58
use of, 21
Michie, D., 5
Mind, concept of, 24, 59, 66
Mind talk, 54
Milner, B., 289, 327, 375
Milner, P., 198
Misanin, J. R., 331
Models of the nervous system, 4, 11, 53
Monod, J., 23
Morphemes, 46, 366
Morrell, F., 389
Moruzzi, G., 165ff.
Mossy fibres, cerebellar, 235ff.
Motivation, concept of, 107
sources of, 242
Motor cortex, 145, 340
Motor integration, 333
Movement, role in visual perception, 261, 263–4
Movement information, for internal representations, 229ff.
Mowrer, O. H., 174

Müller, Johannes, 136

Naming, 40
Need detectors, 127
Negative feedback, 191, 206; *see also* Recurrent inhibition
Neocortex, lambda systems in, 253ff.
structure of, 249ff.
Neural representations, nature of, 32
of outer world, 243
of properties, 217ff.
of relations, 221ff.
Neuroglia, 136
Neurons, structure of, 135ff.
Newton, 5
Nielson, H. C., 331
Nissl, F., 254
Noda, H., 228, 247, 257
Novel stimuli, 169
Novelty of stimuli, 159, 175, 314

O'Brien, J., 185
Occipital lobe, 145
O'Keefe, J., 245
Olds, J. A., 178ff.
Olivary nucleus, 237
One-trial learning, 168
Orban, G., 228
Orbital cortex, 146
Orbitofrontal cortex, 241
Orbitofrontal–insulotemporal complex, 339
Orbitofrontal–insulotemporal cortex, 305
Organic order, 93
OR gates, 186, 192
Orienting reactions, 116, 160, 162ff.
Orienting responses, 314
Orthogonal variables, special sense of, 78
Oscarsson, O., 237
Overdetermination, in shape recognition, 278

Pain, meaning of, 62
pathways of, 323
Papez, J., 244, 325
Parallel fibres, cerebellar, 235
Parietal lobe, 145, 294ff.
Parieto-temporo-frontal relationships, 319
Parmeggiani, P. L., 316
Partial reinforcement, 386

Pavlov, I. P., 109
Penfield, W., 327
Pericellular nests, 140
Perseveration, 279
Phonemes, 46, 366
Place learning, 28
Pleasure centres, see Reward systems
Polymorph cells, 252
Pons, 151
Porter, R. W., 230
Positive feedback, 206
Posterior association areas, 363
Prefrontal lobectomy, 317
Pribram, K. H., 250, 292, 318
Principle of Effects, see Law of Effect
Principle of Expectancy, 113ff., 168
Problem solving, 47
Projected pain, 318, 323, 349
Properties, recognition of, 217ff.
Proprioceptors, 117
Protein synthesis and neural activity, 331
Psychology, the language of, 51
Psycho-physical parallelism, 59
Punishment systems, 177ff., 326
Purkinje cells, 235ff.
Purposive behaviour, 55; see also Goal-directed activity
Purposiveness, in nature, 23
    subjective sense of, 20
    see also Goal-directed activity
Putman, H., 15
Pyramidal cells, 251ff.
Pyramidal motor system, 146

Rational thought, 51; see also Reasoning
Raumschalen, 287
Reafference, 215ff., 272, 273
Reasoning, 49; see also Rational thought
Recognition, 346
Recruiting responses, 342
Recurrent inhibition, 187ff.
    in cerebellum, 240
    in hippocampus, 247
    in neocortex, 253
Red nucleus, 146
Redding, F. K., 244
Reductionism, 19, 74
Refractory period, 138
Regression, statistical, 27
Reinforcement, of responses, 110, 173ff., 182

primary, 167ff.
secondary, 168
Relation, the concept of, 42
Relations, recognition of, 221ff.
Representations, internal, of outer world, 10
Reproductive memory, 208, 351ff.
Response, concept of, 6, 9
Response modulation, 201ff.
Reticular formation, 4, 151, 165, 325, 333, 339, 341, 386, 388
Retroactive interference, 201
Reverberation, 244, 293, 315, 324ff.
Reward systems, 177ff., 326
Rhinencephalon, 241
RNA levels and neural activity, 331
Rosenblatt, F., 4
Rosenblueth, A., 92
Ryle, G., 34, 64

Saccades, 267, 270
Sager, O., 387
Satiety centres, 179, 322
Scale of life, 90
Schilder, P., 295
Science, semantic requirements of, 55
Scotoma, 266
    completion of figures across, 280
Searching, 90, 102
Self, internal representation of, 70
Self-awareness, 69, 71, 350
Self-categorization, 61, 71
Sem-Jacobson, C. W., 293
Sensory pathways, 149, 153
Sentence frame, 372
Septum, 241
Servomechanisms, 10, 117ff.
Shannon, C. E., 58
Shape recognition, problem of, 8
    through central vision, 275ff.
Sharpless, S., 165
Short-circuiting, 180ff.
Shorter, J. M., 353
Significance, of stimuli, 312, 315
'Simple' cells, in visual cortex, 158
Skinner, B. F., 23, 106, 110
Sleep, 342, 348
Smith, W. M., 264
Social conscience, 228
Sokolov, E. N., 162ff., 285
Soma, 138
Somatic cortex, responses in, 393
Soul, concept of, 24

Speech comprehension, 359ff.
Speech perception, phonemes in, 367
Speech production, 355ff.
  phonemes in, 367
Sperry, R. W., 250, 254, 295, 347
Spikes, 137
Spinal cord, 334
Spindle bursts, 161
Spines, dendritic, 140, 198
Spinothalamic tracts, 149
Split-brain preparations, 152, 250, 385
Spontaneous activity, 154
Spreading depression, 330
Stability, of internal models, 283ff.
  of living organism, 86
  of visual scene, 281ff.
Stable images, 33
Stellate cells, cerebellar, 235
  cortical, 251
Stepien, I., 327
Stimulus, concept of, 7, 9
Stimulus generalization, 201
Stochastic models, 191
Stratton, G. M., 267
Stretch reflex, 119, 336
Subgoal, definition of, 99
Substantia nigra, 146
Subthalamic nucleus, 146
Superego, 228
Superior colliculus, 309
Supplementary motor areas, 145
Sutherland, N. S., 271
Synapses, 136ff.
Synaptic changes in learning, 170ff., 198ff., 280
Synaptic potency, 141
Synaptic vesicles, 138

Taylor, W. K., 382
Telekinetic system, 301
Teleology, *see* Goal-directed activity
Temporal lobe, 145ff.
  lesions in, 289ff.
  stimulation of, 293
Temporal sequence recognition, 206ff.
  and cortical networks, 253
Thach, W. T., 239
Thalamic nuclei, 335ff.
Thalamus, 149
Thorndike, E. L., 110
Thought, nature of, 35, 48
Tinbergen, N., 103, 104
Tolman, E. C., 28, 112, 113, 174

TOTE (test–operate–test–exit program segments), 11
Tracer frequencies, 388
Transfer, between hemispheres, 330
  of learning, 28, 103, 303, 310
Transformation expectation, 115
Transposition phenomena, 222
Travis, R. P., 340
Trevarthen, C. B., 385
Trying, 90
Turing, A. M., 5, 15
Turing machine, 5

Uncertainty, in information theory, 378
Unconscious, the (Freudian), 70
Unconsciousness, clinical sense of, 70
Unity of self, 349ff.
Unsuccessful behaviour, 90
Uttley, A. M., 4

Venn diagram, 42
Vigilance, 161
Virtual variations, 75, 94
Visual association areas, 389
Visual cortex, responses in, 9, 158, 265ff., 290
Visual pathways, 156ff.
Vitalism, 74
Voeks, V. W., 172
Voluntary movements, 309

Walter, W. Grey, 57, 89, 293, 316
Warrington, E. K., 244
Watson, J. B., 34, 65
Weingarten, M., 388
Weisskrantz, L., 12
Wernicke's area, 363
What-evaluating systems, 312ff., 315, 387
What-evaluation, 303
What–where separation, 301
Wiener, N., 91
Wigner, E., 67
Woodger, J. H., 89, 98
Word-equivalents, 361–362
Word-modifiers, 44
Word-roots, 362

Yarbus, A. L., 270
Young, J. Z., 4, 95, 271

Zaporozhets, A. V., 270
Zelman, A., 333